PROGRESS IN HEMATOLOGY

PROGRESS IN HEMATOLOGY

VOLUME IV

Edited by

Carl V. Moore, M.D.

and

Elmer B. Brown, M.D.

With 21 Contributors

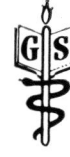

Grune & Stratton   New York and London

1964

Library of Congress Catalog No. 56–5843

Printed in U.S.A. (WP-B)

Contents

v

Contributors

EMILY, M. BARROW, Ph.D., Research Associate, Department of Pathology, University of North Carolina, Chapel Hill, N.C.

GEORGE M. BERNIER, M.D., Research Associate, Department of Biochemistry; Assistant in Medicine, College of Medicine, University of Florida, Gainesville, Fla.

GORDON R. BLOOMBERG, M.D., Instructor in Clinical Pediatrics, Washington University School of Medicine; Assistant Pediatrician, St. Louis Children's Hospital and St. Louis Maternity Hospital, St. Louis, Mo.

ELLEN M. COLLIER, B.S., Chemist, National Institute of Arthritis and Metabolic Diseases, National Institutes of Health, Bethesda, Md.

EMIL FREI, III, M.D., Associate Scientific Director for Experimental Therapeutics, Intramural Research, National Cancer Institute, National Institutes of Health, Bethesda, Md.

EMIL J FREIREICH, M.D., Head, Leukemia Service, Medicine Branch, National Cancer Institute, National Institutes of Health, Bethesda, Md.

JOHN B. GRAHAM, M.D., Professor of Pathology, School of Medicine, University of North Carolina, Chapel Hill, N.C.

S. GRANICK, Ph.D., Professor, The Rockefeller Institute, New York, N.Y.

ROBERT C. GRIGGS, M.D., Department of Medicine, Western Reserve School of Medicine, Cleveland Metropolitan General Hospital, Cleveland, Ohio.

PAUL HELLER, M.D., Professor of Medicine, University of Illinois College of Medicine; Associate Chief of Staff for Research, Veterans Administration West Side Hospital, Chicago, Ill.

MERILYN C. HILLER, M.S., Biologist, National Institute of Arthritis and Metabolic Diseases, National Institutes of Health, Bethesda, Md.

ERNST R. JAFFÉ, M.D., Career Scientist of the Health Research Council of the City of New York (I-169); Associate Professor of Medicine, Albert Einstein College of Medicine, New York, N.Y.

ROBERT D. LANGE, M.D., Associate Professor of Medicine, Medical College of Georgia, Augusta, Ga.

RICHARD D. LEVERE, M.D., Assistant Professor, The Rockefeller Institute, New York, N.Y.

DONALD M. MARCUS, M.D., Assistant Professor of Medicine, Albert Einstein College of Medicine, New York, N.Y.

VICTOR J. MARDER, M.D., Hospital St. Louis, Paris, France; Formerly Clinical Investigator, National Institute of Arthritis and Metabolic Diseases, National Institutes of Health, Bethesda, Md.

VERA PAVLOVIC-KENTERA, M.D., Voluntary Research Fellow in Medicine, Medical College of Georgia, Augusta, Ga.; On leave from Institute for Medical Research, Belgrade, Yugoslavia.

FRANK W. PUTNAM, Ph.D., Professor and Head, Department of Biochemistry, University of Florida College of Medicine, Gainesville, Fla.

GERALD SCHIFFMAN, Ph.D., Associate Professor, Department of Research Medicine, University of Pennsylvania, Philadelphia, Pa.

N. RAPHAEL SHULMAN, M.D., Chief, Clinical Hematology Branch, National Institute of Arthritis and Metabolic Diseases, National Institutes of Health, Bethesda, Md.

ADEL A. YUNIS, M.D., Assistant Professor of Medicine, Director of Hematology Research, University of Miami, Miami, Fla.; Formerly Assistant Professor of Medicine, Washington University School of Medicine, St. Louis, Mo.

Introduction

LEANDRO M. TOCANTINS became a productive, highly respected, and influential member of the academic hematologic community in this, his adopted country. His early work on mammalian platelets, particularly the experimental production of thrombocytopenia by administration of heterologous antiplatelet serum, and his recent studies of problems related to bone marrow transplantation exemplify his accomplishments in the laboratory. His ability to make wise, objective, and impartial judgments caused government and scientific groups to seek his counsel in many ways. Tocantins wrote well. He enjoyed assembling the popular "Panels on Therapy" for *Blood*. He did an excellent job of editing the first three volumes of "Progress in Hematology". His death, at too early an age, is a scientific and personal loss deeply felt by hematologists everywhere. The present editors will consider their job well done if they can select as wisely subjects that are timely for review, and win as completely the cooperation of investigators to undertake the job.

The magnitude of research effort has become so great during the last two decades, and the pace so fast that the problem of communication, of keeping abreast, is now appalling. Scientists have attempted to compensate, at least in part, by exchanging information and ideas through symposia, conferences, and reviews. In selecting subjects to be included in Volume 4 of "Progress in Hematology", therefore, the editors had to be guided not only by recent developments within a given field, but also by the coverage provided elsewhere to each subject. The absence of reviews on hemoglobinopathies and leukocyte kinetics, for instance, can be explained on this basis. The contributors graciously agreed to rather short deadlines so that the time interval between preparation of their reviews and publication could be short, and the material as current as possible. Great appreciation is expressed to each author.

Hematologic progress remains greatest in the area of explaining mechanisms of disease, in providing increased understanding of biological phenomena. Translation of this information to therapeutic advances of great significance will certainly come as it has in the past, but more time is needed. We hope that the selections in this volume of "Progress in Hematology" will in some measure help speed the process.

CARL V. MOORE
ELMER B. BROWN

Heme Synthesis in Erythroid Cells

——— S. GRANICK, AND RICHARD D. LEVERE ———

ABBREVIATIONS USED

AIA	Allyl Isopropyl Acetamide
AIP	Acute intermittent porphyria
ALA	δ-Aminolevulinic acid
ALAase	Enzyme that converts ALA to PBG, i.e. ALA dehydrase
CoA or CoASH	Coenzyme A
COPRO	Coproporphyrin
COPROGEN	Coproporphyrinogen
DNA	Deoxyribose nucleic acid
ϵ_M	Molar extinction coefficient
FMN	Flavin mononucleotide
FAD	Flavin adenine dinucleotide
HEME	Ferrous or ferric porphyrin
α-KG	α-Ketoglutaric acid
Km	Michaelis constant
NAD, NAD⁺, NADH	Nicotinamide dinucleotide, oxidized form, reduced form
NuDP, NuTP	Nucleoside di and tri phosphate, i.e. ADP, ATP; GDP, GTP; IDP, ITP
PBG	Porphobilinogen
PBGase	Enzymes that convert PBG to UROGEN III
PROTO	Protoporphyrin
PROTOGEN	Protoporphyrinogen
Pyridoxal-P	Pyridoxal phosphate
m-RNA	Messenger RNA
RNA	Ribose nucleic acid
R. spheroides	Rhodopseudomonas spheroides, a purple photosynthetic bacterium
TPP	Thiamine pyrophosphate
UDase	Uroporphyrinogen decarboxylase
URO	Uroporphyrin
UROGEN	Uroporphyrinogen

I. INTRODUCTION

STUDIES OF HEME are of interest for two reasons. First, HEME is the agent which makes O_2 available to the cell, activates the O_2 and transfers electrons to O_2. To carry out these functions, HEME is combined with special proteins to form hemoglobin, the various cytochromes and other HEME enzymes. Secondly, because HEME is highly colored, it is possible to follow the differentiation and maturation of a cell by observing changes in its HEME content.

In this review we shall summarize the current data on HEME biosynthesis and attempt to answer the intriguing question of how its synthesis is controlled during cell differentiation and maturation. A number of excellent reviews of HEME biosynthesis are already available[1-11] and should be referred to for

From The Rockefeller Institute, New York 21, N. Y.

Supported in part by U. S. Public Health Service Grant No. GM 04922.

a fuller discussion and more complete bibliography. Here, we shall restrict ourselves to the HEME of the red cell, referring to other cells and tissues only for supplementation or contrast. No attempt will be made to cover the literature. Rather, papers will be selected to illustrate current ideas and hypotheses.

II. SUMMARY OF THE BIOSYNTHETIC CHAIN FORMING HEME

The steps in the synthesis of HEME are presented in Figure 1. This synthesis is beautiful in its essential simplicity. It is as if a molecular engineer had set up the synthesis on an assembly line. First, two ubiquitous, small molecules—glycine and succinate—become attached by one machine (i.e. an enzyme) to form a short chain molecule, δ-aminolevulinic acid (ALA). Next, two ALA molecules are placed side by side on another machine and tied together to form a small, ring-shaped molecule, a monopyrrole, porphobilinogen (PBG). Then, on the next machine, four PBG molecules are tied together in succession to form a large ring, a colorless tetrapyrrole, called uroporphyrinogen (UROGEN). At the next machine, this molecule is trimmed by cutting off successively four carboxyl groups from four acetic side chains that stick out from the edges of the molecule, thus forming coproporphyrinogen (COPROGEN). At the next machine, oxidations with O_2 occur on two of the side chains and protoporphyrinogen (PROTOGEN) is formed. As the colorless molecule issues from the end of the assembly line it is given a paint job by being autoxidized with O_2, and out pops a shiny, red protoporphyrin molecule. Finally, into the center of this molecule is added the engine, the iron atom, to form the molecule HEME or iron protoporphyrin.

Only the first reaction requires energy, i.e. for the activation of succinate (as succinyl-CoA) to combine with glycine to form ALA. All the other reactions, except possibly the conversion of PBG to UROGEN, are downhill or irreversible. They are strongly favored thermodynamically because they involve the formation of resonating pyrrole and porphyrin rings, decarboxylations, and oxidations of propionic acid groups. O_2 is required in two places. One is in the oxidation of citric acid via the cycle to supply succinyl-CoA. The other is in the oxidation of COPROGEN to PROTOGEN. It is interesting to note that both these enzymic oxidations occur in mitochondria.

III. DISTRIBUTION OF ENZYMES OF THE HEME BIOSYNTHETIC CHAIN

All aerobic cells, bacterial as well as plant and animal, have the ability to synthesize HEME. HEME synthesis has frequently been studied in the avian erythrocyte which resembles a late mammalian erythroblast in HEME metabolism. Both cells contain nuclei and mitochondria and can synthesize hemoglobin. When chicken cells, or rabbit reticulocyte cells or red cells from erythroblastosis foetalis are hemolyzed, a number of the enzymes of the HEME biosynthetic chain are found to be soluble and can be separated from each other by zone electrophoresis on starch[12]. The insoluble enzymes are presumably localized in the mitochondria or particles derived from mitochondria (although nuclei have not been ruled out as additional sites).

Figure 2 shows this interesting distribution. The first enzyme, ALA-synthetase, is in the mitochondria; the second, third and fourth enzymes which convert ALA to PBG to UROGEN III and COPROGEN III are soluble and

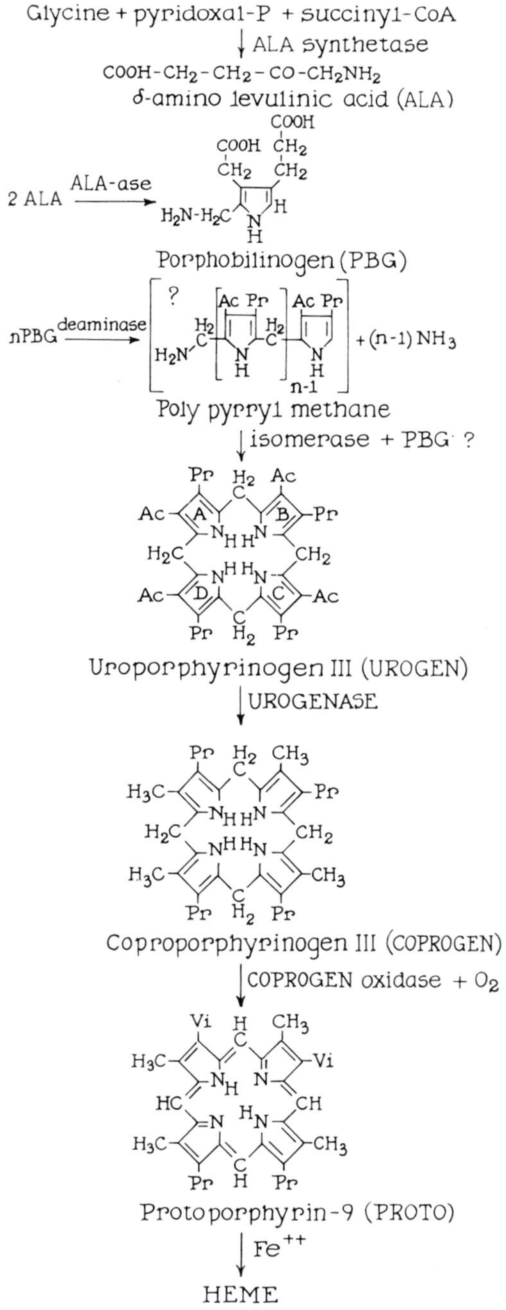

Glycine + pyridoxal-P + succinyl-CoA

$\downarrow$ ALA synthetase

$COOH-CH_2-CH_2-CO-CH_2NH_2$

δ-amino levulinic acid (ALA)

2 ALA $\xrightarrow{\text{ALA-ase}}$

Porphobilinogen (PBG)

nPBG $\xrightarrow{\text{deaminase}}$ $+ (n-1) NH_3$

Poly pyrryl methane

$\downarrow$ isomerase + PBG ?

Uroporphyrinogen III (UROGEN)

$\downarrow$ UROGENASE

Coproporphyrinogen III (COPROGEN)

$\downarrow$ COPROGEN oxidase + O_2

Protoporphyrin-9 (PROTO)

$\downarrow$ Fe^{++}

HEME

Fig. 1.—The general scheme of biosynthesis of HEME. Ac = CH$_2$COOH; Pr = —CH$_2$CH$_2$—COOH; Vi = —CH = CH$_2$. Two moles of ALA are required to form porphobilinogen. Four moles of PBG are required to form uroporphyrinogen. The polypyrrylmethane shown is a hypothetical intermediate. When 4 acetic side chains of uroporphyrinogen III are decarboxylated to methyl (CH$_3$) groups, then coproporphyrinogen III results. Oxidation and decarboxylation of two of the propionic (Pr) acid groups to vinyl (Vi) groups yields protoporphyrin-9. (Reprinted by permission of Granick & Mauzerall. *Metabolic Pathways*, Vol. II, Academic Press, 1960.)

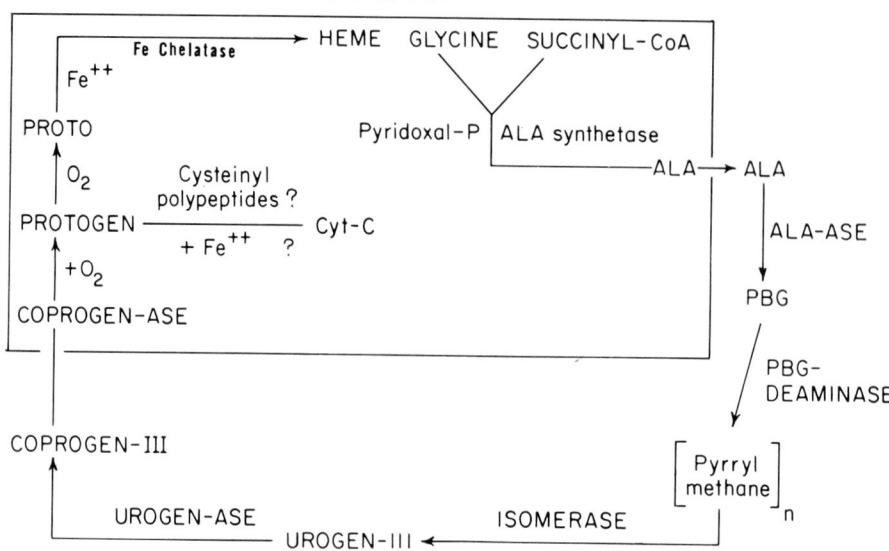

FIG. 2.—Distribution of the enzymes of HEME biosynthesis in the liver cell.[13] The first enzyme ALA-synthetase (ALA-ASE), and the last two enzymes, coproporphyrinogen oxidase (COPROGEN-ASE) and iron chelatase, are localized in the mitochondria and the other enzymes, which are soluble, are localized in the surrounding cytoplasm. (Reprinted with permission of Granick & Mauzerall. *Metabolic Pathways*, Vol. II, Academic Press, 1960.)

reside in the cytoplasm; and the last two which convert COPROGEN to PROTOGEN and PROTO to HEME are insoluble and are localized in the mitochondria[13]. Evidence for this localization will be discussed under the heading for each enzyme.

The separation of the soluble enzymes of rabbit reticulocytes by zone electrophoresis on a starch block is shown in Figure 3. When the supernatant solution of a centrifuged hemolyzate is applied directly to the starch block and electrophoresed, the hemoglobin migrates toward the cathode and small amounts of colorless enzyme fractions migrate toward the anode and are separated. The relative rates of anodic migration of the soluble enzymes of the different species used are: Rabbit: ALAase > UDase > PBGase. Chicken: ALAase > PBGase > UDase. Human: UDase > PBGase > ALAase. By using the new column fractionation methods[14] prior to electrophoresis to enrich the non-hemoglobin proteins, it should be possible to obtain more of these enzymes for study.

IV. HEME SYNTHESIS—GENERAL ASPECTS

In a now classic series of papers, Shemin and Rittenberg[4, 5] demonstrated that labeled glycine, when fed to a human, was incorporated into the HEME of newly formed erythrocytes and was released from these cells about 120 days later, i.e. the average lifetime of the red cell (Fig. 4). These brilliant studies that led to the finding of glycine and succinyl-CoA as the elementary building blocks, with ALA as the product, have been amply reviewed. Other major

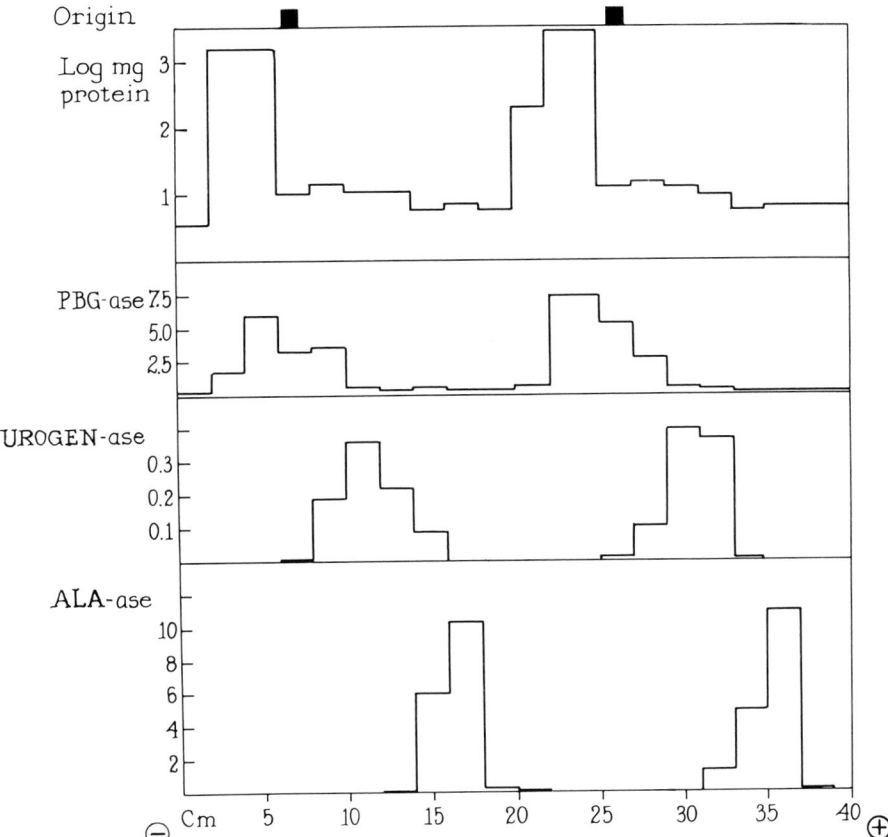

Fig. 3.—Electrophoretic separation on starch of the supernatant fluid from a hemolysate of rabbit reticulocytes.[12] Two streaks of supernatant fluid were applied to a starch plate at 7 cm and 26 cm distance (origin) from the cathode end. The hemoglobin migrated to the left and the colorless proteins including the three enzymes migrated toward the right. The figures on the vertical axis represent the total protein and total activity of eluates from 2 cm-wide segments of the starch block. The ALA-ase activity is expressed in μmoles of PBG formed from added ALA. PBG-ase activity is in μmoles of PBG converted to UROGEN III. UROGEN-ase activity is in μmoles of UROGEN III converted to COPROGEN III. All activities are per hour per eluted fraction. (Reprinted by permission of Granick. J. Biol. Chem. 232: 1119, 1958.)

achievements were the isolation of PBG by Westall[15] from the urine of patients with acute porphyria and the elucidation of its structure by Cookson and Rimington[16].

The intact red cell needs several enzyme systems to make ALA. The formation of succinyl-CoA requires a citric acid cycle, as shown by the tracer studies with acetate and succinate[4, 5] and by inhibition studies with malonate, arsenite, transaconitate and fluoracetate[17]. A cytochrome system that transfers electrons to O_2 is coupled to the citric acid cycle, as shown by inhibition studies with N_2 and CO. Dinitrophenol inhibits ALA synthesis in a manner which is not clearly understood. It may inhibit ALA-synthetase[18] or it may inhibit the formation of ATP which is required to maintain coenzymes or to synthesize succinyl-CoA.

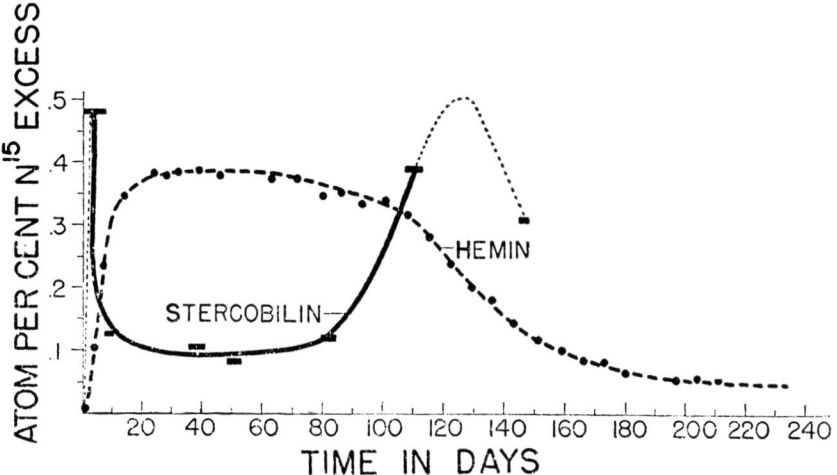

FIG. 4.—N[15] concentration of HEME and stercobilin of a normal man after feeding N[15] labeled glycine for 2 days.[164, 165] The dashed line represents the change in labeling of circulating HEME with time. The smooth line represents labeling of the stercobilin isolated from the feces, with time. (Reprinted with permission of London et al. J. Biol. Chem. 184: 351, 1950.)

As the cells mature, different enzymes of the biosynthetic chain become limiting. The citric acid cycle enzymes and enzymes of the electron transport chain are localized in mitochondria. Reticulocytes still contain some mitochondria. As the mitochondria degenerate in the maturing cells, the ability to synthesize ALA decreases rapidly. However, the enzymes that convert ALA to PROTO disappear more slowly[19]. In mature erythrocytes, only the enzyme activities that convert ALA to COPRO can be detected.

When avian erythrocytes are supplied with glycine (0.05M), PROTO[20], as well as HEME[21], accumulates. Dresel and Falk[22] observed that about two-thirds of the newly formed porphyrin was in the form of PROTO, and the remainder in the form of HEME. Evidently, with supra-normal concentrations of glycine, larger amounts of ALA than normal are produced and the rate-limiting step becomes the one that incorporates iron to form HEME. The addition of ferrous iron (2×10^{-4}M) to these red cells lowered the PROTO only by 10–20%[22]. In whole chicken erythrocytes incubated with glycine aerobically at 37°, the rate of HEME and PROTO synthesis is constant during 24 hours[22]. Dresel and Falk calculated that this rate is about one-fourth that which would occur *in vivo*.

A method based on PROTO determinations was devised by Granick[17] to obtain information on the enzyme systems required to make ALA in the intact cell. The effect of various substrates and inhibitors was compared, using glycine as one substrate and ALA as the other and measuring the PROTO formed by a colorimetric procedure after extracting it with organic solvents. For example, when arsenite was added to the cells together with glycine, PROTO synthesis was blocked because the citric acid cycle was blocked, but PROTO synthesis from ALA remained unaffected.

Addition of various members of the citric acid cycle to whole cells together with glycine is found to enhance the yield of PROTO, indicating that the red cell membrane is partially permeable to these compounds[17]. In the synthesis of PROTO from glycine and α-KG, a marked temperature effect is noted in the range 32–38°, corresponding to a Q-10 of about 10. This result suggests a permeability effect, e.g. a change in a lipid phase in the membrane or the activation of several rate-limiting processes or an active transport process.

With hemolyzed chicken erythrocytes, the synthesis of PROTO is markedly depressed. The steps in ALA synthesis appear to be affected primarily by a dilution of the available coenzymes, such as pyridoxal-P, FMN, NAD and CoA. Steps from ALA to PROTO are not greatly affected[17]. When Dresel and Falk added a boiled yeast extract to the hemolyzed red cells they observed as much as a 6-fold stimulation of PROTO synthesis from glycine and α-KG. Using frozen and thawed chicken erythrocytes, Granick[17] found that PROTO synthesis from glycine and α-KG was restored to 60% of the yield from intact cells by the addition of pyridoxal-P, coenzyme A, glutamine, ribose 5-P, NAD and a mixture of nucleotides; restoration to 80% of activity was obtained by the addition of an acid deproteinized pig liver fraction which probably contained a mixture of nucleotides and coenzymes. These additives maintained a metabolism in the hemolyzed preparation sufficient for steady PROTO formation during a 15-hour incubation period.

V. Synthesis of δ-Aminolevulinic Acid

The labeleing experiments of Shemin and coworkers[4, 5] led to the recognition that ALA was the first product of the biosynthetic chain of heme. ALA is formed from glycine and succinyl-CoA according to reaction I.

I Succinyl-CoA + Glycine $\xrightarrow[\text{Pyridoxal-P}]{\text{δ-ALA-synthetase}}$ δ-Aminolevulinic acid + CO_2 + CoA

II Acetyl-CoA + Glycine $\xrightarrow[\text{Pyridoxal-P}]{\text{AA-synthetase}}$ Aminoacetone + CO_2 + CoA

Studies by Schulman and Richert[23] on vitamin B_6 and pantothenic acid- deficient ducklings showed that pyridoxal-P and coenzyme A are required for this reaction. Similarly, Lascelles[24] showed that porphyrin synthesis in *Tetrahymena vorax*, a protozoan, requires both of these vitamins. Wintrobe and coworkers[25] found that pigs deficient in B_6 produced small, pale, red cells deficient in HEME and very low in free protoporphyrin. The low HEME content is due to the low activity of ALA-synthetase which requires pyridoxal-P as its prosthetic group. The smallness of the cells indicates a low protein content which may occur because pyridoxal-P is also required for transamination reactions to supply some amino acids that are used for protein synthesis.

Localization of ALA-synthetase in mitochondria

ALA-synthetase is found in the insoluble fraction[26, 27] of red cell hemolysates obtained from chickens that have been treated with phenylhydrazine. This insoluble or particle fraction consists of nuclei, mitochondria and cell membranes. Arsenite poisons the ability of these particles to make succinyl-CoA via the citric acid cycle which is localized exclusively in mitochondria. ALA-synthetase is also found in mitochondria obtained from guinea pigs with chemically induced porphyria[27]. Thus, both ALA-synthetase and the mechanism for making its substrate, succinyl-CoA, are present in mitochondria.

Succinyl-CoA synthesis

Neuberger's laboratory was the first to demonstrate that succinyl-CoA is one of the substrates of ALA-synthetase[18]. The particles from the chicken red cells form ALA when incubated in air with glycine, α-KG, CoA, Mg^{++} and pyridoxal-P. The intact particles are, however, impermeable to succinyl-Co A. Freeze-drying renders them permeable to this compound. The disrupted particles form ALA from glycine and added or generated succinyl-CoA. Gibson et al.[18] also showed that the disrupted particles, in addition to ALA-synthetase, contain α-ketoglutarate dehydrogenase and glutamic dehydrogenase.

In order to demonstrate the ALA-synthetase in the disrupted particles, Gibson et al. generated succinyl-CoA from α-KG using an oxidase from pig heart as shown in the following series of reactions III. Glutamic dehydrogenase and ammonia were added to regenerate the NAD^+.

III a) α-KG + TPP + NAD^+ + CoA + lipoic oxidase (pig heart) $\rightarrow$ succinyl-CoA + Co_2 + NADH + H^+.

b) NADH + NH_3 + α-KG + glutamic dehydrogenase $\rightarrow$ NAD^+ + glutamic acid.

c) Succinyl-CoA + glycine + pyridoxal-P + ALA-synthetase (disrupted particles from chicken reticulocytes) $\rightarrow$ ALA + CO_2 + Co A

Succinyl-CoA may be formed in several ways. In erythrocytes, the main pathway appears to be via the enzyme complex α-KG-oxidase and the citric acid cycle. It is usually assumed that α-KG-oxidase is localized only in the mitochondria. This complex has a molecular weight of about 2 million and contains 5 enzyme activities. Massey[28] succeeded in obtaining a soluble complex, mol. wt. 260,000, which contained TPP, lipoic acid and FAD. The steps in the oxidation of α-KG are given in a series of reactions IV.

IV a) α-KG (K_m = 1.3 $\times$ 10^{-5} M) + TPP $\rightarrow$ succinyl-TPP + CO_2

b) succinyl-TPP + $\begin{array}{c} S \\ | \\ \text{lipoyl enzyme} \\ | \\ S \end{array}$ $\rightleftharpoons$ succinyl $\begin{array}{c} S \\ \diagup \\ \text{lipoyl enzyme} \\ \diagup \\ HS \end{array}$ +

TPP

c) succinyl $\overset{\displaystyle S}{\underset{\displaystyle HS}{\diagup\diagdown}}$ lipoyl enzyme + CoA-SH $(K_m = 10^{-7}$ M$) \rightleftharpoons$ succinyl-

S-Co A + $\overset{\displaystyle HS}{\underset{\displaystyle HS}{\diagdown\diagup}}$ lipoyl enzyme

d) $\overset{\displaystyle HS}{\underset{\displaystyle HS}{\diagdown\diagup}}$ lipoyl enzyme + $\left|\overset{\displaystyle S}{\underset{\displaystyle S}{\diagup\diagdown}}\right.$ FAD enzyme $\rightleftharpoons$ $\left|\overset{\displaystyle S}{\underset{\displaystyle S}{\diagup\diagdown}}\right.$ lipoyl enzyme + $\overset{\displaystyle HS}{\underset{\displaystyle HS}{\diagdown\diagup}}$ FAD enzyme

e) $\overset{\displaystyle SH}{\underset{\displaystyle SH}{\diagdown\diagup}}$ FAD enzyme + NAD$^+$ $(K_m = 4.5 \times 10^{-6}$ M$) \rightleftharpoons$ $\left|\overset{\displaystyle S}{\underset{\displaystyle S}{\diagup\diagdown}}\right.$ FAD enzyme

+ NADH + H$^+$

The succinyl-S CoA reacts with a nucleoside diphosphate to form a nucleoside triphosphate as shown in reaction V.

V. Succinyl-S-CoA + NuDP + Pi $\underset{\longleftarrow}{\overset{\longrightarrow}{\text{succinyl-CoA synthetase}}}$ Succinate + NuTP + Co A-SH

The reversibility of this reaction was suggested by the studies of Shemin and Kumin[29]. They blocked succinate oxidation in intact duck erythrocytes with 0.02 M malonate so that very little α-KG would be generated from the citric acid cycle. When they now added methylene-labeled succinate the label was incorporated into newly formed HEME. From this experiment it was inferred that about 30–50% of the succinyl-CoA could be derived directly from added succinate.

Reactions IV and V also occur in liver and have been studied in liver mitochondria obtained from chemically porphyric animals that have a relatively high ALA-synthetase activity[27]. To distinguish between the extent of the forward and reverse reactions the mitochondria were poisoned with arsenite. With α-KG and glycine as substrates it was estimated that 85% of the succinyl-CoA which was used for ALA synthesis was derived from the oxidation of α-KG, and 15% from succinate by the reverse of reaction V. When succinate and glycine were substrates under the same conditions, 35–60% of the succinyl-CoA was derived from succinate.

ATP when added to hemolyzed chicken erythrocytes enhanced ALA synthesis 3-fold only when succinate was substrate[30], a result that also suggests the physiologic importance of the reverse of reaction V.

The properties of succinyl-CoA synthetase have been reviewed by Hager[31]. The enzyme is specific for succinate. The equilibrium constant is 3.7 and the free energy 750 cal. and, therefore, the reaction is thermodynamically easily reversible. For the kidney enzyme the Km for succinate is 5×10^{-3}M. The animal synthetase requires either GTP or ITP whereas the enzyme from spinach requires ATP[32].

Burnham[33] has obtained a purified succinyl-CoA synthetase from *Rhodopseudomonas spheroides* which should be useful to provide continuous generation of succinyl-CoA in further studies of ALA synthetase.

A third type of reaction for succinyl-CoA synthesis is the one from propionyl CoA. The propionyl-CoA reacts with CO_2 and a biotin enzyme to form methylmalonyl-CoA. The latter is converted by a soluble enzyme containing B_{12} to succinyl-CoA[34]. These reactions provide a pathway for the conversion of propionic acid into a compound of the citric acid cycle. This method of succinyl-CoA formation appears to be especially important in sheep and other ruminants which use the propionic acid produced in the rumen as an energy source. The B_{12} reaction has not been shown in erythrocytes. B_{12} deficiency does not result in an inability of red cells to form HEME but rather in an increased level of circulating methyl malonic acid which may possibly be related to the neurological symptoms associated with this deficiency.

A fourth method of succinyl-CoA synthesis is via a CoA transferase from acetoacetyl-CoA to succinate. This enzyme has low activity in liver[35].

The available data indicate that mitochondria are the principal site of ALA synthesis because succinyl-CoA is formed via α-KG-oxidase, a mitochondrial enzyme complex and because ALA-synthetase is present in mitochondria. In erythrocytes, the presence of mitochondria correlates well with the ability to synthesize HEME. The reticulocyte lacking a nucleus but containing some mitochondria can form some HEME and globin. Recently, hemoglobin synthesis has been claimed for nuclei of avian erythrocytes[36]. It will now be necessary to inquire whether enzymes for HEME synthesis are present in these nuclei or whether HEME is supplied to the nuclei via the cytoplasm.

Properties

ALA-synthetase of erythrocyte particles or liver mitochondria is inhibited by a number of substances such as cysteine, CoA-SH and L-penicillamine. These probably react with the aldehyde group of the pyridoxal-P coenzyme on the enzyme to form a thiazolidine ring, or with HCN to form a cyanohydrin[8, 18]. Aminomalonate is also a good inhibitor (Ki = 2×10^{-5}M)[37].

ALA-synthetase from the purple photosynthetic bacterium *R. spheroides* has been obtained in a soluble form by Kikuchi et al.[38]. Shemin has described the preparation of the enzyme[39]. The enzyme occurs in the chromatophores. The ALA-synthetase has been localized in the solubilized fraction which precipitates with 30% ammonium sulfate. The mechanism of action proposed for ALA-synthetase (Fig. 5) is the condensation of pyridoxal-P with glycine to form a Schiff-base on the enzyme En, thus forming a stabilized carbanion with loss of a proton. This is followed by condensation in which the acyl-C atom of succinyl-CoA acts as an electron acceptor. The decarboxylation occurs simul-

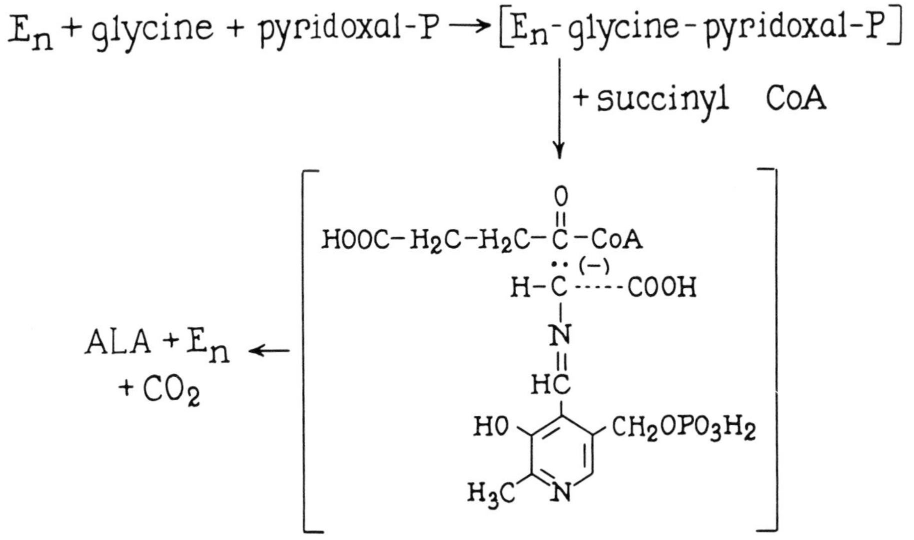

$$E_n + glycine + pyridoxal\text{-}P \rightarrow [E_n\text{-}glycine\text{-}pyridoxal\text{-}P]$$

$$+ succinyl\ CoA \downarrow$$

$$ALA + E_n + CO_2 \leftarrow \left[\begin{array}{c} O \\ \| \\ HOOC\text{-}H_2C\text{-}H_2C\text{-}C\text{-}CoA \\ H\text{-}\overset{\cdot\cdot}{C}\text{-----}COOH \\ (-) \\ | \\ N \\ \| \\ HC \\ HO\diagdown\diagup CH_2OPO_3H_2 \\ H_3C\diagdown N\diagup \end{array} \right]$$

Fig. 5.—Mechanism of ALA synthesis.[38] (Reprinted by Permission of Shemin et al. J. Biol. Chem. 233: 1214, 1958.)

taneously or shortly thereafter. Enzyme activity is maximal at pH 6.9. The Km for pyridoxal-P is 5×10^{-6}M, for succinyl-CoA is 2.2×10^{-5}M and for glycine 3×10^{-3}M. Inhibitors of this enzyme material indicate that SH groups are required for activity. The enzyme is inhibited 50% by ALA itself at 5×10^{-2}M. α-KG is a competitive inhibitor of glycine utilization which may explain the fact that in erythrocytes, concentrations of α-KG above 0.001 M inhibit ALA synthesis.

α-Aminoketones other than ALA can be formed by the condensation of glycine with a number of acyl-CoA compounds. Gibson et al.[18] found that in particles from chicken reticulocytes, the order of reactivity of acyl-Co A compounds with glycine is succinyl-CoA > acetyl-CoA > propionyl-CoA > glutaryl-Co A. Studies with liver mitochondria indicate that ALA-synthetase is specific for succinyl-CoA. The formation of aminoacetone from acetyl-CoA and glycine (reaction II) is brought about by another enzyme[40].

Iron deficient bird erythrocytes have a diminished rate of ALA synthesis[41]. When such erythrocytes are incubated for 30 minutes with Fe^{++} the rate of ALA synthesis increases 2–3 times. Similarly, the iron chelating agent o-phenanthroline (1×10^{-3}M) decreases by half the PROTO synthesis of chicken erythrocytes[17, 18]. Neither hemolysates nor cell particles from iron deficient cells respond to addition of iron. Some hypotheses to explain this effect are: Iron may induce the synthesis of an iron enzyme, induce the synthesis of ALA synthetase, or stabilize the enzymes.

Degradation of ALA via a succinate-glycine cycle

It was proposed by Shemin and Russell[42] that ALA not only gives rise to the porphyrins but can be oxidized back to succinic acid. The oxidation can then provide a pathway for glycine oxidation. Another pathway proposed by Shemin, which uses aminoacetone, is probably of greater significance in glycine oxidation than is the one from ALA[40]. The evidence for a cycle via ALA was based on whole animal experiments, and quantitative estimates of their significance could not be obtained. The data provided by Shemin and co-workers[43] showed that the ALA-carbon derived from glycine could form formate and enter the ureido group of a purine in red cells, and in addition, if the animal was poisoned with malonate, some ALA was excreted as succinate.

In the succinate-glycine cycle the first step postulated is the deamination of ALA. A transaminase which is slightly active in erythrocytes although more active in other tissues has been reported by Kowalski et al.[44]; it transaminates the amino groups of ALA to pyruvate. However, Gibson et al.[37] have found that the transaminase reaction favors the formation of ALA rather than its deamination, as shown in their system with 1-alanine or β-alanine as donor and α-dioxovaleric acid as acceptor.

Ninety per cent of the ALA added to hemolyzed chicken erythrocytes is converted to porphyrins[22]. This result suggests that once ALA is formed in the erythrocytes, little of it is oxidized. Rather, because of the relatively active ALA-dehydrase enzyme it is readily converted to PBG.

ALA-determination

The synthesis of ALA is best followed by its reaction with acetylacetone to form a pyrrole and the determination of the pyrrole colormetrically with Ehrlich's reagent (p-dimethylamino benzaldehyde in acid)[45]. Methods for the separation and determination of ALA, PBG and aminoacetone have been developed[40].

VI. CONVERSION OF δ-AMINOLEVULINIC ACID TO PORPHOBILINOGEN BY ALA-DEHYDRASE (PBG-SYNTHETASE)

ALA and the class of α-aminoketo compounds to which it belongs are, in general, stable in acid but rapidly and reversibly self-condensed to dihydropyrazines in alkaline solution (pH 8) as shown in Figure 6. The dihydropyrazines autoxidize in air to form aromatic pyrazines.

ALA-dehydrase has been partially purified from ox liver[46], rabbit reticulocytes[12] and from R. spheroides[47]. The Km for these enzymes is, respectively, 1.4×10^{-4}M, 5×10^{-4}M and 3×10^{-4}M. The optimal pH is about 6.7 for the the animal enzymes and 8.6 for the R. spheroides enzyme. The enzyme requires activation by SH compounds such as glutathione or cysteine. Metals inhibit roughly in the order of the solubility products of their sulfides. The enzyme will only accept ALA as substrate. Inhibitor studies[12] suggest that a carbonyl group γ to an ionized carboxyl group, but not an amino group, is required for binding of the substrate to the enzyme. Kinetic studies[12] suggest the following mechanism (Fig. 6). Both molecules of ALA are bound by the enzyme, the first at least 10 times more firmly than the second. The binding of the second ALA may involve spontaneous formation of the ketimine at B. The presence of a metal at C (as Lewis acid) would favor the formation of an enolate ion, but no metal was found. The aldol condensation requires that an enolate ion attack the carbonyl of the adjacent ALA molecule at A. The condensation at A with resultant hydrogen shift would then result in pyrrole

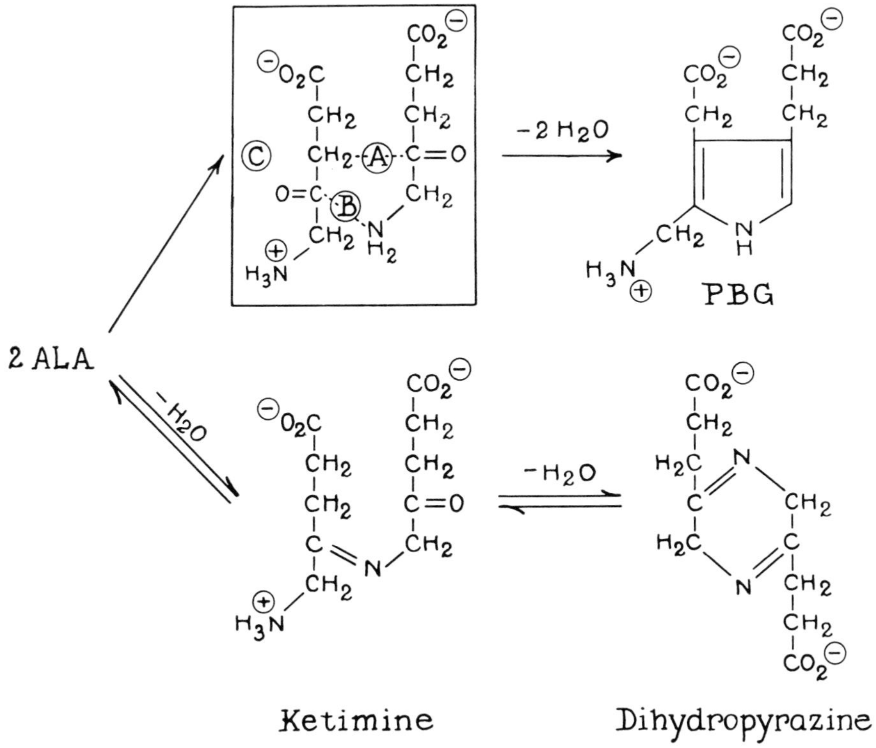

FIG. 6.—The condensation of two ALA molecules by ALA-dehydrase to PBG is shown. Also shown is the condensation of two ALA molecules non-enzymically to a ketimine and thence to a dihydropyrazine. (Reprinted by permission of Granick & Mauzerall. *Metabolic Pathways*, Vol. II, Academic Press, 1960.)

formation. The enzyme is inhibited by EDTA "uncompetitively." Both the liver and reticulocyte enzymes are inhibited at low concentrations (Ki = 10^{-5}M)[12, 46]. The enzyme from chicken erythrocytes is only partly inhibited at 10^{-5}M EDTA and the inhibition is not increased even at 10^{-2}M[12]. Possibly, a change in configuration of the enzyme or removal of a metal or both are involved in this peculiar effect. The *R. spheroides* enzyme, on the other hand, is not inhibited by EDTA[47].

VII. CONVERSION OF PORPHOBILINOGEN TO UROPORPHYRINOGEN III

This reaction requires two enzymes, as was first recognized by their differential susceptibility to heat. When an enzyme preparation is incubated with PBG, UROGEN III is formed. If the preparation is heated to 60° for 15 minutes, only UROGEN I is formed. Preparations from Chlorella cells[10, 48], erythrocytes[49] and *R. spheroides*[50] behave in the same way.

The four possible isomers of uroporphyrinogen are shown in Figure 7. Only isomers I and III are ever encountered in nature. A stepwise condensation of 4 PBG molecules with the elimination of NH_3 at each step would give rise to isomer I. However, for isomer III to be formed one of the pyrrole residues must be "flipped over" during the condensation. This problem and the many

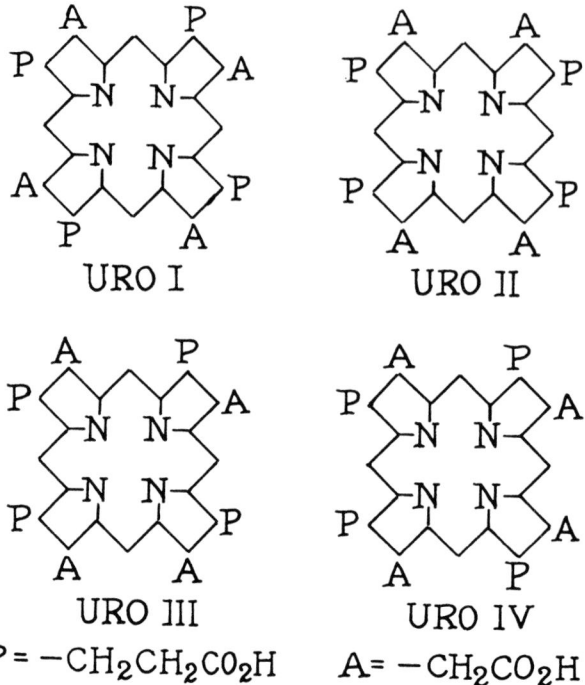

FIG. 7.—Schematic representation of the four isomers of uroporphyrin. Isomer III differs from I in that one pyrrole ring (in the lower left-hand corner of the porphyrin ring) has been "flipped over." (Reprinted by permission of Granick & Mauzerall. *Metabolic Pathways*, Vol. II, Academic Press, 1960.)

mechanisms that have been offered in explanation have been discussed in detail by Bogorad[10]. Here we mention only the ingenious hypothesis of Mathewson and Corwin[51]. They suggest that PBG condenses to a protonated tetramer (Fig. 8, No. 3) which retains the α-hydrogen atoms, thus allowing for greater flexibility of the molecule. The tetramer contains three pyrrolenine rings and may cyclize in one of three ways. It may cyclize directly to form UROGEN I, with the splitting out of NH_3. Or, it may cyclize, then open and recyclize to form either UROGEN III or a corrin ring precursor of B_{12}. In the formation of UROGEN III the $—CH_2NH_3{}^+$ group of one pyrrole "d" attacks not at the α position of pyrrole "a" containing the H atom (as for UROGEN I synthesis) but rather at the α-position which contains a $—CH_2—$.

Bray and Shemin[52] have found that the main skeleton of the corrin structure of B_{12} is derived from the condensation of 8 ALA molecules in a manner similar to porphyrin biosynthesis. The six "extra" methyl groups are derived from the methyl group of methionine probably via adenosyl methionine[52]. Bonnet[53] has recently reviewed the chemistry of B_{12}.

Bogorad has investigated the two enzyme activities required for the synthesis of UROGEN III in plant material. Using an acetone powder of spinach he obtained an extract which, when heated to 60° had only Uroporphyrinogen I synthetase activity (i.e. PBG deaminase)[56]. This enzyme converts 4 PBG

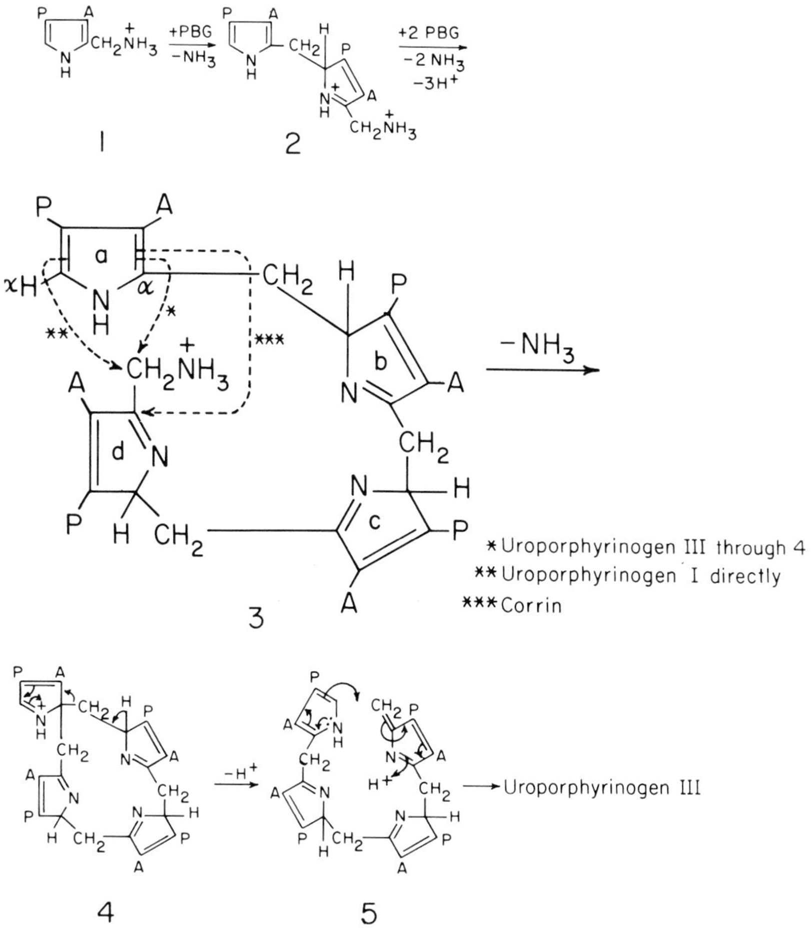

FIG. 8.—Mechanism of Mathewson and Corwin[51] for the synthesis of uroporphyrinogen isomers I and III and the corrin ring of Vit. B_{12}. (Reprinted by permission of Mathewson & Corwin. J. Am. Chem. Soc. 83: 135, 1961.)

quantitatively under anaerobic conditions to UROGEN I as indicated by the reaction:

$$4 \text{ PBG} \rightarrow 1 \text{ UROGEN I} + 4 \text{ NH}_3$$

The Km at pH 8.2, 37° is 7×10^{-5}M. The enzyme requires SH groups for activity. It will act only on PBG. It will not act on isoporphobilinogen (in which the acetic and propionic acid groups are exchanged) nor with opso-pyrroledicarboxylic acid (PBG in which H is substituted for $CH_2NH_3^+$). The latter two compounds act as competitive inhibitors[10, 54, 55]. Dipyrrylmethanes with two $CH_2NH_3^+$ side chains, or with none, are not used by the enzyme.

Intermediates accumulate when PBG is condensed enzymatically in the presence of NH_2OH or NH_3^{+}[10, 56]. The second enzyme, uroporphyrinogen III-cosynthetase (PBG isomerase) was isolated by Bogorad from an aqueous extract of wheat germ[56]. This enzyme does not act directly on PBG. However,

UROGEN III is formed when both enzymes are incubated together with PBG. The overall Km at pH 8.2, 37° is 1×10^{-4} M. Hydroxylamine is a powerful inhibitor of UROGEN III formation. UROGEN I is not converted to URO-GEN III by the enzyme. The lack of inhibition of sulfite or dithionite ions suggests that the condensations occur at the methane (i.e. fully reduced) not methene level[57]. Probably PBG is condensed by the first enzyme to a trimer, and the second enzyme acts with another PBG to form UROGEN III.

Although two enzyme activities must be present, electrophoresis of hemolysates of red cells from 3 different species indicates that only one zone contains activity to convert PBG to UROGEN III[12]. There is no zone with activity to form only UROGEN I. This suggests that both enzymes may be associated in some kind of complex.

VIII. CONVERSION OF UROPORPHYRINOGEN TO COPROPORPHYRINOGEN BY UROPORPHYRINOGEN-DECARBOXYLASE

The porphyrinogens are colorless tetrapyrrylmethanes containing 6 more H atoms than the porphyrins (Fig. 9). Fischer had early reported their occurrence in biological material. He obtained COPROGEN from the congenital porphyria patient, Petry[58]. Watson, Schwartz and coworkers reported that COPROGEN was present in the urine of porphyria patients[59]. Suspicions arose that these porphyrinogens were the actual intermediates in porphyrin biosynthesis when it was observed that the porphyrins URO and COPRO could not be used for HEME or chlorophyll synthesis by cells. The structure of PBG gave further indirect evidence for this view since the condensation of this pyrrole produces UROGEN. In 1955 Bogorad[60] obtained COPRO by

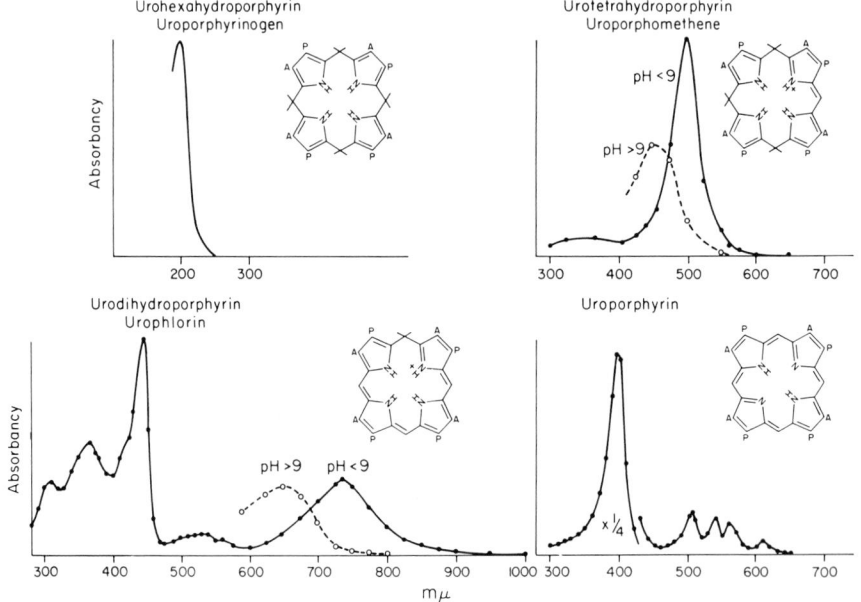

FIG. 9.—Formulas and absorption spectra of different oxidized states of uroporphyrinogen.[12, 62, 63] (Reprinted by permission of Granick. J. Biol. Chem. 232: 1119, 1958.)

incubation of a chlorella preparation with UROGEN, and Neve, Labbe and Aldrich[61] found that the addition of UROGEN to hemolyzed red cells increased the incorporation of Fe^{59} into HEME.

The porphyrinogens of URO and COPRO are most readily prepared by shaking the porphyrin with sodium amalgam in the dark in the absence of air[57]. Traces of the colored porphyrins markedly sensitize the autoxidation of the porphyrinogens in air. The spectra of the porphyrinogen (hexahydroporphyrin), the tetrahydroporphyrin (with a strong absorption band at 500 mμ), the dihydroporphyrin or phlorin (with a band at 735 mμ) and the porphyrin itself are shown in Fig. 9 and were obtained by Mauzerall[62]. The mechanism of autocondensation of PBG in acid and neutral solutions to form various UROGEN isomers was also delineated by the brilliant work of Mauzerall[63].

An enzyme preparation was obtained from rabbit reticulocytes by zone electrophoresis on starch. The enzyme has a high affinity for substrate (Km 5×10^{-6}M) and a pH optimum of 6.8[57]. It acts only on UROGEN to decarboxylate the 4 acetic side chains to —CH_3. URO is not acted on. Sulfite or dithionite ions which only complex tightly with di- or tetrahydroporphyrins at methene bridge C atoms do not inhibit the enzymatic decarboxylation. The decarboxylation proceeds stepwise but the intermediate 7 to 5 carboxyl-containing porphyrinogens, although they can be detected, are converted rapidly to the 4 carboxyl-containing COPROGEN. The enzyme decarboxylates all four isomers of UROGEN in the order III > IV > II > I. Isomer III reacts at twice the rate of isomer I.

The decarboxylase is assumed to be a single enzyme since electrophoresis of the red cell hemolysates of three different species yields only one zone with the enzyme activity, in each instance. It is inferred from the lack of isomer specificity that the enzyme decarboxylates the side chains at random and thus a large number of intermediates may exist, all of which, on continued decarboxylation, yield the appropriate isomer of COPROGEN.

IX. Conversion of Coproporphyrinogen to Protoporphyrinogen by Coproporphyrinogen-Oxidase

The formation of PROTO from COPROGEN has been observed in preparations from chicken erythrocytes[64], *Euglena*[65] and beef liver mitochondria[13]. In contrast to the non-specific nature of UROGEN decarboxylase for isomer types, the oxidase enzyme is highly specific. It attacks COPROGEN III, not I[65]. With a *Euglena* preparation neither isomer I or II are substrates. Isomer IV undergoes oxidative decarboxylation only one-tenth as fast as isomer III[66]. Porra and Falk have also reported a slight activity with isomer IV[67].

This high specificity for COPROGEN III is the main reason for the ubiquitous distribution of PROTO of series III and the absence of PROTO of series I. However, two other enzymes of the biosynthetic chain of HEME have discriminated in favor of isomer III. One is the UROGEN-cosynthetase, the action of which results in the formation of over 99.9% of UROGEN III and only traces of isomer I, as judged by the amounts of isomer I found in normal urine. UROGEN-decarboxylase also favors isomer III, acting 2–3 times as fast on III as on I.

The coproporphyrinogen oxidase has a greater activity in liver and bone marrow than in other tissues[13]. It has a Km of about $2 \times 10^{-5}M$ and pH optimum of 7.7. Only two of the four propionic acid groups are oxidatively decarboxylated. Specifically, those at side chain positions 2 and 4 form vinyl groups (Fig. 1). During the reaction, an intermediate that has one vinyl and three propionic acid groups appears and then disappears. Available evidence indicates that the oxidation of the propionic acid proceeds by hydride ion removal, with CO_2 leaving simultaneously. Cyanide does not inhibit the enzyme. No substitute for O_2 as oxidant has been found that would oxidize the propionic acid groups yet not oxidize the porphyrinogen as well. Even H_2O_2 cannot replace O_2 as oxidant with this enzyme. The impure enzyme preparation from guinea pig liver contains a flavin.

Methods for the preparation and determination of porphyrinogen have been described by Mauzerall and Granick[57]. The porphyrinogens are best determined by oxidation to the porphyrins with I_2 at neutral pH, avoiding excess I_2. However, protoporphyrinogen must be photo-oxidized or autoxidized because it is destroyed by I_2[13]. The number of carboxyl groups on a porphyrin is readily determined by paper chromatography with a lutidine-NH_3-H_2O system[68]. The specific isomers of COPRO are best analyzed by paper chromatography with the same system[68, 69]. To determine the isomers of URO, they must first be decarboxylated to the respective COPRO isomers[70].

X. PROTOPORPHYRIN OF ERYTHROCYTES AND OTHER TISSUES

Protoporphyrin is a red pigment that fluoresces red. It is present in only trace amounts in mature, normal erythrocytes, but in larger amounts in reticulocytes. Younger erythrocytes, i.e., normoblasts, contain still more. The pigment from normal erythrocytes was identified as PROTO-9, i.e. the natural type III isomer, by Grotepass in 1937[71].

Many factors affect the amount of free erythrocyte protoporphyrin (E.P.). There may be 20–40 $\mu g/100$ ml in normal RBC and ten times more in iron deficiency anemia or after acute hemorrhage[25, 72, 73].

In general, factors such as acute hemorrhage that cause reticulocytes to be shed into the blood stream at a rate greater than normal will increase the free E.P. in the blood stream.

Various factors that prevent iron incorporation into PROTO may cause a high E.P. Such factors are: deficiency of iron in the body because of diet; defective absorption of iron; defective mobilization of iron from body stores as in anemias of infection, nephritis, lymphoma and leukemia; defective mechanisms for iron absorption by the developing erythrocyte; defective transfer of iron from the red cell surface as possibly in lead poisoning; defective incorporation of iron into PROTO by the iron incorporating enzyme. In lead poisoning of rabbits the E.P. may be as high as 500 $\mu g\%$. In phenylhydrazine poisoning both the PROTO and COPRO are high[75].

E.P. is low in pyridoxine deficiency because this vitamin is required to form the prosthetic group of ALA-synthetase; its lack prevents ALA synthesis and therefore PROTO synthesis. E.P. is also low in folic acid deficiency, but this must be a rather indirect effect.

Relatively high concentrations of PROTO are found in certain tissues of some animals, but in only trace amounts in a wide variety of cells. The Harderian eye gland of the rat contains a high concentration. PROTO is deposited in various bird egg shells at the time the shell is forming[76]. The brown egg shells of Plymouth Rock hens fluoresce red under ultraviolet light. PROTO is also present in egg yolk. In the incubated egg, PROTO develops not only the embryo but increases in the egg white by excretion from the embryo so that about 130 μg are present in the egg white of a nearly fully developed embryo.

XI. Iron Transfer to Erythroid Cells

During maturation the erythroid cells of the bone marrow must acquire sufficient iron for hemoglobin synthesis. The amount of iron required per cell is over 100 times that needed by other kinds of cells. It is evident that special mechanisms have been developed to accumulate the relatively large amount of iron and yet avoid excess. Brown[77] has recently reviewed two known pathways for iron transfer to red cells. The major one is via transferrin. The other pathway is by a process of pinocytosis from reticuloendothelial cells.

Iron transfer by transferrin

The outstanding studies of Jandl et al.[78] have elucidated the mechanism of iron transfer from transferrin to erythroid cells (Fig. 10). Transferrin is a serum β_1 globulin with a molecular weight of 90,000. There are two independent sites on its surface[79] which can chelate with one ferric ion and bind the ion very tightly. Jandl et al.[78] demonstrated (using crystalline transferrin) that the reticulocyte membrane contains specific sites for the reversible attachment of transferrin. Trypsin can digest away these sites. When transferrin is less than 20% saturated with iron it can compete with the bone marrow for iron. Between 20–60% of saturation, i.e. the physiological limits, iron is transferred at a maximal rate to the reticulocytes. Above 60% of saturation the iron may be unloaded onto tissues such as liver that have comparatively less affinity for it.

Iron-rich transferrin is bound to the reticulocyte membrane 4–5 times as strongly as iron-poor transferrin. After transferrin attaches to the membrane of the reticulocyte, the iron becomes bound to the membrane and the transferrin leaves. This transfer process appears to be aided by ascorbic acid and to require ATP because dinitrophenol (10^{-4}M) inhibits it. Lead poisoning prevents the iron from migrating into the cell; this fact suggests that some transport mechanism, possibly involving SH groups, may be required for this step. Once the iron is inside the cell it may migrate into the mitochondrion and be used directly for incorporation into protoporphyrin to form HEME, or it may be temporarily stored in the form of ferritin. The exchange of iron between transferrin and reticulocytes is represented diagrammatically in Figure 10.

Iron transfer by rhopheocytosis

The process by which erythroblasts acquire iron from reticuloendothelial cells has been elucidated by Bessis and coworkers[80] (Fig. 11). They observed in the bone marrow large reticuloendothelial or "nurse" cells, which are closely surrounded by a group of erythroblasts. The central reticuloendothelial cell

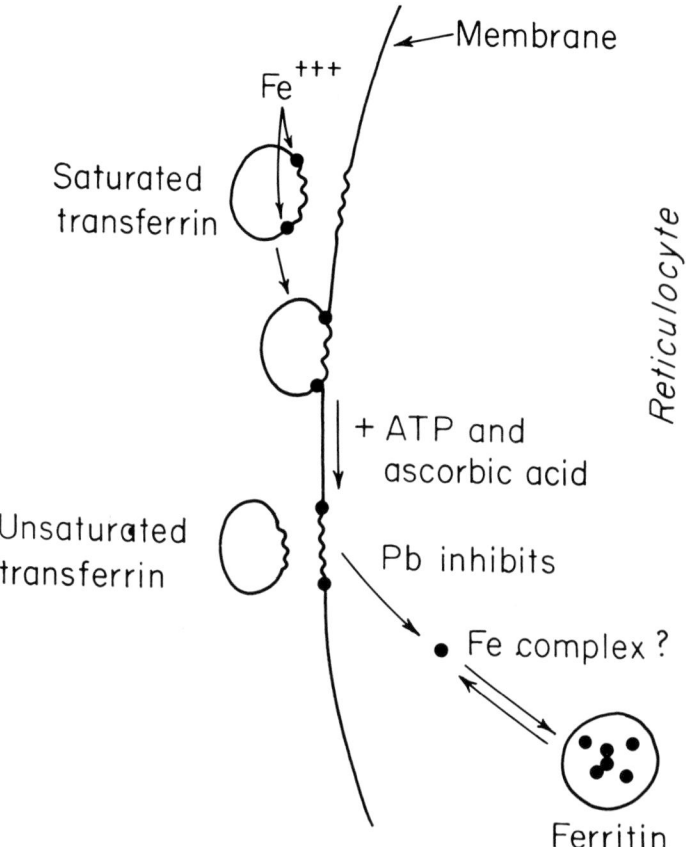

FIG. 10.—Iron transfer between transferrin and reticulocytes. Saturated transferrin is bound to the reticulocyte membrane at specific sites.[78] Iron transfer to the membrane is dependent on ATP and ascorbic acid. Since lead causes accumulation of iron on the membrane it is possible that SH containing substances (glutathione, cysteine) form transient complexes with iron to allow its transport into the cytoplasm.

sends delicate protoplasmic blebs into the erythroblasts. These blebs are studded on their inner surface with ferritin molecules. The erythroblasts pinch off the blebs as vesicles, and the vesicles migrate toward the inside of the erythroblasts and eventually break down, releasing the ferritin. The reticulo-endothelial cells may obtain their iron from transferrin, and also by phago-cytosis of effete red blood cells.

In thalassemia and in sideroachrestic anemias huge amounts of iron accumulate in the immature red cells. The iron may be present as siderotic granules and as ferritin; often, degenerating mitochondria are filled with ferritin.

XII. INSERTION OF FERROUS IRON INTO PROTOPORPHYRIN. THE IRON CHELATASE ENZYME

Attempts to isolate a ferrous iron chelating enzyme have been hampered by the relative ease of the non-enzymic incorporation of iron into porphyrins.

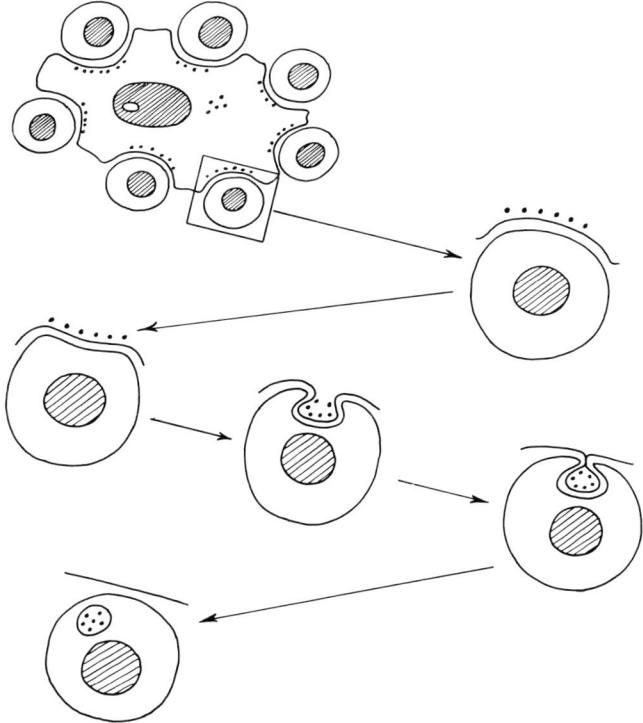

Fig. 11.—Above, left, is depicted a reticuloendothelial "nurse" cell surrounded by erythroblasts. The process of rhopheocytosis is diagramatically represented in the next series of drawings which show the area of contact between the "nurse" cell and erythroblast in more detail.[77, 80]

Conditions which enhance the chelation of porphyrins with iron by enzymes also enhance the non-enzymic chelation. These conditions are: the maintenance of iron in the ferrous form by anaerobiosis or by reducing agents such as ascorbic acid, cysteine or glutathione; the avoidance of buffers such as those containing phosphate or amines that complex with iron; the solubilization of highly insoluble or colloidal PROTO by means of various detergents so that PROTO may become available in a monomolecularly dispersed form.

The enzyme catalyzing the chelation of iron to form HEME has been found in liver mitochondria and in particles from hemolyzed chicken or duck erythrocytes. The enzyme seems to be localized in mitochondria. However, the nuclei of avian erythrocytes have not yet been eliminated as another site of this enzyme.

Labbe and Hubbard[81] studied the chelatase enzyme from rat liver mitochondria and from duck erythrocytes. Tween 20 was employed as the solubilizing agent in their system. They suggested that SH groups are needed by the enzyme to bind the porphyrin. Both Fe^{++} and Co^{++} can be inserted into the porphyrin by the enzyme; other metals are inhibitory. Dicarboxylic porphyrins but not tetracarboxylic porphyrins are used by the enzyme. The rate of iron incorporation by the enzyme is more than ten times the non-enzymic rate[82]. Labbe and Hubbard considered that the enzyme is more selective with respect to the kind of metal, than to the kind of porphyrin, because the enzyme in the cell is presented with only one porphyrin, PROTO, but needs to select Fe^{++} from among a number of other metal ions.

Oyama et al.[83] obtained a solubilized preparation from duck erythrocytes using sodium cholate; their preparation incorporated ferrous, zinc, and cobalt ions into the porphyrin in a ratio of 100:10:2.

Porra and Jones[84] isolated a chelatase enzyme from pig liver mitochondria. Their test system contained a detergent to render the porphyrin more soluble. GSH was also added and O_2 removed to maintain the iron in the ferrous state. SH groups were required to keep the iron reduced, not to activate the enzyme. Only the dicarboxylic porphyrins like proto-, meso-, deutero- and hemato- were substrates but not tetracarboxylic porphyrins like copro-. The pH curve of the reaction had two maxima of activity, suggesting the presence of two enzymes. At pH 7.8 and 37°, their enzyme preparation exchanged 1.25% of the iron between protoheme and labeled ferrous citrate in the presence of dithionite in one hour.

Neve[85] prepared a Tween 40 extract from chicken erythrocyte particles and fractionated it with ammonium sulfate. Lead acetate ($10^{-5}M$) inhibited the chelatase activity of this preparation by 65%. Schwartz et al.[86] found that in the presence of globin the incorporation of iron into PROTO by their preparation of enzyme was increased 3-fold, but Yoneyama et al.[87] found globin inhibitory.

XIII. Hemoglobin Synthesis, Heme, and the Folding of the Globin Polypeptide

Hemoglobin formation is usually considered to take place by the insertion of HEME into a highly hydrophobic pocket of the globin, with the vinyl groups of the HEME buried in the pocket and the propionic acid groups projecting from near the surface of the globin. There are about 90 van der Waal's contacts between the HEME group and the histidine plus other residues lining the pocket[88] which all add up to stabilize the globin configuration around the HEME. The iron of the HEME makes contact with the imidazole-N of a histidine residue of the globin and, if the iron is in the ferrous form, the HEME will now have the ability to accept O_2 reversibly.

Native globin may be prepared from hemoglobin. When native globin is combined with ferrous protoporphyrin-CO (i.e. in an atmosphere containing CO) a two-step reaction is observed. One occurs with a first order rate constant of 3×10^{-6}/mole/sec.[89, 90] and the second step, which gives the hemoglobin-CO complex, occurs in about 10^{-2}/sec. A globin-protoporphyrin molecule may be formed as readily as hemoglobin. Therefore, the iron is apparently not essential for the firm binding or for forming a stable molecule. The order of binding to globin is Fe PROTO > Fe meso- > Fe deutero- > Fe hematoporphyrin. The very slight but significant reversibility of the binding of HEME to globin is inferred from the fact that the (Fe^{++} HEME·CO) attached to globin can be made to exchange with another HEME-protein in a half time of the order of hours, in the absence of O_2[91].

When globin is formed on polysomes it is assumed that the three-dimensional folding takes place spontaneously because it is thermodynamically the most stable configuration. Such spontaneous folding has been demonstrated for ribonuclease, the lysozyme of egg white, trypsin and taka-amylase A[92] where the folding is aided by the formation of S-S bridges.

A different assumption is that HEME is required for the folding of globin. It is known that the hemoglobin from which HEME is removed is a highly unstable protein. The idea that HEME may bring about the appropriate folding and provide a stable molecule before the heme-globin molecule leaves the polysome may be worth investigating. In favor of this possibility are the tracer studies with labeled glycine added to reticulocytes which show that the HEME and globin are produced in a 1:1 ratio. On the other hand, the studies of Morell et al.[93] suggest that cobalt poisoning of cells depresses the synthesis of HEME but not of protein (assumed to be globin).

Polypeptide synthesis has been shown to begin at the amino end of the chain. It is possible to imagine a spontaneous coiling of the polypeptide starting from the amino end as it grows out from the polysome even in the absence of HEME. However, Kendrew[88] has pointed out that the first two helices of the globin at the amino end are at right angles to each other and therefore do not interact; thus no stability is gained at this early stage of polypeptide synthesis. If folding could begin at the carboxyl end, then stability would accrue because there are two helices at this end which sit more or less parallel to each other and interact. However, if folding did not begin until the carboxyl end had been completed, a polypeptide, 150 amino acids long, would be dangling from the polysome.

XIV. Synthesis of Heme Proteins Other Than Hemoglobin

The proerythroblast contains HEME enzymes similar to those found in other aerobic cells. All the HEMES are derivatives of the type III isomer (Section VIII). The enzymes include cytochrome-b and catalase which, like hemoglobin, contain iron protoporphyrin as the prosthetic group. Crytochrome oxidase has a modified iron porphyrin in which side chain position 2 is [—CHOH—CH$_2$—(CH$_2$·CH$_2$·CH(CH$_3$)·CH$_2$)$_3$H] in place of a vinyl group, and position 8 has a —CHO group in place of a —CH$_3$[94]. The above HEMES can be readily removed from their respective proteins by organic solvents.

Cytochrome-c, on the other hand, contains a HEME which is bound through each vinyl side chain to a cysteine residue forming a thioether bond at the 2 and the 4 positions. This HEME, because it is covalently linked to the protein, cannot be removed with organic solvents. The mechanism assumed for cytochrome-c formation is an enzymatic reaction of apocytochrome-c with iron protoporphyrin through the vinyl groups. Recently, a different mechanism has been suggested[13] based on the fact that SH compounds readily react with vinyl groups of reduced porphyrins. Sano et al.[95] have shown that apocytochrome-c reacted readily with reduced protoporphyrin to form thioether bonds. The iron was then inserted into the ring to produce a molecule resembling cytochrome-c. Perhaps cytochrome-c is formed enzymatically in cells by a similar mechanism.

XV. NUCLEAR HEMOGLOBIN

The presence of hemoglobin in erythroblast nuclei

Various investigators have inferred that avian and mammalian normoblast nuclei contain hemoglobin (or HEME) on the basis of staining techniques[96, 97, 98], absorption microspectroscopy[99] and electron density[100, 101] studies. Stein and co-workers[102] have unequivocally demonstrated hemoglobin in avian erythrocyte nuclei isolated by the Behren's non-aqueous technique. Schmid et al.[103] found intense porphyrin fluorescence in the nuclei of many of the developing normoblasts in the bone marrow of patients with congenital erythropoietic porphyria. They also noted benzidine postive inclusions in the nuclei of some of these normoblasts, indicative of heme or hemoglobin.

The present authors, employing a new fluorescent technique to visualize HEME[104] have been able to confirm the presence of HEME (presumably hemoglobin) in normal avian and human normoblasts. The blood or bone marrow smear is flooded with 1.5N perchloric acid containing 0.2 M mercapto-ethanolamine hydrochloride, covered with a cover-slip and examined under a fluorescence microscope. After 10–60 seconds of ultraviolet light (380–410 mμ) irradiation of the slide while on the microscope stage, red fluorescence appears in cellular areas containing HEME or HEME proteins. The treatment with perchloric acid followed by ultraviolet light irradiation causes fixation of the cells, reduces and removes the iron from the porphyrin ring and converts the porphyrin to its acid form. The acid porphyrin fluoresces, emitting light at 600 and 660 mμ. Figure 12—1b and 2b are black and white fluorescence photographs of normoblasts from normal human bone marrow which was so treated. Porphyrin fluorescence, equally distributed between the cytoplasm and nucleus, is intense in polychromatic and orthochromatic normoblasts. Both the cytoplasm and nucleus of myeloid cells exhibit a very faint fluorescence. In the cytoplasm this is undoubtedly due to cytochromes. The HEME components of the white cell nuclei are as yet unidentified. Normoblast stages preceding the polychromatic normoblast also demonstrate fluorescence, however, the fluorescence is no greater than that due to cytochromes alone as seen in the myeloid cells. Though it is not clearly shown in the photographs, the perchlorate-induced porphyrin fluorescence is not uniformly distributed in the normoblast nucleus. There are regions almost devoid of fluorescence intermixed with regions of intense fluorescence, creating a pattern similar to the spaces produced by the clumping of heterochromatin seen with Wright's stain.

Nuclear synthesis of hemoglobin

Hammell, Rasmussen and Bessman[36] have described hemoglobin synthesis by isolated pigeon erythrocyte nuclei. Their nuclear fraction was obtained by hemolysis of whole cells with saponin and contained cell membranes and cytoplasmic particles in addition to nuclei. Using whole pigeon erythrocytes which were pulse labeled with C^{14} leucine and incubated for 5 minutes, these authors reported that hemoglobin was formed in the nucleus and then migrated out into the cytoplasm.

Studies on isolated thymocyte nuclei by Allfrey and Mirsky[205] have shown that these nuclei possess an active ATP generating system which would enable

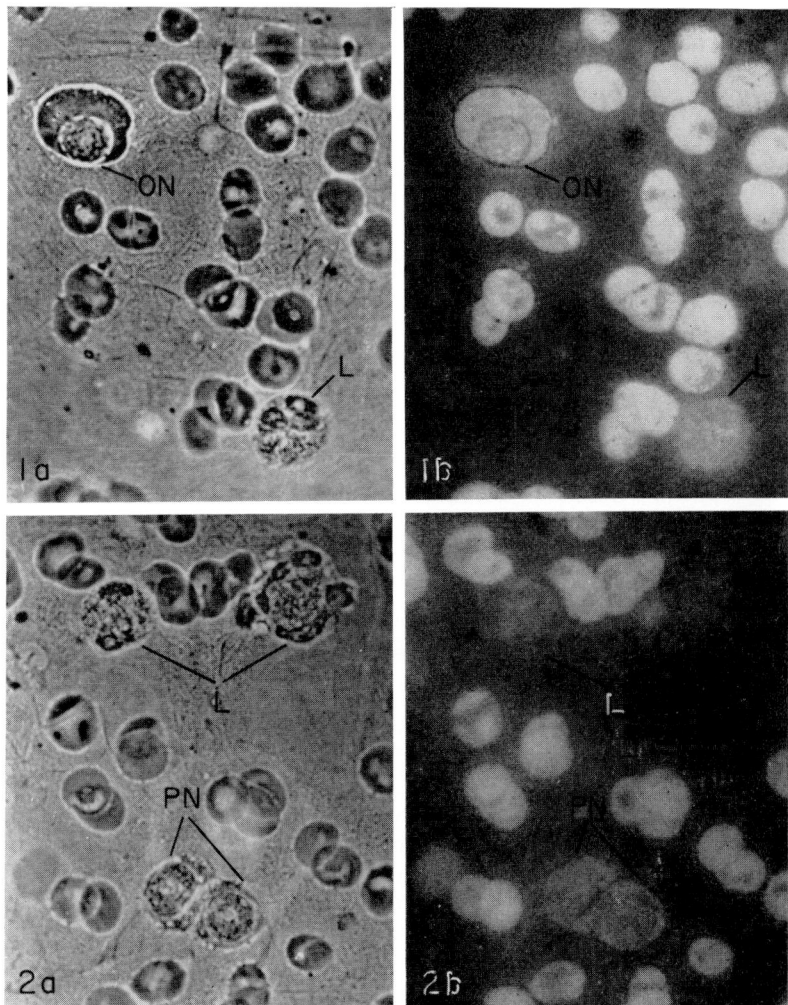

FIG. 12.—1a) Phase contrast photograph of normal human bone marrow showing an orthochromatic normoblast (ON), neutrophil (L), and many mature erythrocytes. Unstained. Mag. × 1000.

1b) Black and white fluorescence photograph of the same field as shown in 1a after treatment with 1.5N HClO₄ and U.V. light irradiation. Red fluorescence is recorded as white. The orthochromatic normoblast (ON) reveals intense cytoplasmic and nuclear fluorescence, while fluorescence in the neutrophil (L) is faint. The induced porphyrin fluorescence is most marked in the mature erythrocytes. Mag. × 1000.

2a) Phase contrast photograph of a normal human bone marrow smear showing two early polychromatic normoblasts (PN) and two neutrophils (L). Mag. × 1000.

2b) Black and white fluorescence photograph of the same field as shown in 2a after treatment with 1.5N HClO₄ and U.V. light irradiation. The polychromatic normoblasts (PN) reveal equal nuclear and cytoplasmic fluorescence. Fluorescence in the neutrophils (L) is barely detectable. Mag. × 1000.

them to synthesize proteins. An ATP generating system for red cells, apart
from the Embden-Meyerhof pathway is indicated by the presence of succinic
dehydrogenase in chicken erythrocyte nuclei. This was shown by the reduction of tetrazolium dyes to insoluble formazans just inside the nuclear membrane in the presence of succinate[106]. On the basis of this evidence it may be
tentatively considered that both the nucleus and cytoplasm are sites of hemoglobin synthesis.

Nuclear heme and "early-labeled" bilirubin

Intranuclear hemoglobin and porphyrins may play a role in the origin of
the "early-labeled" fraction of bile pigment. In normals, following the administration of C^{14}-glycine, 80–90 percent of the C^{14}-labeled fecal urobilinogen
is derived from the hemoglobin of erythrocytes ending their normal life span
of 120 days[107, 108]. The remaining 10–20 percent of the C^{14} appears in the
bile within 20 days after administration of the labeled glycine and comes
from sources other than senescence of circulating erythrocytes. In congenital
erythropoietic porphyria this "early-labeled" fraction of urobilinogen may
account for as much as 80 percent of the administered glycine[107]. It is possible
that a fraction of this "early-labeled" bile pigment is due to degradation of
other HEME proteins, i.e., cytochrome, myoglobin, peroxidase and catalase.
Other possibilities include: intramarrow hemolysis of cells prior to their release into the circulation ("ineffective erythropoiesis"); direct synthesis of
urobilinogen from HEME not derived from HEME-protein; the breakdown
of circulating erythrocytes with a shortened life span. In the light of the presence of hemoglobin in the normoblast nucleus, it is attractive to hypothesize
that a portion of "early-labeled" urobilinogen appearing within the first 2 to
4 days after C^{14}-glycine administration, may be derived from the hemo-
globin-containing nucleus following its normal extrusion from the cell.

XVI. ERYTHROID DIFFERENTIATION AND MATURATION

In this section we wish to summarize the concurrent changes in DNA, RNA,
protein and HEME that appear as the relatively undifferentiated hemocyto-
blast changes into a mature red cell. This will serve as a background for the
discussion, in the following section of the mechanisms that control hemoglobin
synthesis.

Two processes go on simultaneously during this transformation, that of cell
division and differentiation. The changes in differentiation occur over a period
of 4–6 days and through approximately three to four cell divisions.

During the transformation, a relatively undifferentiated cell (the hemo-
cytoblast) is converted into a pronormoblast and through further changes, into
a red blood cell. These changes are thought to represent the inactivation of
certain genes, and the activation of other genes, especially those concerned with
HEME and globin formation. Because the cell can multiply for a limited
number of divisions, the ability to duplicate its DNA (replication) is not
changed. Yet the ability to form different messenger RNAs (transcription) is
changed; this constitutes the differentiation process.

DNA.—As summarized in Fig. 13D the DNA content and, therefore, the number of genes remains unchanged until the late polychromatic or orthochromatic normoblast stage[109]. Because cells undergoing division have a period in the interphase (8 hours) during which DNA is replicating, such cells will usually contain more DNA than that equivalent to 2n chromosomes. When the cells cease dividing at the polychromatic normoblast stage, they will have the 2n equivalent of DNA. Finally, the nucleus is lost; either *in toto* or in a stepwise fashion by extrusion of fragments.

RNA synthesis (Fig. 13C) is at a maximum in the pronormoblast, declines continuously during maturation, and stops either at the polychromatic[109] or early orthochromatic stage[110]. No RNA synthesis occurs in reticulocytes[109],

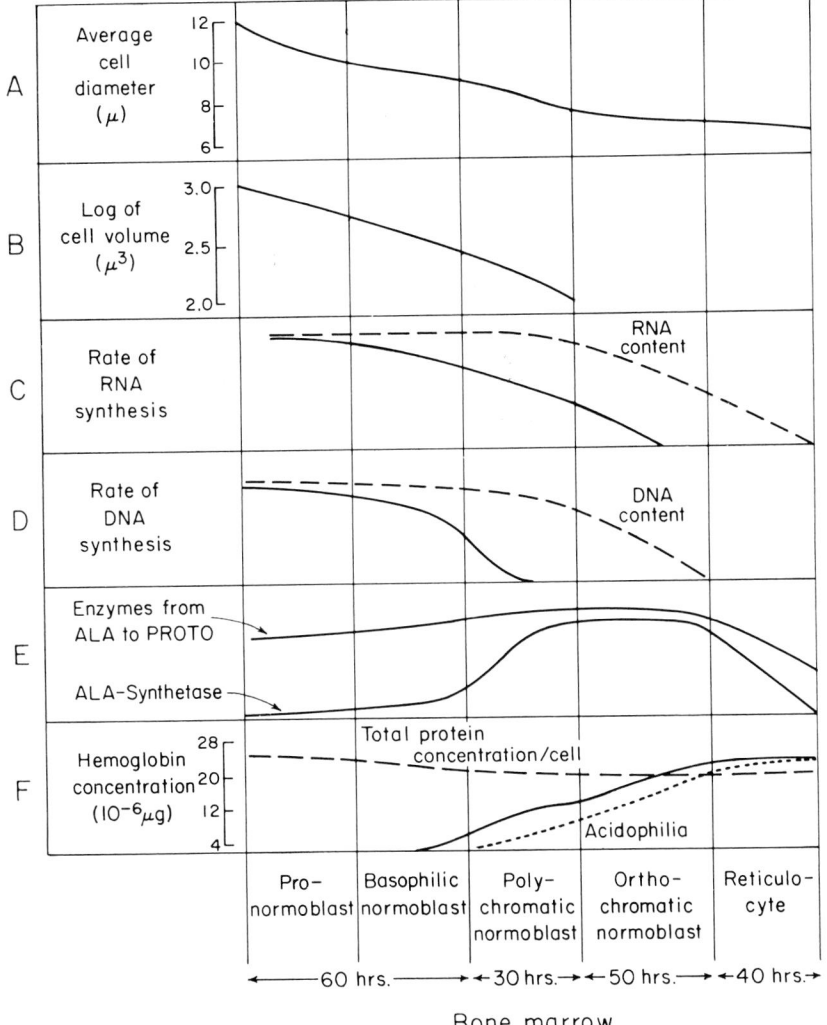

Fig. 13.—Changes of various substances during erythroid differentiation and maturation. Substances listed in left-hand column are represented by corresponding solid black lines. Unless specified, graphs represent relative values.

[110, 111]. The major fraction of RNA is in the form of ribosomes with smaller amounts present as amino acid transfer RNA and messenger RNA. (In bacteria the weight ratio of ribosomes to transfer RNA to messenger RNA is 80:15:5, resp.). In the normoblast the majority of the messenger RNA is probably concerned with globin synthesis. In addition to the cytoplasm, the nucleus appears to be a site for globin synthesis[112]; therefore, functional ribosomes and messenger RNA must be present in both cytoplasm and nucleus. Studies by Borsook[113] with Actinomycin-D have provided evidence that the RNA synthesis is dependent on the presence of DNA.

It is interesting to note that the cytoplasmic RNA concentration falls at a time when maximal hemoglobin synthesis begins. Grasso[109] suggests that only the RNA and ribosomes necessary for hemoglobin synthesis are then retained. Hemoglobin synthesis in reticulocytes, where there is no DNA and RNA synthesis, appears to occur on preformed m-RNA. This synthesis is not inhibited by RNA base analogs[114].

Protein synthesis proceeds at a rather steady rate throughout all stages of erythroid maturation including the reticulocyte. In pronormoblasts and basophilic normoblasts there is synthesis of non-hemoglobin protein, comprised mainly of enzymes which turn over and do not accumulate in the cytoplasm[110]. The rate of hemoglobin synthesis depicted in Fig. 13F probably is low in basophilic normoblasts reaching peak levels in the polychromatic normoblast. It continues at this level throughout the orthochromatic stage. Hemoglobin synthesis takes place in reticulocytes but production here, under non-stress conditions, probably accounts for only ten percent of the total hemoglobin produced during maturation. However, this indicates that hemoglobin synthesis can occur in the absence of a nucleus. Synthesis of the polypeptide chains of globin occurs on polysomes[115]. These are ribosome aggregates apparently held together by messenger RNA. Specific messenger RNAs direct the synthesis of specific polypeptide chains (α, β, γ or δ). Only the polysome aggregates, not individual ribosomes, are active in hemoglobin synthesis. In reticulocytes, the polysomes disaggregate, resulting in a decrease in rate of hemoglobin synthesis, although total ribosomal RNA decreases more slowly[110]. In the absence of nuclear DNA there is no synthesis of new messenger-RNA for globin production, and globin synthesis can be expected to fall rapidly as the preformed messenger-RNA is lost through attack by nucleases. One of the possible mechanisms through which HEME synthesis comes to a stop simultaneously with the cessation of globin production is by the covering up of genes, i.e. heterochromatin formation.

Heterochromatin.—Progressive maturation of the erythroid cell is associated with a continued increase in the clumping of nuclear DNA. This is seen morphologically in the "checkerboard" appearance of late stage nuclei and the dense staining reaction of the orthochomatic nucleus. These condensed portions of chromosomes are referred to as heterochromatin and the extended, more diffusely staining segments as euchromatin. Heterochromatin is most marked in those cells which are highly specialized in function, i.e. they synthesize relatively large amounts of only a small number of different proteins. Apart from erythroid forms, the extensive condensation of chromatin is typically seen in lymphocytes, plasma cells and thymocytes. In thymocytes, condensed DNA makes up 80 percent of the total nuclear DNA. Frenster, Allfrey and Mirsky[116] showed that the heterochromatin fraction of calf thymocytes is only $\frac{1}{3}$ to $\frac{1}{8}$ as active as the euchromatin fraction in the synthesis of DNA, RNA and protein. Euchromatin is analogous to the "puff" regions of the polytene chromosomes of Diptera. These "puff" regions are extended areas of chromosomal DNA and are more active in RNA and protein synthesis during interphase than the condensed chromosomal regions[117]. The induction of "puffing" in these chromosomes by the molting hormone—ecdysone—is an excellent example of extrinsic control on genetic activity to produce messenger-RNA. On the basis of this information, we should consider the heterochromatin of normoblasts as repressed genetic material. At the level of the orthochromatic normoblast the chromatin has become completely repressed (pyknotic). Nuclear extrusion ensues.

The close physical association of histones with nuclear DNA has suggested that these basic proteins may play an important role in the regulation of genetic activity[118]. The positively charged histone molecules in the nucleus are attached to the chromosomes through salt-like linkages with the negatively charged phosphate groups of DNA. It is not yet known whether histone is arranged in a co-lineal or cross-stranded relationship with the DNA helix. There is recent evidence[119] to indicate that euchromatin may have a lower ratio of histone to DNA than heterochromatin. When trypsin is added to nucleohistone to digest the histone, the DNA becomes more active in RNA synthesis indicating that DNA has become derepressed or uncovered. In late stage nucleated erythrocytes, the weight ratio of histone to DNA is one. It would be of interest to learn how this ratio changes during red cell differentiation. Although the idea that histone plays a primary role in genetic regulation is an attractive hypothesis, the chemical bond between DNA bases and histones is non-specific. Therefore, it is not clear how this linkage can be directed so as to block the expression of only specific portions of genomic material.

Tooze and Davies[120] have suggested that hemoglobin, positively charged at the pH of the cell, acts like histone in causing complete condensation of nuclear DNA. This is supported by the presence of hemoglobin in the nuclei of normoblasts (See previous section) and the ability of globin to combine with DNA *in vitro*. Thus, hemoglobin, when present in large amounts, may act by a negative feedback mechanism to shut off all HEME and globin synthesis.

HEME.—The stages of differentiation can be followed more readily in red cells than in most other cells because of their internal content of porphyrin and HEME pigments. These pigments are produced in relatively large amounts in the red cells and have properties by which they can be readily detected. The porphyrins and HEMES have an intense absorption band ($\epsilon_M > 10^5$), especially in the 400 mμ region (the Soret band). HEME may be detected by its peroxidase activity with the benzidine-H_2O_2 test. HEME may also be converted to porphyrin by removal of the iron from the molecule and the protoporphyrin can then be detected in minute quantities by its fluorescence in ultraviolet light (see section XV).

In both chick blastoderms and liver cells the enzymes of the biosynthetic chain that convert ALA to HEME are present in non-limiting amounts. The limiting enzyme is the one that synthesizes ALA from succinyl-Co A and glycine. The rate of HEME synthesis is proportional to the acitivty of this ALA-synthetase which appears to reside only in mitochondria[27].

In order to study the early stages of hemoglobin development the present authors[121] have examined chick blastoderm cells prior to the initial appearance of hemoglobin. At this early stage the cells may be in a latent phase that may divide without further differentiation[122]. Cells at this early level of differentiation, comparable to the human hemocytoblasts, contain all of the enzymes of the HEME biosynthetic chain from ALA to HEME in non-limiting amounts (Fig. 13). Only when the blastoderm has formed erythroid tissue and is capable of producing globin does the ALA-synthetase enzyme appear with high activity so that large amounts of HEME can be made (Fig. 13). Saillen's work[123] indicates that in myeloid cells HEME synthesis is also limited by the activity of ALA-synthetase. It is suggested in the section on control mechanisms that it is globin synthesis which provides the induction stimulus for the synthesis of more ALA-synthetase and therefore for more HEME.

End product inhibition

There are two general ways to limit the activity of ALA-synthetase. One is by end product inhibition, i.e. the product of the biosynthetic chain, HEME, inhibits the first enzyme of that chain, ALA-synthetase. This mechanism has been demonstrated only for the bacterium *R. spheroides*, but not yet for animals. Burnham and Lascelles[124] found that the ALA-synthetase of this bacterium was inhibited reversibly by 10^{-6}M HEME. As shown in figure 2, the enzyme that synthesizes ALA and the one that forms HEME are both localized in the mitochondria of liver cells, thus making such an end product inhibition at least spatially possible. If end product inhibition occurs in animal cells it seems to be only partially effective.

End product repression

Repression of the synthesis of ALA-synthetase possibly at the gene level may be the more important way in which HEME synthesis is controlled. Studies on chemical porphyria[125] have shown that a drug like allyl-isopropyl-acetamide will bring about an increase in ALA-synthetase. For this increase DNA must be intact. In *R. spheroides*, Lascelles[126] has shown that HEME added to the cells represses the synthesis of this enzyme 3 to 5-fold, an observation which suggests that HEME may be involved in the repressor mechanism.

XVII. Control Mechanisms of Hemoglobin Synthesis

This section contains a number of hypotheses. It is addressed primarily to the experimentalist who knows the difference between fact and fancy and how to appreciate both.

Based on information obtained from bacterial genetics, Jacob and Monod have formulated various ingenious models of genetic regulation which they have recently reviewed[127]. Although differentiation is undoubtedly more complex in multicellular organisms than in bacteria, these models offer an excellent starting point for an investigative approach to the mechanisms of erythroid differentiation. The models for regulation of genetic expression contain the following four fundamental characters:

1. Structural gene—a deoxynucleotide (DNA) segment of the chromosome which gives rise to a short-lived ribonucleic acid, messenger ribonucleic acid (m-RNA). M-RNA brings the specific information of DNA to the ribosomes (nuclear or cytoplasmic protein-forming particles) for the synthesis of a specific protein.

2. Operon—a region of DNA consisting of an operator gene, one or more adjacent structural genes, permease genes, etc. The operator gene is responsible for the initiation of m-RNA synthesis from the genes of the operon.

3. Regulator gene—a DNA segment responsible for the production of a *repressor* which has the ability to block reversibly the activity of a specific operator gene.

4. Effectors—these are usually molecules smaller than proteins which are capable of reversibly combining with repressors to prevent their inhibition of operator gene activity. An effector may also combine with an aporepressor to form a repressor.

In multicellular organisms we must expect many factors, both intracellular and environmental, to interact in the control of cytodifferentiation. Products of one biosynthetic chain may act as *effectors* in other synthetic processes. *Effector* activity may also be found in hormones and the metabolites of neighboring cells.

What control mechanism may be operative in the regulation of the biosynthesis of HEME and globin? Fig. 14 is a hypothetical schema for the control of hemoglobin synthesis which is based on some established facts and a good deal of speculation. This schema attempts to account for the 1:1 correspondence between HEME and globin-polypeptide in the hemoglobin monomer. The schema assumes; a) that globin genes are turned on independent of HEME synthesis; b) that because of globin synthesis the rate of HEME synthesis is increased; c) that no globin polypeptide is completed in the absence of HEME.

Prior to the initiation of hemoglobin synthesis, the operon responsible for globin synthesis is activated but kept repressed by its cooresponding regulator gene as depicted in step 1. The operon concerned with the synthesis of ALA-synthetase, the limiting enzyme in the HEME biosynthetic chain, is also repressed. However, here it is assumed that the aporepressor produced by regulator gene 1 requires HEME for effectively repressing the operon for ALA-synthetase (step 2). With the entrance of specific *effector* substances into the cell the *repressor* of the globin operon is rendered inactive (step 3), allowing globin synthesis to commence. Erythropoietin or possibly metabolites from neighboring cells are substances which might act in this manner to initiate globin synthesis. The globin thus formed now utilizes any available free HEME for hemoglobin formation (step 4) depriving the repressor of the ALA-synthetase operon of its effectiveness and allowing the synthesis of this enzyme to proceed at a maximal rate. Since the other enzymes in the HEME

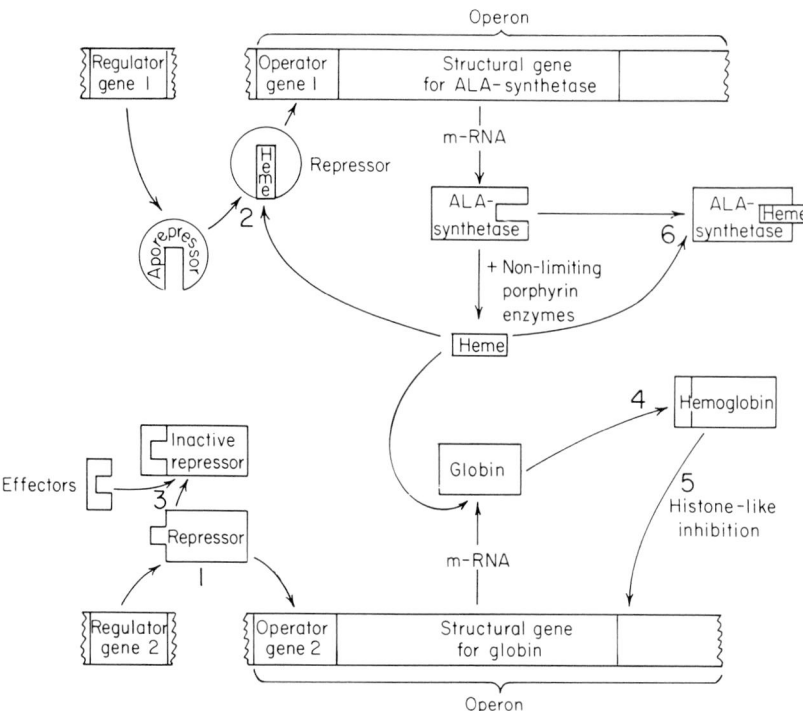

Fig. 14.—Hypothetical schema for control of hemoglobin synthesis.

biosynthetic chain are already present in non-limiting amounts, hemoglobin production is at this point limited only by the availability of substrates.

To explain the 1:1 ratio of the HEME to globin monomer formed by the red cells it is postulated that the globin will not come off the polysome unless it has been correctly folded around the HEME (See section XIII). Rich[128] has suggested that when two adjacent monomers are completed they will come off the polysome together as a dimer. Hammel and Bessman[112] found that HEME stimulates globin synthesis when added to a preparation of hemolyzed avian erythrocytes which consisted mostly of nuclei. This supports the hypothesis that HEME is required for globin synthesis.

Increasing concentrations of hemoglobin in the normoblast nucleus act like histone to combine with, condense, and inactivate DNA (step 5). Globin synthesis can now continue only on preformed m-RNA and stops when this m-RNA is depleted. This DNA inhibition by hemoglobin will also prevent the formation of new ALA-synthetase. However, even with cessation of the synthesis of this enzyme, HEME formation could continue for many hours after globin production has stopped by utilization of the preformed ALA-synthetase. This would lead to an overproduction of HEME and porphyrins. Since, under normal conditions, this overproduction does not occur there must be an additional control mechanism to regulate the synthesis of ALA. It is postulated in step 6 that the free HEME, appearing after the termination of globin synthesis, acts directly to inhibit ALA-synthetase and prevent an overproduction of porphyrins. The presence in the mitochondria of both the first and last enzymes in the HEME biosynthetic chain (Fig. 2) lends support to such an end product inhibition in the control of HEME synthesis.

Other avenues of control would include the availability of substrates, co-enzymes and metal ions. As most of the enzymes of the HEME biosynthetic chain require SH groups for activity, the cellular levels of reduced glutathione might also participate in the control of their activity.

XVIII. Diseases of Porphyrin Metabolism

A full undertanding of the metabolic lesions present in the experimental and inherited forms of porphyria will be of great importance in the elucidation of control mechanisms operative in the biosynthesis of HEME. This section is not meant to be a review of the porphyria diseases but rather a consideration of the biochemical aspects of these disorders as they pertain to normal HEME metabolism. In some of these disorders, specific enzymatic blocks serve to dramatize the normal biosynthetic pathway. In others, where porphyrins are synthesized in overabundance, we can learn much about the manner in which HEME synthesis is normally regulated. Some of the pertinent features are summarized in Table I. The postulated biochemical lesions are outlined in Figure 15.

Erythropoietic porphyrias

Congenital Erythropoietic Porphyria.—This disease usually makes its clinical appearance at birth or during the first two years of life[129, 130, 131] and is inherited as an autosomal recessive with an equal incidence in males and females. Photosensitivity is one of the cardinal manifestations of this disease and usually appears shortly after birth. A similar congenital disease has been described in cattle. These animals exhibit photosensitivity and here too, the disease is inherited as an autosomal recessive character[132, 133, 134, 135]. The disease also occurs in swine, but differs from the bovine and human forms in that there is no photosensitivity and the inheritance is dominant in type[133, 134]. These patterns of inheritance suggest a regulator gene abnormality in the human and bovine forms; and an operator gene defect in the dominant porcine type.

The porphyrin abnormalities in congenital erythropoietic porphyria are outlined in Table I. The outstanding biochemical disturbance is the marked elevation of URO-I and COPRO-I in the circulating erythrocytes and bone marrow. Elevations of porphyrin levels in the liver and spleen are secondary to destruction of the porphyrin-laden erythrocytes[136]. Incubation of hemolysates of red cells from patients with congenital erythropoietic porphyria with ALA or PBG results in the production of a mixture of type I and III porphyrins. In contrast, similar incubations using normal erythrocytes produce predominantly Series III isomers[49, 137].

The overproduction of type I porphyrins can best be explained on the basis of a genetically determined defect in the enzyme PBG-isomerase which, with PBG-deaminase, is necessary for the synthesis of URO-III from PBG. With a defect in PBG-isomerase, URO-I is synthesized from PBG. The mechanism of action of these enzymes has been described in section VII. Obviously,

TABLE I.—*Heme Precursors In Diseases of Porphyrin Metabolism*

Condition	Inheritance	Age of Clinical Onset	Organ Primarily Involved	Compounds* In Urine Per Day	Compounds* Excreted Per GM. Feces (Dry Wgt.)	Compounds* Per 100 ml. RBC	Photosensitivity
Normal	—	—	—	URO-(15-30 µg) I > III COPRO-(60-250 µg) I > III PBG-(<1 mg) ALA-(<3 mg)	COPRO I-(~7 µg) PROTO IX-(~23 µg)	COPRO-(1-2 µg) PROTO-(10-60 µg)	—
Congenital Erythropoietic Porphyria	Recessive	Birth to 5 yrs.	Erythropoietic	URO I-3+ (~100 mg) COPRO I-2+ (~10 mg)	URO-2+ (~2 mg) I ≫ III COPRO-3+ (~130 mg) I ≫ III PROTO-N	URO I-3+ COPRO I-2+ PROTO-N to 1+	Present (Severe)
Erythropoietic Protoporphyria	Dominant	Usually childhood	Erythropoietic	URO III-N COPRO III-2+ (~500 µg)	COPRO III-2+ (20-80 µg) PROTO-2+ (20-100 µg)	URO-N COPRO III-N to 1+ PROTO-2 to 3+	Present (Moderate)
Acute Intermittent Porphyria	Dominant	15-40 years	Liver	Acute Phase PBG-3+ (40-200 mg) ALA-2+ (20-40 mg) Remission PBG-N to 1+ (~20 mg) ALA-N to 1+ (~20 mg)	Acute Phase Porphyrins-N to 1+ Remission Porphyrins-N	N	Not Present

Cutaneous Hepatic Porphyrias	Dominant	20–50 years	Liver	Acute Phase PBG- 1 to 3+ (~20–200 mg.) ALA- 1 to 2+ (~8–64 mg.) URO I & III- N to 2+ COPRO- variable Remission PBG & ALA-N Porphyrins- N to 1+	Acute Phase URO III- 1 to 3+ COPRO III- 2 to 3+ (~650 µg) PROTO- 2 to 3+ (~900 µg) Remission URO III- 1 to 2+ COPRO III- 1 to 3+ (~400 µg) PROTO- 1 to 3+ (~650 µg)	N	Present (mild to severe)
Toxic Porphyrias	Acquired	—	Liver	ALA- N to 2+ (1–47 mg) PBG- N to 1+ (3–16 mg) COPRO- 2+ (1–2 mg) URO- 1 to 3+ (up to 2.5 mg)	COPRO- 1 to 2+ PROTO- N to 2+	N	Present (mild to severe)

N-normal amount; 1+-slightly increased amount; 2+-moderately increased amount; 3+-markedly increased amount.
* Porphyrins expressed as total of porphyrins and porphyrinogens.

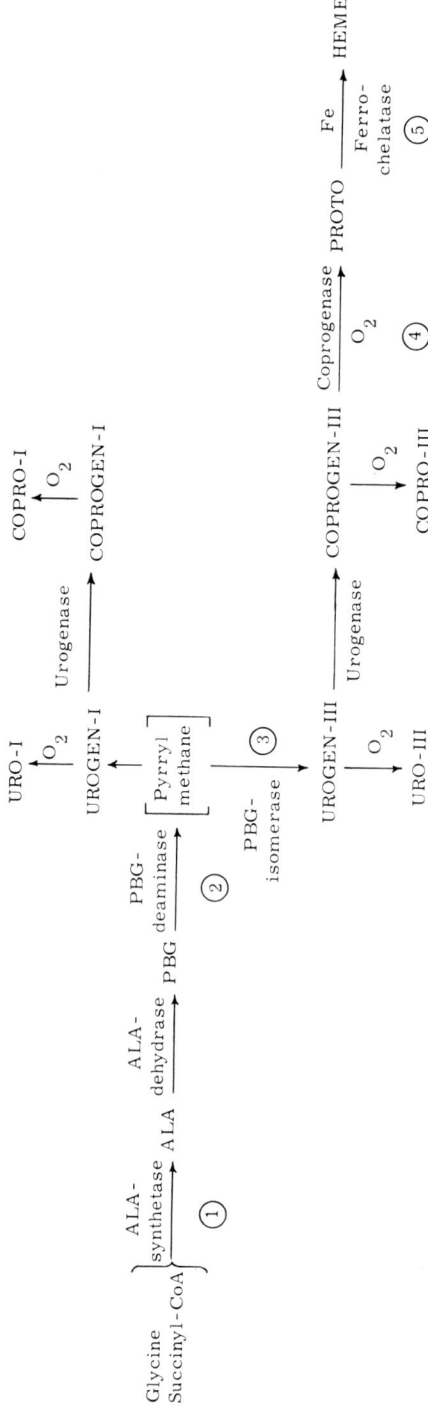

FIG. 15.—Hypothesis For the Lesions in the Porphyrias.

I Erythropoietic—In both congenital porphyria and congenital protoporphyria, it is postulated that the basic defect is an overproduction of ALA in the red cell due to increased activity of ALA-synthetase (1). In congenital porphyria the activity of PBG-isomerase (3) is decreased and in the presence of excess substrate there is an overproduction of type I isomers. In congenital protoporphyria there is no defect at (3) and this allows for oversynthesis of type III isomers. PROTO then accumulates when the iron-inserting capabilities of ferro-chelatase (5) are exceeded.

II Hepatic—Here the loss of control of step (1) is limited to hepatic tissue where there is a subsequent overproduction of ALA and PBG. The overproduction then brings latent genetic enzyme defects to light. In acute intermittent porphyria, if PBG-deaminase (2) is limiting, ALA and PBG will accumulate and be excreted. Enzyme defects at (4) and (5) would lead to elevated levels of type III isomers as seen in the cutaneous hepatic porphyrias.

the defect in PBG-isomerase is not complete, for this situation would be incompatible with life as the type I isomers do not form PROTO. Because of the heat lability of PBG-isomerase[48], it is of interest to note that when normal erythrocytes are heated prior to incubation with ALA or PBG, they also lose their ability to form predominantly type III porphyrins[49].

Since the hemoglobin concentration per red cell is normal in face of the enzyme defect and the increased erythropoiesis, it is logical to assume that the total porphyrin synthesis is several times greater than normal. Under these circumstances, it is attractive to postulate that the basic inherited abnormality may be a loss of normal control mechanisms at steps prior to the formation of PBG. For example, increased activity of ALA-synthetase would lead to the overproduction of PBG from glycine and succinate. This would present the enzyme PBG-isomerase with increased amounts of substrate and possibly reveal what might otherwise be a latent enzyme defect.

Congenital Erythropoietic Protoporphyria.—This is a recently described inborn error of porphyrin metabolism first characterized by Magnus and co-workers[138] in 1961. The family study by Haeger-Aronson[139] provides evidence to suggest that erythropoietic protoporphyria is inherited as a Mendelian dominant character.

Clinically, this disease is characterized by mild photosensitivity as manifested by erythema, edema, and urticaria of exposed skin areas. The skin lesions are much less severe than those of congenital erythropoietic porphyria and vesicle and bulla formation are not characteristic. There is a marked increase in the PROTO concentration of circulating erythrocytes and many of these cells exhibit fluorescence. In addition, the bone marrow PROTO levels are increased and fluorescent normoblasts have been noted. The localization of the fluorescence within these cells has not been described. Fecal PROTO and COPRO-III concentrations are elevated (see Table I). In contrast to congenital erythropoietic porphyria there is no increase in the levels of fecal or urinary URO (I or III). The plasma levels of PROTO are also elevated. Anemia has not been noted except in one of the brothers described by Porter and Lowe[140].

The biochemical mechanisms leading to the excess PROTO levels in erythropoietic protoporphyria have not been fully elucidated. The PROTO which is present in elevated levels in this disorder has been found to be identical with PROTO-9[138, 141] and is not an isomer which is unable to combine with iron to form HEME. Ferrokinetic studies with Fe^{59} done on one patient[138] have produced normal results, indicating no abnormality in iron incorporation. Detailed studies by Porter[141] using an *in vitro* system, have shown that the bone marrow of patients with this disorder is capable of normal incorporation of iron into PROTO. However, he found porphyrin synthesis from glycine and α-ketoglutarate to be 10 to 20 times greater than that produced by marrow of individuals with sickle cell anemia. In view of this marked *in vitro* porphyrin synthesis one may ask why the erythrocyte PROTO levels, as compared to total HEME production, are so low.

These data provide strong evidence that the basic defect in this congenital disorder is an overproduction of PROTO-9 rather than a block in iron incorporation for HEME formation. One must consider that this overproduction represents the result of the loss of normal cellular regulation of porphyrin synthesis. As mentioned in the previous section, the step in the biosynthetic chain from glycine and succinyl-Co A to ALA would appear to be the most likely place for such a loss of control to be expressed. It is tempting to speculate that the overproduction of porphyrins may have a parallel in chemical porphyria where there appears to be a *de novo* increase in the enzyme ALA-synthetase leading to excessive synthesis of porphyrins. The increase in ALA-synthetase activity in congenital erythropoietic protoporphyria may be due to increased levels of this enzyme or may represent a failure of normal control mechanisms to decrease the enzyme activity as the erythroid cell reaches its normal complement of hemoglobin (see Fig. 14).

Hepatic porphyrias

Acute Intermittent Porphyria (Swedish type).—This is the commonest of the inherited porphyrin diseases. Waldenström[142] was the first unequivocally to demonstrate that acute intermittent porphyria was an inherited disease and to suggest that it was transmitted as a dominant character. It is now generally accepted that a single abnormal gene is sufficient for expression of the clinical syndrome. With the more sensitive tests for urinary PBG and ALA, a latent state has frequently been detected in relatives of afflicted individuals. This suggests that the abnormal gene is variable in its expression and that relatives who have been found to excrete no excesses of PBG or ALA might still be heterozygous for this disorder of porphyrin metabolism[130].

Acute abdominal pain is the most frequently occurring manifestation of acute intermittent porphyria (AIP)[143]. Neurologic manifestations are also an important feature of the disease and have been extensively reviewed by Goldberg[56, 143, 144] and Waldenström[145]. Photosensitivity is not present.

While the factors associated with the emergence of AIP from sub-clinical to clinical levels are not understood, there are certain conditions which are known to precipitate acute attacks. Waldenström[142] was the first to demonstrate that barbiturate administration may be directly related to the initiation of an acute episode. This finding has now been confirmed repeatedly, so that one may emphatically state that barbiturates are contraindicated in patients with AIP. Goldberg and Rimington[130] feel that this prohibition should include the members of the patient's family. The mode of action of barbiturates in inducing acute attacks will be considered in the section dealing with experimental porphyria.

Various infectious diseases have also been described as producing the onset of clinical symptoms. In addition, alcohol[143] stilbestrol[146, 147], parturition and sulfonamides have been implicated in the precipitation of an acute attack.

Characteristic of the acute attack is the excretion in the urine of large quantities of PBG and ALA (see Table I). The traces of porphyrins present in the urine of patients with acute intermittent porphyria are derived primarily from the non-enzymic condensation of PBG. Since PBG is colorless, the freshly voided urine is usually normal in color. Upon standing, particularly in the light, it turns red with the formation of porphyrins and porphobilin from

PBG. Porphobilin appears to be a dipyrrylmethene derived from the condensation of two molecules of PBG. During remissions, the PBG and ALA levels fall but usually remain slightly elevated[148]. Fecal porphyrins are only minimally elevated.

There is good evidence presently available to support the concept that the excess ALA and PBG levels found in this disorder result from hepatic overproduction of these compounds rather than from a block in their utilization. Based on studies of chemical porphyria, it now seems most likely that the basic defect is an abnormality in the mechanisms controlling HEME biosynthesis. This will be discussed in the section dealing with chemical porphyria.

Cutaneous Hepatic Porphyria (South African type, porphyria variegata).—The highest incidence of this disease is found in the white South African population. However, the disease is not limited to this ethnic group and has been described from all parts of the world. Inheritance occurs as a non-sex-linked Mendelian dominant character[149]. Unlike acute intermittent porphyria, photosensitivity is one of the major manifestations of this disorder. Acute attacks, with abdominal pain and neurologic abnormalities, are seen in addition to the photosensitivity[150].

Apart from photosensitivity, the pattern of porphyrin excretion in the urine and feces helps to distinguish this form of porphyria from acute intermittent porphyria, (Table I). During remissions the urinary levels of PBG, ALA and porphyrins are within normal limits. However, the fecal concentrations of COPRO and PROTO are elevated even during these periods and latent cases can frequently be detected by examination of the feces for URO, COPRO, and PROTO. These porphyrins are of the type III isomers.

In the acute phase of the disease the urine contains both URO and COPRO in large quantities. Urinary PBG and ALA levels are also elevated[151] during this phase of the disease.

The excess porphyrin production, as in acute intermittent porphyria, is due to abnormal hepatic ALA production. Erythrocyte and bone marrow PBG and porphyrins are within normal limits[136, 146].

Acquired Hepatic Porphyria.—Many hundreds of examples of this disorder have been described among the Bantus of South Africa[152]. The major clinical manifestation is photosensitivity. Acute attacks, like those seen in AIP are rare. No familial pattern has been detected. The urine contains markedly increased levels of URO and COPRO, the former predominating (Table I). In some cases, slight elevations of PBG and ALA are also noted. Fecal COPRO and PROTO, on the other hand, are only minimally elevated[153]. The etiologic agent, or agents responsible for the disease have not been specifically identified. It is known, however, that hemosiderosis and hepatic insufficiency are common in the Bantu. In addition, alcoholic consumption among this group is high and, as pointed out by Barnes[153], much of this alcohol is adulterated and toxic.

An acquired disease of porphyrin metabolism has also been noted in Turkey[76]. Schmid[77] has also reviewed these cases and in addition, has reported on the biochemical abnormalities in detail. Consumption of wheat that had been treated with the fungicide hexachlorobenzene prior to planting was found to be the common etiologic agent[154, 155]. Chemical induction of porphyria in animals has since been found to be possible utilizing this chemical (see below).

Elevations in urinary URO and COPRO concentrations, associated with mild photosensitivity, are also seen in occasional cases of alcoholic cirrhosis. Less commonly, increased levels of urinary PBG can be found. However, the fact that this syndrome is so rare in such a common disorder as Laennec's cirrhosis raises the question, as suggested by Watson[146], of whether in these individuals the acquired liver disease is bringing a latent genetic defect to the level of clinical detection.

Porphyrinuria

Elevated urinary porphyrins, unassociated with photosensitivity, may be found during the course of many systemic diseases. Increased renal excretion of COPRO has been observed to accompany Hodgkin's disease, aplastic anemia, infectious hepatitis, acute myocardial infarction, carcinomatosis, acute rheumatic fever, pyogenic infections, poliomyelitis and Hartnup disease[129, 130, 156].

In lead poisoning there are marked elevations of urinary and serum ALA and COPRO III. In addition, erythrocyte PROTO and COPRO (during the initial stages) are elevated. The abnormal porphyrin metabolism appears to be due to the effect of lead on the HEME biosynthetic path in the red cell. The subject of lead intoxication has recently been extensively reviewed by Chisolm[157]. From animal studies it has been demonstrated that lead inhibits both the conversion of ALA to PBG and the incorporation of iron into PROTO. ALA-dehydrase, an SH-containing enzyme and the insertion of iron into PROTO, also requiring-SH groups, are inhibited by lead. Inhibition of ALA-dehydrase has been reported in erythrocytes of lead poisoned children[158]. The basophilic stippled red cells, which are characteristic of plumbism, contain mitochondria and iron granules. These cells have a greater than normal aerobic metabolism, probably due to the persistance of mitochondria.

Experimental Porphyria (Chemical Porphyria)

The first description of chemical porphyria was made by Stokvis, in 1895, who observed that excretion of "hematoporphyrin" could be produced in rabbits by sulfonal poisoning. In 1942, Schmid and Schwartz[159] reported that a disease resembling AIP could be produced by treating animals with Sedormid. Now, a number of chemicals of diverse structure are known which will cause similar effects in animals. The disease has been chemically induced in rabbits, rats, guinea pigs, chickens and chick embryos. A few of the more recent comprehensive reviews on this subject are those by Waldenström[160], Schmid[131], Goldberg and Rimington[130], Granick and Mauzerall[1], Granick and Urata[27] and Barnes[161]. Animals poisoned with these inducing drugs excrete large quantities of COPRO, URO, PBG and ALA in the urine. Fecal PROTO and COPRO are also elevated. These porphyrins are all type III isomers. The livers contain excess amounts of porphyrins, PBG and ALA and elevations of these compounds in other organs are secondary to primary hepatic synthesis.

Two explanations can be offered to explain the increased ALA present in the liver. Either this is an excessive production of ALA or ALA is normally produced at a high rate, but then not broken down rapidly enough in the Shemin cycle.

In 1963, Urata and Granick[40] found that guinea pig liver normally produced very little ALA. Rather, it was another aminoketone, aminoacetone, that was formed in appreciable amounts according to reaction II. As proposed by Elliot[162], the aminoacetone was found to turn over rapidly in a series of reactions similar to those of the Shemin cycle. To account for the high ALA levels found in chemical porphyria, it is therefore necessary to postulate that excessive amounts are being produced.

To study the cause of the excessive amounts of ALA formed by the liver, Granick and Urata[27] produced a chemical porphyria in guinea pigs with the collidine chemical, diethyl-1,4-dihydro-2,4,6-trimethyl pyridine-3,5-dicarboxylate (DDC), a compound first used by Solomon and Figge[163]. On examination of the enzymes of the porphyrin biosynthetic chain in the liver it was found that only the first enzyme, ALA-synthetase, was affected by treatment with DDC. In the untreated guinea pig, the activity of this enzyme was only barely detectable. They found, after feeding DDC, that the enzyme activity had increased forty-fold. The other enzymes of the biosynthetic chain from ALA to PROTO were normally highly active and this activity was not appreciably changed after feeding DDC. These findings indicate that the rate of hepatic porphyrin synthesis is limited primarily by the activity of ALA-synthetase.

An increase in ALA-synthetase activity might result from activation of an inactive enzyme or as a result of *de novo* synthesis of the enzyme. Granick observed no increase in ALA-synthetase activity when DDC was incubated with normal liver homogenates or mitochondria. In an attempt to investigate the possibility of *de novo* synthesis of ALA-synthetase, Granick[124] set up a technique for growing chick embryo liver cells in tissue culture. Excess porphyrin production was then induced in these cells by adding chemicals like DDC and AIA to the incubation medium. With this *"in vitro* porphyria" technique it was shown that porphyrin production in these fetal liver cells also was limited by ALA-synthetase. Induction of increased porphyrin production could be blocked by adding inhibitors of protein synthesis, like Mitomycin or Actinomycin, to the cell medium concomitant with the introduction of the inducing chemical. Since porphyrin formation was blocked by Mitomycin or Actinomycin it could be concluded that DNA was required for the increased ALA-synthetase activity and that this increase was secondary to *de novo* synthesis of the enzyme.

This increased synthesis of ALA-synthetase in liver cells, induced by chemicals, suggests that there is a mechanism for the control of this enzyme by repression of its formation. As previously mentioned, in *R. spheroides*, a photosynthetic purple bacterium, Lascelles[126] has shown that HEME can repress the formation of ALA-synthetase 3 to 5-fold. Granick[124] found no evidence with his tissue culture method that HEME repressed the induction of porphyrin synthesis by AIA. However, this negative result may be due to the impermeability of the cells to the added HEME. Assuming that HEME is necessary for repression (Fig. 14) then compounds which interact with HEME or prevent HEME from "sitting on" the aporepressor might derepress.

A simple hypothesis to explain the enhanced porphyrin synthesis present in both acute intermittent porphyria and cutaneous hepatic porphyria is that the regulatory control mechanism governing the activity of the structural gene for ALA-synthetase is defective and does not sufficiently repress the formation of this enzyme. Because these diseases require only one defective allele, it is possible that the defect lies in the operator of the structural gene. In the recessive erythropoietic porphyrias, an abnormality of the regulator genes is more probable since in the heterozygote one normal regulator would be sufficient for repression.

It is possible that in both acute intermittent porphyria and cutaneous hepatic porphyria there is an identical genetic lesion which is then expressed on different genetic backgrounds (see Fig. 15). A reasonable hypothesis is that in acute intermittent porphyria, where ALA and PBG are excreted, the enzyme condensing PBG to UROGEN may be limiting under the stress condition of excessive ALA formation. On the other hand, in the cutaneous hepatic porphyrias, where COPRO and PROTO are the main porphyrins excreted, the limiting enzymes may be those that convert COPROGEN to PROTO and PROTO to HEME. In acute intermittent porphyria the disease is intermittent. Perhaps the control mechanism is so poorly balanced in these individuals that even small amounts of drugs like barbiturates (or toxins from bacteria?) may derepress and lead to a massive abnormal synthesis of ALA.

The neurological involvement that accompanies AIP is not explained by these simple hypotheses, nor is the delay in manifestations of the disease until early adulthood or middle age. Abnormal hepatic porphyrias have still more to teach us about the normal.

ACKNOWLEDGMENTS

We wish to acknowledge our gratitude to Dr. Miriam Jacob for editing this paper and making it more readable and to Dr. D. Mauzerall for his criticism. We should also like to express our appreciation and the indebtedness of ourselves and other researchers in the field of the porphyrins to Dr. S. F. MacDonald of the National Research Council of Canada, who has, over the years, most generously provided many of us with difficultly synthesized and authentic samples of dipyrrylmethanes and isomeric porphyrins which have been used in the enzyme studies on HEME biosynthesis.

REFERENCES

1. Granick, S., and Mauzerall, D.: Metabolism of heme and chlorophyll. In *Pathways of Chemical Metabolism*. D. Greenberg (ed.) Vol. II pg. 526–606, Academic Press New York 1960.
2. Rimington, C.: Biosynthesis of haemoglobin. Brit. M. Bull. 15: 19–26, 1959.
3. Rimington, C.: Haem pigments and porphyrins. Ann. Rev. Biochem. 26: 561–586, 1957.
4. Shemin, D.: The biosynthesis of porphyrins. Harvey Lectures 50: 258–284, 1954–55.
5. Shemin, D.: The biosynthesis of porphyrins. Ergeb. Physiol. 49: 299–326, 1957.
6. Marks, G. S.: Biosynthesis of porphyrins. Annual Reports Chem. Soc. 59: 385–399, 1962.
7. Margoliash, E.: Porphyrins and hemoproteins. Ann. Rev. Biochem. 30: 549–578, 1961.
8. Neuberger, A.: Aspects of the metabolism of glycine and porphyrins. Biochem. J. 78: 1–10, 1961.

9. Falk, J. E.: Chemistry and biochemistry of porphyrins and metalloporphyrins. In *Comprehensive Biochemistry*. 9: 3–33 M. Florkin and E. H. Stotz (eds.) 1963.

10. Bogorad, L.: The biosynthesis of protochlorophyll. In *Comparative Biochemistry of Photoreactive Systems*. M. B. Allen (ed.) p. 227–256. Academic Press N.Y. 1960.

11. Lascelles, J.: Tetrapyrrole synthesis in microorganisms. In *The Bacteria* 3: 335–72 (1962) I. C. Gunsalus and R. Y. Stanier (eds.) Academic Press, N.Y.

12. Granick, S. and Mauzerall, D.: Enzymes converting δ-aminolevulinic acid to coproporphyrinogen. J. Biol. Chem. 232: 1119–1140 (1958).

13. Sano, S. and Granick, S.: Mitochondrial coproporphyrinogen oxidase and protoporphyrin formation. J. Biol. Chem 236: 1173–1180 (1961).

14. Hennessey, M. A., Waltersdorph, A. M., Huennekins, F. M., and Gabrio, B. W.: Separation of erythrocyte enzymes from hemoglobin. J. Clin. Invest. 41: 1257–1262 (1962).

15. Westall, R. G.: Isolation of porphobilinogen from the urine of a patient with acute porphyria. Nature 170: 614–616 (1952).

16. Cookson, G. H. and Rimington, C.: Porphobilinogen. Biochem. J. 57: 476–484 (1954).

17. Granick, S.: Formation of δ-amino-levulinic acid in erythrocytes. J. Biol. Chem. 232: 1101–1117 (1958).

18. Gibson, K. D., Laver, W. G. and Neuberger, A.: Initial stages in the biosynthesis of porphyrins 2. The formation of δ-amino-levulinic acid from glycine and succinyl-coenzyme A by particles from chicken erythrocytes. Biochem. J. 70: 71–81 (1958).

19. Feldman, F. and Lichtman, H. C.: *In-vitro* porphobilinogen and porphyrin synthesis in Thalassemia Major and sickle cell anemia. N.Y. Acad. Sci. Conference on Problems of Cooley's Anemia. Dec. 5–7, 1963.

20. Bernard, H., Gajdos, A. and Gajdos-Torök, M.: Action de certains activateurs et inhibiteurs sur la biosynthése de la protoporphyrine hémoglobinique par les globules rouges périphériques. Compt. Rend. Soc. Biol. 145: 538–540, 1951.

21. Shemin, D., London, I. M., and Rittenberg, D.: The in vitro synthesis of heme from glycine by the nucleated red blood cell. J. Biol. Chem. 173: 799–800, 1948.

22. Dresel, E. I. B. and Falk, J. E.: Studies on the biosynthesis of blood pigments 2. Haem and porphyrin formation in intact chicken erythrocytes. Biochem. J. 63: 72–79, 1956.

23. Schulman, M. P. and Richert, D. A.: Heme synthesis in vitamin B_6 and pantothenic acid deficiencies. J. Biol Chem. 226: 181–189 (1957).

24. Lascelles, J.: Synthesis of porphyrins by cell suspensions of Tetrahymena vorax: Effect of members of the Vitamin B group. Biochem. J. 66: 65–72 (1957).

25. Wintrobe, M. M.: Factors and mechanisms in the production of red blood cells. Harvey Lectures 45: 87–126 (1950).

26. Laver, W. G., Neuberger, A., and Udenfriend, S.: Initial stages in the biosynthesis of porphyrins I. Formation of δ-AL by particles obtained from chicken erythrocytes. Biochem. J. 70: 4–14 (1958).

27. Granick, S., and Urata, G.: Increase in activity of δ-amino-levulinic acid synthetase in liver mitochondria induced by feeding of 3,5-dicarbethoxy-1,4-dihydrocollidine. J. Biol. Chem. 238: 821–827 (1963).

28. Massey, V.: The composition of the ketoglutarate dehydrogenase complex. Biochem. Biophys. Acta. 38: 447–460 (1960).

29. Shemin, D., and Kumin, S.: The mechanism of porphyrin formation. The formation of a succinyl intermediate from succinate. J. Biol. Chem. 198: 827–837, 1952.

30. Brown, E. G.: The relationship of the tricarboxylic acid cycle to the synthesis of δ-amino-levulinic acid in avian erythrocyte preparations. Biochem. J. 70: 313–321, 1958.

31. Hager, L. P.: Succinyl-CoA synthetase. In *The Enzymes* P. D. Boyer, H. Lardy and K. Myrrback (eds.) pg. 387–398, Vol. 6, 1962.

32. Sanadi, D. R., Gibson, D. M., Ayengar, P. and Jacob, M.: α-Ketoglutaric dehydrogenase. V Guanosine diphosphate in coupled phosphorylation. J. Biol. Chem. 218: 505–520, 1956.

33. Burnham, B. F.: Purification and characterization of succinyl coenzyme A synthetase from Rhodoseudomonas spheroides. Acta. Chem Skand. 17: S 123–128, 1963.

34. Stadtman, E. R., Overath, P., Eggerer, H., and Lynen, F.: The role of biotin and Vitamin B_{12} coenzyme in propionate metabolism. Biochem. and Biophys. Res. Comm. 2: 1–7 (1960).

35. Stern, M. J., Del Campillo, A.: Enzymes of fatty acid metabolism IV Preparation and properties of coenzyme A transferase. J. Biol. Chem. 221: 15–31 (1956).

36. Hammel, C. L., Rasmussen, P. and Bessman S. P., Hemoglobin synthesis. A nuclear function in the avian erythrocyte. J. Cell Biol. Abstracts 19: 31A 1963.

37. Gibson, K. D., Matthew, M., Neuberger, A., and Tait, G. H.: Biosynthesis of porphyrins and chlorophylls. Nature 192: 204–208 (1961).

38. Kikuchi, G., Kuman, A., Talmage, P., and Shemin D.: The enzymatic synthesis of δ-amino-levulinic acid. J. Biol. Chem. 233: 1214–1219 (1958).

39. Shemin, D.: δ-amino-levulinic acid dehydrase from Rhodopsuedomonas spheroides. In *Methods in Enzymology* V 883–884. S. P. Colowick and N. O. Kaplan (eds.) Academic Press (1962).

40. Urata, G. and Granick. S.: Biosynthesis of aminoketones and the metabolism of amino-acetone. J. Biol. Chem. 238: 811–820 (1963).
41. Vogel, W., Richert, D. A., Pixley, B. Q., and Schulman, M. P.: Heme synthesis in iron deficient duck blood. J. Biol. Chem. 235: 1769–1775 (1960).
42. Shemin, D., and Russell, C. S.: δ-amino-levulinic acid, its role in the biosynthesis of porphyrins and purines. J. Am. Chem. Soc. 75: 4873–4874, 1953.
43. Nemeth, A. M., Russell, C. S. and Shemin, D.: The succinate-glycine cycle. II Metabolism of δ-aminolevulinic acid. J. Biol. Chem. 229: 415–422, 1957.
44. Kowalski, E. Dancewicz, A. M., and Szot, Z.: δ-amino levulinic-säuretransaminase, ein neues Enzyme. In proceed. IV Internat. Congress Biochem. Vienna 1958 and 4–65 p. 46 N.Y. 1959 Pergamon Press Inc.
45. Mauzerall, D., and Granick, S.: The occurrence and determination of δ-amino-levulinic acid and porphobilinogen in urine. J. Biol. Chem. 219: 435–446, 1956.
46. Gibson, K. D., Neuberger, A. and Scott, J. J.: The purification and properties of δ-amino levulinic acid dehydrase. Biochem. J. 61: 618–629, 1955.
47. Shemin, D.: δ-amino levulinic acid dehydrase from Rhodopseudomas Spheroides. In Methods in Enzymology Colowick, S. P. and Kaplan, N. O. (eds.) Academic Press, 1962.
48. Bogorad, L., and Granick, S.: The enzymatic synthesis of porphyrins from porpho-bilinogen. Proc. Nat. Acad. Sci. 39: 1176–1188, 1953.
49. Booij, H. L., and Rimington, C.: Effect of pre-heating on porphyrin synthesis by red cells. Biochem. J. 65: 4P., 1957.
50. Heath, H., and Hoare, D. S.: The biosynthesis of porphyrins from porphobilinogen by Rhodopsuedomonas spheroides. Biochem. J. 72: 14–22, 1959.
51. Matheweson, J. H., and Corwin, A. H.: Biosynthesis of pyrrole pigments: A mechanism for porphoblinogen polymerization. J. Amer. Chem. Soc. 83: 135–137 (1961).
52. Bray, R. C., and Shemin, D.: On the biosynthesis of Vitamin B$_{12}$ J. Biol. Chem. 238: 1501–1508 (1963).
53. Bonnett, R.: The chemistry of the Vit. B$_{12}$ group. Chem. Rev. 63: 573–605 (1963).
54. Carpenter, A. T. and Scott J. J.: Relationship of opsopyrroldicarboxylic acid to the biosynthesis of porphyrins. Biochem. J. 71: 325–333 (1959).
55. Hoare, D. S. and Heath H.: Dipyrromethanes and the biosynthesis of porphyrins. Bio-chem. Biophys. Acta 39: 167–169 (1960).
56. Bogorad, L.: Porphyrin Synthesis I. Uroporphyrinogen I synthetase. In Methods in Enzymology V 885–895 Colowick, S. P. and Kaplan, N. O. (eds.) Academic Press 1962.
57. Mauzerall, D. and Granick, S.: Porphyrin biosynthesis in erythrocytes III. Uropor-phyrinogen and its decarboxylase. J. Biol. Chem. 232: 1141–1162 (1958).
58. Fischer, H. and Orth, H.: Die Chemie des Pyrrols. Leipzig 1937 Akad. Verlag. 2: part 1 pg. 472.
59. Watson C. J., Pimento de Mello, R., Schwartz, S., Hawkinson, V. E., and Bossenmaier, I.: porphyrin chromogens or precursors in urine, blood bile and feces. J. Lab. and Clin. Med. 37: 831–842, 1951.
60. Bogorad, L.: Intermediates in biosynthesis of porphyrins from porphobilinogen. Science 121: 878–879, 1955.
61. Neve, R. A., Labbe, R. F., and Aldrich, R. A.: Reduced uroporphyrin III in the bio-synthesis of heme. J. Am. Chem. Soc. 78: 691–692, 1956.
62. Mauzerall, D.: The photo-reduction of porphyrins. Structure of the products. J. Am. Chem. Soc. 84: 2437–2445, 1962.
63. Mauzerall, D.: The condensation of porphobilinogen to uroporphyrinogen. J. Am. Chem. Soc. 82: 2605–2609, 1960.
64. Granick, S., and Mauzerall, D.: Enzymes of porphyrin synthesis in red blood cells. Ann. N.Y. Acad. Sci. 75: 115–121, 1958.
65. Granick, S., and Mauzerall, D.: Enzymatic formation of protoporphyrin from copro-porphyrinogen. Fed. Proc. 17: 233, 1958.
66. Granick, S., and Mauzerall, D.: unpublished data.
67. Porra, R. J. and Falk, J. E.: The enzymatic conversion of coproporphyrinogen III into protoporphyrin IX. Biochem. J. 90: 69–75, 1964.
68. Falk, J. E.: Chromatography of porphyrins and metalloporphyrins. J. Chromat. 5: 277–299, 1961.
69. Mauzerall, D.: The thermodynamic stability of porphyrinogens. J. Am. Chem Soc., 82: 2601–2605, 1960.
70. Edmundson, P. R., and Schwartz, S.: Studies of uroporphyrins. III An improved method for the decarboxylation of uroporphyrin. J. Biol. Chem. 205: 605–609, 1953.
71. Grotepass, W.: Porphyrins in normal blood cells. Ned. Tijdschr. Geneesk., 81: 362–366, 1937.
72. Watson, C. J., and Larson, E. A.: The urinary coproporphyrins in health and disease. Physiol. Rev. 24: 478–510, 1947.
73. Cartwright, G., and Wintrobe, M. M.: Hematopoiesis. Ann. Rev. Physiol. 11: 335–354, 1949.

74. Wintrobe, M. M.: Factors and mechanisms in the production of red corpuscles. Harvey Lectures 45: 87–126, 1950.
75. Schmid, R., Schwartz, S., and Watson, C. J.: Porphyrins in the bone marrow and circulating erythrocytes in experimental anemias. Proc. Soc. Exp. Biol. and Med. 75: 705–708, 1950.
76. Voelker, O.: Die Verbreitung von Porphyrin in Volgeleischalen. J. Ornithologie 88: 604–611 (1940).
77. Brown, E. B.: The utilization of iron in erythropoiesis. Am. J. Clin. Nutrit. 12: 77–87, 1963.
78. Jandl, J. H., Inman, J. K., Simmons, R. L., and Allen, D. W.: Transfer of iron from serum iron-binding protein to human reticulocytes. J. Clin. Invest. 38: 161–185, 1959.
79. Windle, J. J., Wiermsa, A. K., Clark, J. R. and Feeney, R. E.: Investigation of the iron and copper complexes of avian conalbumin and human transferrin by electron paramagnetic resonance. Biochemistry 2: 1341–1345 (1963).
80. Bessis, M. C.: Cytological aspects of hemoglobin production. pp. 125–156. The Harvey Lectures. series 58. Academic Press New York, 1963.
81. Labbe, R. F., and Hubbard, N.: Metal specificity of the iron protoporphyrin chelating enzyme from rat liver. Biochem. Biophys. Acta 52: 130–135, 1961.
82. Labbe, R. F.: An enzyme which catalyzes the insertion of iron into protoporphyrin. Biochem. Biophys. Acta 31: 589–590, 1959.
83. Oyama, H., Suzita, Y., Yoneyama, Y., Yoshikaya, H.: Stoichiometry of heme synthesis by partially purified enzyme preparation from duck erythrocytes. Biochem. Biophys. Acta. 47: 413–414, 1961.
84. Porra, R. J. and Jones, O. T. G.: An investigation of the role of ferrochelatase in the biosynthesis of various haem prosthetic groups. Biochem. J. 87: 186–192, 1963.
85. Neve, R. A.: The enzymatic incorporation of iron into protoporphyrin, In *Hematin Enzymes* Vol. 2: 207–210, 1961 (J. E. Falk, R. Lemberg and R. K. Morton eds.) Pergamon Press.
86. Schwartz, H. C., Goudsmit, R. Hill R. I., Cartwright, S. F., and Wintrobe, M. M.: The biosynthesis of hemoglobin from iron protoporphyrin and globin. Jour. Clin. Invest. 40: 188–195, 1961.
87. Yoneyama, Y., Okyama, H., Sugeta, Y., and Yoshikawa, H.: Formation *in vitro* of hemoglobin and myoglobin from iron protoporphyrin and globin in the presence of an iron chelating enzyme. Biochem. Biophys. Acta 74: 635–641, 1963.
88. Kendrew, J. C.: Recent work on myoglobin. In Arden House Conference on Hemoglobin. pg. 2–10 Columbia University 1962.
89. Gibson, Q.: Reaction of various hemes with globin. Correlation with x-ray structure. p. 10–13. In Arden House Conference of Hemoglobin. Columbia U. 1962.
90. Gibson, Q. H., and Antonini E.: Rates of reaction of native human globin with some hemes. J. Biol. Chem. 238: 1384–1388 (1963).
91. Rossi-Fanelli, A. and Antonini, E.: Dissociation of Hematin from hemoproteins at neutral pH. J. Biol. Chem. 235: P. C. 4 (1960).
92. Anfinsen, C. B., Macromolecular considerations of cellular organization. In Canadian Cancer Conference 5: 3–9 (1963) Academic Press.
93. Morell, H., Savoie, J. C. and London, J. M.: The biosynthesis of heme and the incorporation of glycine into globin in rabbit bone marrow *in vitro*. J. Biol. Chem. 233: 923–929 (1958).
94. Grassi, M., Gerti, A., Coy, U. and Lynen F.: Zur chemischen Konstitution des Cytohämins. Biochem Zeit. 337: 35–47 (1963).
95. Sano, S.: Personal communication.
96. De Carvalho, S.: Cytochemie de l'hémoglobine. Demonstration de l'existance de cette substance dans les nojoux des érythro-blastes. Compt. rend. Soc. biol. 145: 607–608, 1951.
97. O'Brien, B. R. A.: The presence of haemoglobin within the nucleus of the embryonic chick erythroblast. Exp. Cell. Res. 21: 226–228, 1960.
98. Wilt, F. H.: The ontogeny of chick embryo hemoglobin. Proc. Nat. Acad Sci. 48: 1582–1590, 1962.
99. Wilkins, M. H. F., and De Carvalho, S: The violet light microscope. A method for visual estimation of haem in living cells. Blood, 8: 944–946, 1953.
100. Davies, H. G.: Structure in nucleated erythrocytes. J. Biophysic. and Biochem. Cytol. 9: 671–687, 1961.
101. Grasso, J. A., Swift, H., and Ackerman, G. A.: Observations on the development of erythrocytes in mammalian fetal liver. J. Cell, Biol. 14: 235–254, 1962.
102. Stern, N., Allfrey, V., Mirsky, A. E., and Saetren, H.: Some enzymes of isolated nuclei. J. Gen. Physiol. 35: 559–578, 1951.
103. Schmid, R., Schwartz, S, and Sondberg, R. D.: Erythropoietic (congenital) porphyria: a rare abnormality of the normoblasts. Blood 10: 416–428, 1955.
104. Granick, S., and Levere, R.: Visualization of heme in cells by a fluorescence technique; the presence of heme in nuclei of human erythroblasts. Fed. Proc. 23: 222, 1964.
105. Allfrey, V. G., and Mirsky, A. E.: Protein synthesis in isolated cell nuclei: Nature 176: 1042–1049, 1955.

106. Defendi, V., and Pearson, B.: Histochemical demonstration of reductase activity in the nucleus of the chicken erythrocyte. Experientia 11: 355–356, 1955.
107. Neuberger, A., Muir, H. M., and Gray, C. H.: Biosynthesis of porphyrins and congenital porphyria. Nature 165: 948–950, 1950.
108. London, I. M., West, R., Shemin, D., and Rittenberg, D.: Porphyrin formation and hemoglobin metabolism in congenital porphyria. J. Biol. Chem. 184: 365–371, 1950.
109. Grasso, J. A., Woodard, J. W., and Swift, N.: Cytochemical studies of nucleic acids and proteins in erythrocyte development. Proc. Nat. Acad. Sci. 50: 134–140, 1963.
110. Borsook, H.: DNA, RNA and protein synthesis after acute, severe blood loss: a picture of erythropoiesis at the combined morphological and molecular levels. Trans. N. Y. Acad. Sci. In press.
111. Pinheiro, P., Le Blond, C. P., and Droz, B.: Synthetic capacity of reticulocytes as shown by radioautography after incubation with labelled precursors of protein or DNA. Exp. Cell. Res. 31: 517–537, 1963.
112. Hammel, C. L., and Bessman, S. P.: Porphyrin effects in avian erythrocyte nuclei. Fed. Proc. 23: 317, 1964.
113. Borsook, H.: personal communication
114. O'Brien, B. R. A.: Development of haemoglobin by de-embryonated chick blastoderms cultured *in vitro* and the effect of abnormal RNA upon its synthesis. J. Embryo. Exp. Morph. 9: 202–221, 1961.
115. Rich, A.: Multiple ribosomal structure in hemoglobin synthesis. *Arden House Conf. on Hemoglobin.* Columbia Univ. Nov., 1962.
116. Frenster, J., Allfrey, V. G., and Mirsky, A. E.: Repressed and active chromatin isolated from interphase lymphocytes. Proc. Nat. Acad. Sci. 50: 1026–1032, 1963.
117. Edström, J. E., and Beerman, W.: The base composition of nucleic acids in chromosomes, puffs, nucleoli, and cytoplasm of *Chironomus* salivary gland cells. J. Cell. Biol. 14: 371–380, 1962.
118. Allfrey, V. G., and Mirsky, A. E.: Evidence for the complete DNA-dependence of RNA synthesis in isolated thymus nuclei. Proc. Nat. Acad. Sci. 48: 1590–1596, 1962.
119. Frenster, J. H., Allfrey, V. G., and Mirsky, A. E.: personal communication.
120. Toole, J. and Davies, H. G.: The occurrence and possible significance of haemoglobin in the chromosomal regions of mature erythrocyte nuclei of the newt. *Triturus Cristatus Cristatus* J. Cell. Biol. 16: 501–511, 1963.
121. Levere, R. D., and Granick, S.: unpublished observations.
122. Grobstein, C.: Cytodifferentiation and its controls. Science 143: 643–650, 1964.
123. Saillen, R.: Biosynthèse du système porphyrique dans les myéloblastes. Helv. Med. Acta. 30: 208–223, 1963.
124. Burnham, B. F., and Lascelles, J.: Control of porphyrin biosynthesis through a negative-feedback mechanism. Biochem. J. 87: 462–472, 1963.
125. Granick, S.: Induction of the synthesis of δ- aminolevulinic acid synthetase in liver parenchyma cells in culture by chemicals that induce acute porphyria. J. Biol. Chem. 238 PC 2248–2249 (1963).
126. Lascelles, J.: The synthesis of enzymes concerned in bacteriochlorophyll formation in growing cultures of *Rhodopseudomonas spheroides.* J. Gen. Microbiol. 23: 487–498, 1960.
127. Jacob, F., and Monod, J.: Genetic repression, allosteric inhibition and cellular differentiation. pgs. 30–57. In *Cytodifferentiation* and *macromolecular synthesis* M. Locke (ed.) Academic Press, N. Y., 1963.
128. Rich, A.: unpublished
129. Watson, C. J.: Porphyria pp. 235–299. In *Advances in Internal Medicine.* Dock, W. and Snapper, I. (Eds.) Year Book Publishers, Chicago, 1954.
130. Goldberg, A., and Rimington, C.: *Diseases of Porphyrin Metabolism.* Charles C. Thomas, Springfield, Ill. pp. 231, 1962.
131. Schmid, R.: The Porphyrias, pp. 939–1021. In *The Metabolic Basis of Inherited Disease.* Stanbury, J. B., Wyngaarden, J. B., and Fredricksen, D. S. (Eds.) McGraw-Hill, New York, 1960.
132. Rimington, C.: Haems and porphyrins in health and disease. Acta. Med. Scand. 43: 177–196, 1952.
133. Jørgensen, S. K., and With, T. K.: Congenital porphyria in swine and cattle in Denmark. Nature 176: 156–157, 1955.
134. Jørgensen, S. K., and With, T. K.: Porphyria in domestic animals: Danish observations in pigs and cattle and comparison with human porphyria. Ann. N. Y. Acad. Sci. 104: 701–709, 1963.
135. Fourie, P. J. J.: The occurrence of congenital porphyrinurea (pink tooth) in cattle in South Africa (Swaziland) Onderstepoort J. Vet. Sci. 2: 535–540, 1936.
136. Schmid, R., Schwartz, S., and Watson, C. J.: Porphyrin content of bone marrow and liver in the various forms of porphyria. AMA Arch. Int. Med. 93: 167–190, 1954.
137. Rimington, C., and Booij, H. L.: Porphyrin biosynthesis in human red cells. Biochem J. 65: 3P, 1958.
138. Magnus, I. A., Jarrett, A., Prankerd, T. A. J., and Rimington, C.: Erythropoietic

protoporphyria. A new porphyria syndrome with solar urticaria due to protoporphy-rinemia. Lancet 2: 448–451, 1961.

139. Haeger-Aronson, B.: Erythropoietic proto-porphyria. A new type of inborn error of metabolism. Am. J. Med. 35: 450–454, 1963.

140. Porter, F. S., and Lowe B. A.: Congenital erythropoietic protoporphyria. I. Case reports, clinical studies and porphyrin analysis in two brothers. Blood 22: 521–531, 1963.

141. Porter, F. S.: Congenital erythropoietic protoporphyria. II. An experimental study. Blood 22: 532–544, 1963.

142. Waldenström, J.: Studien über porphyrie. Acta Med. Scand. Suppl. 82, 1937.

143. Goldberg, A.: Acute intermittent porphyria. Quart. J. Med. 28: 183–209, 1959.

144. Gibson, J. B., and Goldberg, A.: The neuropathology of acute porphyria. J. Path. and Bact. 71: 495–509, 1956.

145. Waldenström, J.: Neurological symptoms caused by so-called acute porphyria. Acta psychiat. et neurol. 14: 375–379, 1939.

146. Watson, C. J.: The problem of porphyria—some facts and questions. New Eng. J. Med. 263: 1205–1215, 1960.

147. Watson, C. J., Runge, W., and Bossenmaier, I.: Increased urinary PBG and URO after administration of stilboestrol in a case of latent porphyria. Metabolism 11: 1128–1133, 1962.

148. Watson, C. J.: Observations on urine Ehrlich's reactions pp. 45–49, in *Les Maladies du Métabolisme des Porphyrines*. Presse Universitaires de France, Paris, 1962.

149. Dean, G., and Barnes, H. D.: The inheritance of porphyria. Brit. Med. J. 2: 89–94, 1955.

150. Eales, L., and Linder, G. C.: Porphyria—the acute attack. S. Afr. Med. J. 36: 284–292, 1962.

151. Dean, G., and Barnes, H. D.: Porphyria in Sweden and South Africa. S. Afr. Med. J. 33: 246–253, 1959.

152. Barnes, J. D.: Porphyria in the Bantu races on the Witwatersrand. S. Afr. Med. J. 29: 781–784, 1955.

153. Barnes, H. D.: The excretion of porphyrins and porphyrin precursors by Bantu cases of porphyria. S. Afr. Med. J. 33: 274–278, 1959.

154. Cam, C., and Nigososyan, G.: Acute toxic porphyria cutanea tarda secondary to hexachlorobenzene, 348 cases. J.A.M.A. 183: 88–91, 1963.

155. Schmid, R.: An outbreak of cutaneous porphyria, pp. 3–43 in *Les Maladies du Métabolisme des Porphyrines*. Presse Universitaries des France, Paris, 1962.

156. Martin, W. J., and Heck. F. J.: The porphyrins and porphyria. A review of eighty-one cases. Am. J. Med. 20: 239–250, 1956.

157. Chisolm, J. J.: Disturbances in the biosynthesis of heme in lead intoxication. J. Ped. 64: 174–187, 1964.

158. Lichtman, H. C., and Feldman, F.: *In vitro* pyrrole and porphyrin synthesis in lead poisoning and iron deficiency. J. Clin. Invest. 42: 830–839, 1963.

159. Schmid, R., and Schwartz, S.: Experimental porphyria. III Hepatic type produced by sedormid. Proc. Soc. Exp. Biol. and Med. 81: 685–689, 1952.

160. Waldenström, J.: The porphyrias as inborn errors of metabolism. Am. J. Med. 22: 758–773, 1957.

161. Barnes, H. D.: Porphyria. Int. Rev. Trop. Med. 2: 197–230, 1963.

162. Elliott, W. H.: Aminoacetone: its isolation and role in metabolism. Nature 183: 1051–1052, 1959.

163. Solomon, H. M., and Figge, F. H. J.: Disturbance in porphyrin metabolism by feeding diethyl-1,4,-dihydro- 2,4,6,-trimethyl-pyridine-3,5- dicarboxylate. Proc. Soc. Exp. Biol. and Med. 100: 583–586, 1959.

164. Shemin, D., and Rittenberg, D.: The biological utilization of glycine for the synthesis of the protoporphyrin of hemoglobin. J. Biol. Chem. 166: 621–627, 1946.

165. London, I. M., West, R., Shemin, D., and Rittenberg, D.: On the origin of bile pigment in normal man. J. Biol. Chem. 184: 351, 1950.

Methemoglobinemia in Man[1]

────────ERNST R. JAFFÉ and PAUL HELLER────────

METHEMOGLOBIN (ferrihemoglobin, hemiglobin, ferriprotoporphyrin IX-globin) is hemoglobin in which the ferrous iron of heme is in the ferric form. Methemoglobin is incapable of binding molecular oxygen reversibly because the sixth coordination position of iron, normally available to oxygen, has lost its unpaired electron and is occupied by water. Because of the additional positive charge on the ferric iron, the water is readily replaced by cyanide or other anions (ligands). Methemoglobin and cyanmethemoglobin are stable molecules which have characteristic absorption spectra (see Figure 4). These spectral properties are utilized in clinical hemoglobinometry and in the determination of methemoglobin by the method of Evelyn and Malloy[31].

Approximately one per cent of the total hemoglobin in normal human erythrocytes is in the form of methemoglobin. This constant concentration is maintained as the result of the equilibrium between the rate at which hemoglobin is oxidized and the rate at which methemoglobin is reduced to hemoglobin. This equilibrium is shown schematically in Figure 1. The oxidation of hemoglobin is represented by arrow 'a'. Arrow 'a-b' indicates the rate of oxidation which may be decreased by mechanisms within erythrocytes that protect the hemoglobin. An increase in the concentration of methemoglobin can result from exposure to noxious agents which increase the rate of oxidation and which may overwhelm the protective mechanisms. Once methemoglobin is formed within erythrocytes, it can be reduced to hemoglobin by enzymatic or other processes that are represented by arrow 'c'. This capacity to reduce methemoglobin may be impaired by abnormalities in the reducing systems of the erythrocyte or in the hemoglobin molecule itself (hemoglobin M). A decrease in the ability to reduce methemoglobin will also result in an increase in the concentration of methemoglobin.

Oxidation of Hemoglobin to Methemoglobin

The presence of a constant, small amount of methemoglobin in normal human blood is compatible with the thesis that oxidation of hemoglobin does occur *in vivo*. Further support for this concept is derived from the observations that methemoglobin reappears at a linear rate of 0.5 to 3 per cent of the total hemoglobin per day in the erythrocytes of patients whose cells are incapable of reducing methemoglobin to hemoglobin, after all of the methemo-

From the Department of Medicine, Albert Einstein College of Medicine, New York and the Department of Medicine, University of Illinois College of Medicine, Chicago, Illinois.

Supported by grants from the U. S. Public Health Service, the Atomic Energy Commission, the Office of Naval Research and the Health Research Council of the City of New York (U-1315) (E.R.J.); and Veterans Administration Medical Research funds and, in part, by a grant from the Hematology Research Foundation, Chicago, Illinois, (P.H.).

[1] The reference citations are not intended to present a complete bibliography. In several instances, only a recent paper or a review article has been cited as a source of references to preceding publications by an author or about a particular topic.

globin has been reduced by appropriate therapy[30, 61, 120]. The rate of oxidation of hemoglobin to methemoglobin *in vitro* is slow. Intact human erythrocytes, incubated at 37°C in the absence of added substrate, contain 70 per cent methemoglobin after 7 days, while a solution of crystalline human hemoglobin is completely oxidized in the same length of time[64]. In hemolyzed erythrocytes, oxidation proceeds to completion in about 5 days[30].

The oxidation of hemoglobin to methemoglobin is still incompletely understood. Spontaneous autoxidation of hemoglobin occurs, perhaps through the formation of intermediates of oxyhemoglobin or deoxygenated hemoglobin[83]. Such intermediate compounds have been separated by electrophoresis during partial oxidation of carbonmonoxyhemoglobin[57].

The ferrous iron of heme may be oxidized directly by a number of agents: ferricyanide, ferric tartrate, bivalent copper, chlorate, certain quinones, alloxans and some dyes with a high oxidation-reduction potential[83]. Methemoglobin is formed when hemoglobin is treated with an excess of chromate, but not with chromic ion[29]. The mechanism by which nitrite, a powerful reducing agent and one of the most widely used methemoglobin-forming compounds, produces methemoglobin has not been elucidated.

More complex reactions have been postulated to explain the methemoglobin-forming properties of certain dyes, ascorbic acid, naphthoquinones, thiols and other compounds[13, 48, 83, 114]. In these reactions, hemoglobin appears to participate as a reducing agent and becomes oxidized. For example, methylene blue can be reduced by hemoglobin to leukomethylene blue and methemoglobin is formed. Leukomethylene blue may be reoxidized to methylene blue by atmospheric oxygen and can catalyze the oxidation of more than a stoichiometric amount of hemoglobin. The equilibirum of these reactions is determined by the concentrations of the four reactants. In the presence of an increased concentration of methemoglobin, leukomethylene blue will reduce methemoglobin. Hydrogen donors, such as phenylhydrazine, leukomethylene blue or ascorbic acid, may also undergo autoxidation with the formation of hydrogen peroxide, a potent oxidizing agent, or an equivalent free radical[83, 97]. This free radical can oxidize hemoglobin directly or form an intermediate with oxyhemo-

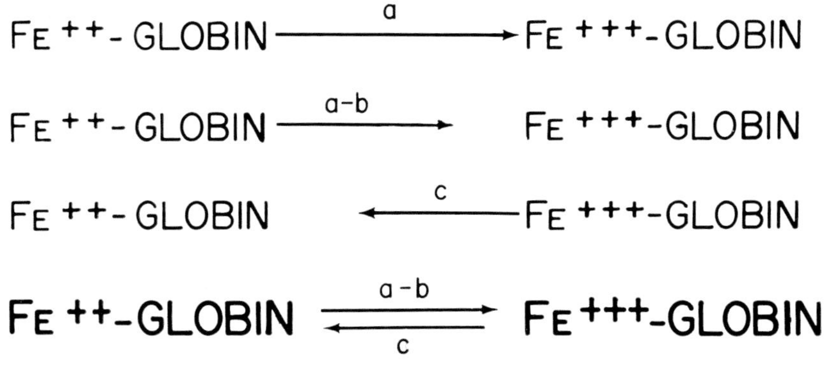

$$\text{Fe}^{++}\text{- GLOBIN} \xrightarrow{ a } \text{Fe}^{+++}\text{-GLOBIN}$$

$$\text{Fe}^{++}\text{- GLOBIN} \xrightarrow{ a\text{-}b } \text{Fe}^{+++}\text{-GLOBIN}$$

$$\text{Fe}^{++}\text{- GLOBIN} \xleftarrow{ c } \text{Fe}^{+++}\text{-GLOBIN}$$

$$\text{Fe}^{++}\text{-GLOBIN} \underset{c}{\overset{a\text{-}b}{\rightleftharpoons}} \text{Fe}^{+++}\text{-GLOBIN}$$

FIG. 1.—Schematic representation of the intracellular equilibrium between hemoglobin (Fe++-globin) and methemoglobin (Fe+++-globin) in which 'a' represents the rate at which hemoglobin is oxidized, 'b' the factors which protect against oxidation and 'c' the rate at which methemoglobin is reduced to hemoglobin.

globin which subsequently decomposes to yield methemoglobin. Aromatic amino and nitro compounds which form methemoglobin only to a limited extent *in vitro* are often very active methemoglobin formers *in vivo*[13]. These compounds, as well as metabolic products of bacteria and tissues, may be converted to metabolites which either act as direct oxidants or participate in the coupled oxidation of hemoglobin with a reducing agent in the presence of atmospheric oxygen. Additional damage, leading to the formation of irreversibly denatured hemoglobins (choleglobin, verdohemoglobin, sulfhemoglobin), may also result from such coupled oxidations[83, 97]. Several investigators[2, 14, 45, 83] have suggested that methemoglobin is a necessary intermediate stage in the degradation of hemoglobin. The results of recent experiments, however, have been interpreted as indicating that methemoglobin formation is a possible, but not essential, step in the breakdown of hemoglobin[11].

Protection of Hemoglobin against Oxidation

Hemoglobin within intact erythrocytes is less susceptible to oxidation than when present in hemolysates or in the purified state, probably because of the existence of intracellular protective mechanisms. Oxyhemoglobin is less susceptible to autoxidation than is reduced hemoglobin, for the rate of autoxidation is proportional to the concentration of deoxygenated heme[16, 92]. This decrease in susceptibility to oxidation upon oxygenation may be related to the changes in the structure of hemoglobin which occur during oxygenation[90]. There also is an electron hiatus between molecular oxygen and intracellular electron donors, such as heme, in mature mammalian erythrocytes because they lack cytochrome oxidase and an intact cytochrome system[98]. This electron hiatus may prevent oxidation by molecular oxygen when oxyhemoglobin is formed.

Active metabolic processes which may protect hemoglobin against oxidation appear to exist in mammalian erythrocytes. Glutathione peroxidase activity can catalyze the decomposition of hydrogen peroxide to water with the oxidation of reduced glutathione (GSH) to oxidized glutathione (GSSG). This enzyme system has been demonstrated in rat and bovine erythrocytes[88] and appears to be present in the non-hemoglobin protein fraction of human erythrocytes[52]. Perfusion of hydrogen peroxide through suspensions of normal human erythrocytes fails to lower the concentration of GSH and fails to cause the formation of methemoglobin as long as glucose is present[21]. A marked decrease in the concentration of GSH and an increase in the concentration of methemoglobin occurs under similar experimental conditions in human erythrocytes deficient in glucose-6-P dehydrogenase activity. These enzyme-deficient cells are unable to regenerate TPNH required for the maintenance of the GSH necessary for the activity of this peroxidase. Human erythrocytes also contain catalase which can decompose hydrogen peroxide. It has been suggested that catalase functions to protect hemoglobin against oxidation[83], but such protection is not observed when hydrogen peroxide is generated slowly by glucose oxidase *in vitro*[69]. Human erythrocytes in which catalase activity is blocked by azide do not show an increase in the concentration of methemoglobin in the presence of an adequate supply of glucose[21]. These latter observations have led to the suggestion that catalase activity is physiologically unimportant in preventing the oxidation of hemoglobin. However, erythrocytes obtained from subjects with hereditary acatalasemia are much more susceptible to the formation of methemoglobin upon the addition of hydrogen peroxide or upon x-ray irradiation than are normal human erythrocytes, despite normal glutathione peroxidase and methemoglobin reductase activities[1, 50]. If formation of hydrogen peroxide is essential for the oxidation of hemoglobin to methemoglobin, the activity of glutathione peroxidase and, perhaps of catalase, might serve to remove this oxidant whenever it is formed. Because the formation of hydrogen peroxide does not appear to occur during autoxidation of hemoglobin[68], the importance of these enzymatic mechanisms under physiological conditions is unclear. The contribution of glutathione peroxidase to protection against drug-induced destruction of hemoglobin *in vitro* seems to have been demonstrated more definitively[21, 52].

It is not certain if GSH, independent of its role as cofactor for glutathione peroxidase, can protect hemoglobin against oxidation[60]. The finding that methemoglobin can be formed without a decrease in the concentration of GSH has led to the suggestion that the oxidation of hemoglobin protects the erythrocyte against depletion of GSH[26, 46]. Further investigations are required to resolve these contradictory points of view.

Ergothioneine, another sulfhydryl compound, is present in normal human erythrocytes in a concentration of about 10 mg per 100 ml of erythrocytes[117]. Erythrocytes obtained from rabbits depleted of ergothioneine by dietary restriction are more susceptible to the methemoglobin-forming effect of nitrite than are erythrocytes from non-depleted rabbits, even without changes in the concentration of GSH[113]. The roles of ergothioneine and of cysteine, another sulfhydryl compound, in human erythrocytes have not been fully defined.

TPN and TPNH, but not GSH, are able to maintain the stability of glucose-6-P dehydrogenase and they can protect hemoglobin in hemolysates against denaturation to choleglobin by ascorbic acid[116]. The pyridine nucleotides may, therefore, afford limited direct protection against oxidation of hemoglobin without mediation through enzymatic mechanisms.

Reduction of Methemoglobin to Hemoglobin

The metabolic processes which are involved in the reduction of methemoglobin to hemoglobin in normal human erythrocytes have been reviewed in detail recently[60] and are summarized only briefly here (Figure 2). Reduction of methemoglobin is dependent upon the structural integrity of the erythrocyte, is associated with carbohydrate metabolism and requires the regeneration of reduced pyridine nucleotides. Kiese[70] and Gibson[38, 39] have suggested that there are two pathways by which electrons can be transferred from reduced pyridine nucleotides to the ferric iron of the heme in methemoglobin.

From his studies and because direct reduction of methemoglobin by DPNH is extremely slow, Gibson has postulated that an intermediate carrier (coenzyme factor I, "diaphorase" or DPNH-methemoglobin reductase) exists in normal human erythrocytes[39]. Scott and his associates[103] have confirmed Gibson's postulate by demonstrating an enzyme system in normal human

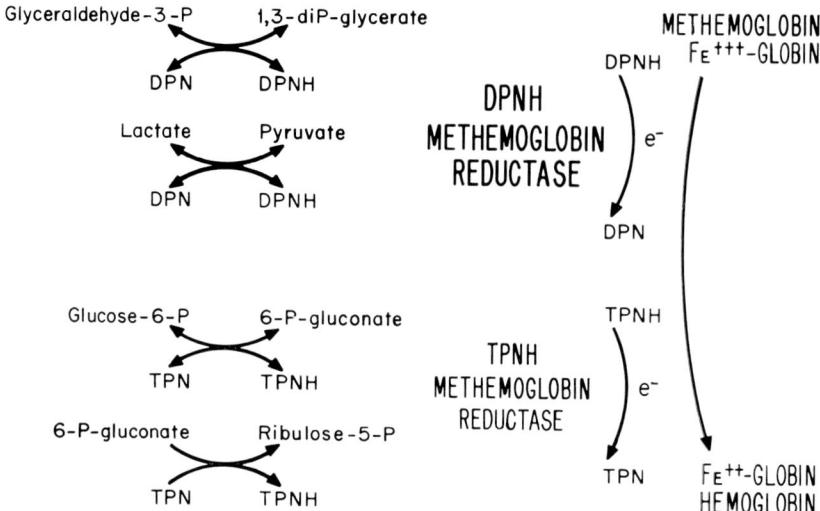

F<small>IG</small>. 2.—Pyridine nucleotide-dependent metabolic pathways involved in the reduction of methemoglobin to hemoglobin in human erythrocytes.

erythrocytes which reduces methemoglobin without requiring an artificial electron carrier. Because the rate at which this enzyme system reduces the dye, 2,6-dichlorobenzenone indophenol, is so much faster than the rate at which it reduces methemoglobin, the reduction of the dye has been utilized to measure the activity of this system in hemolysates of nitrite-treated erythrocytes. A severe deficiency in the activity of this system is found in the erythrocytes of many patients with hereditary methemoglobinemia (vide infra) [18, 59, 93, 100]. Because the precise nature of this system has not been defined and because of its preferential utilization of DPNH, this enzyme system should be designated as DPNH-methemoglobin reductase.

The second pathway has been suggested by Kiese[70, 73] and by Gibson[39] on the basis of their observations on the effect of methylene blue on the reduction of methemoglobin. They have postulated that this dye opens up a new pathway for the reduction of methemoglobin. This pathway is thought to require TPNH and a different intermediate carrier (coenzyme factor II, Hämiglobinreduktase or TPNH-methemoglobin reductase). Huennekens and his associates[55] have isolated an enzyme system from human erythrocytes that can reduce methemoglobin to hemoglobin in the presence of TPNH and an autoxidizable dye, such as methylene blue. They have suggested that this enzyme has two prosthetic groups. One, an unknown carrier, perhaps ferric iron, may be detached upon hemolysis and purification, but can be substituted for by an autoxidizable dye. The existence of a second group, a tightly bound iron-porphyrin moiety, has been questioned[108]. This system is thought to require the transfer of electrons from TPNH to methylene blue or the unknown natural cofactor and then to the enzyme. The reduced enzyme can then reduce methemoglobin or another electron acceptor. The rapid rate at which leukomethylene blue reduces methemoglobin to hemoglobin has led Beutler and Baluda[12] to suggest that this methemoglobin reductase may exert its effect before methylene blue is reduced. This system should be referred to as TPNH-methemoglobin reductase.

Ascorbic acid can reduce methemoglobin to hemoglobin *in vivo* and *in vitro*, probably without intervention of an enzyme system[39, 58, 70]. DPNH and TPNH, and the sulfhydryl compounds, GSH and cysteine, reduce isolated methemoglobin slowly *in vitro*[13, 54, 83, 102]. An ergothioneine-dependent oxidation of TPNH by hemolysates of human erythrocytes has been described[75] and such a reaction might be capable of promoting the reduction of methemoglobin.

The relative importance of the various mechanisms for the reduction of methemoglobin to hemoglobin has been evaluated from several lines of evidence which have been summarized elsewhere[60]. The DPNH-methemoglobin reductase system appears to be the major pathway by which methemoglobin is reduced in normal human erythrocytes. The DPNH required is generated by glyceraldehyde-3-P dehydrogenase activity or, in the presence of excess lactate, by lactic dehydrogenase activity (Figure 2). Reduction of methemoglobin by ascorbic acid and by GSH may become significant under conditions where the capacity of this mechanism is exceeded. The role of the hexose monophosphate shunt pathway in the reduction of methemoglobin has been attributed to the non-enzymatic reduction of methemoglobin by GSH[115]. DPNH-methemoglobin reductase may serve as a reserve system which requires an artificial electron carrier, such as methylene blue, to become fully effective in reducing methemoglobin to hemoglobin. The necessary TPNH is generated by the first two reactions of the hexose monophosphate shunt pathway (Figure 2).

Physiological and Clinical Consequences of Methemoglobin

Cyanosis, not accompanied by obvious cardiac or pulmonary abnormalities, should suggest the possibility of methemoglobinemia. Although it is more precise to refer to this condition as methemoglobincythemia because the altered hemoglobin is present within the erythrocyte and is not free in the plasma, convention dictates the designation methemoglobinemia. This disorder may result from: A) exposure to toxic agents which enhance the oxidation of hemoglobin, B) genetically determined abnormalities in the metabolism of the erythrocyte which impair the ability of the cells to reduce methemoglobin, and C) genetically determined abnormalities in the structure of the hemoglobin molecule (hemoglobin M) which increase the susceptibility to oxidation and decrease the susceptibility to reduction.

Methemoglobin imparts a reddish brown or brown color to blood which persists after vigorous shaking with air. A concentration of 1.5 to 2.0 gm of methemoglobin per 100 ml of blood will produce visible cyanosis, while about 5 gm of deoxygenated (reduced) hemoglobin per 100 ml of blood is required to produce the same degree of cyanosis[32, 80]. Man can tolerate a moderate degree of methemoglobinemia with only mild symptoms attributable to the lowered oxygen-carrying capacity of the blood. Subjects with hereditary methemoglobinemia experience only slight exertional dyspnea, easy fatigability and occasional headaches[13, 30, 32, 58]. A mild compensatory erythrocytosis may occur in patients with long-standing methemoglobinemia. The minimal symptoms are in striking contrast to the prominent cyanosis associated with methemoglobin concentrations of 20 to 45 per cent. Similar concentrations, resulting from the administration of certain drugs, can be tolerated with only moderate exertional dyspnea[10, 13]. The lethal concentration of methemoglobin in man is unknown, but is probably over 70 per cent[13, 17].

In addition to preventing reversible binding of oxygen, methemoglobin may alter the affinity of the remaining hemoglobin for oxygen. Darling and Roughton[24] have reported that drug-induced methemoglobinemia produces a shift to the left of the oxygen dissociation curve with decreased release of oxygen to the tissues at low partial pressures of oxygen. Such abnormal oxygen dissociation curves have been described in studies of four patients with hereditary methemoglobinemia[4, 39, 40]. Essentially normal curves, however, have been obtained with blood from six other cases of hereditary methemoglobinemia[30, 81, 85, 120] and from subjects with nitrite-induced methemoglobinemia[10]. It has been suggested that when a displacement of the dissociation curve does occur, only some of the heme moieties of each hemoglobin molecule have been oxidized[39]. Such partial oxidation might then alter the heme-heme interaction of the remaining unoxidized heme groups to increase their affinity for oxygen.

Methemoglobin, as an isolated alteration, does not appear to have an adverse effect on the structural integrity of human erythrocytes. The presence of methemoglobin does not increase the degree of spontaneous hemolysis[58] or the osmotic fragility[67] of erythrocytes. Erythrocytes of subjects with hereditary methemoglobinemia survive normally in the circulation of a normal recipient and in the patient's own circulation[49]. A slight increase in the apparent life span of erythrocytes of patients with sickle cell disease in whom concentrations of more than 20 per cent methemoglobin were maintained by the administration of sodium nitrite has been reported[10]. Methemoglobin S is not susceptible to sickling. Its presence decreases the amount of deoxygenated hemoglobin S at a given oxygen tension and diminishes the tendency of the erythrocyte to be deformed.

Reports about the content of methemoglobin in old, as compared to young, human erythrocytes have been contradictory. These findings are summarized elsewhere[60]. Several investigators have found a higher methemoglobin content in the denser or more osmotically fragile older erythrocytes, either with normal total methemoglobin concentrations or after drug-induced methemoglobinemia. Other investigators have failed to observe such differences. Numerous studies, however, have demonstrated that the capacity to reduce methemoglobin to hemoglobin decreases with aging of mammalian erythrocytes *in vivo*.

Thus, the exact relationship of methemoglobin formation to the destruction of human erythrocytes upon exposure to certain drugs or at the end of the normal life span of these cells remains to be determined. Since erythrocytes of subjects with hereditary methemoglobinemia appear to have a normal life span, the formation of methemoglobin by itself may be of little importance. Perhaps the formation of methemoglobin takes place coincidentally with irreversible alterations in essential structures of the erythrocyte membrane or of enzymes within the cell.

A. *Toxic Methemoglobinemia*

Toxic methemoglobinemia can result from exposure to many drugs and chemicals. A complete review of the pharmacology and toxicology of these agents is beyond the scope of this discussion and the reader is referred to the publications by Bodansky[13] and Finch[32]. A few examples, however, are discussed here.

The inadvertent ingestion of as little as 200 mg of sodium nitrite can produce marked methemoglobinemia in an adult and may contribute to death[44]. Nitrates have been incriminated frequently in toxic methemoglobinemia, probably because they can be reduced to nitrites in the gastrointestinal tract by micro-organisms. So-called "enterogenous cyanosis" has been attributed to such a mechanism[32]. An unusually large number of cases of toxic methemoglobinemia has been reported in infants who have been fed formulas prepared with well-water containing high concentrations of nitrate. More than 700 instances have been reported, and the mortality has been as high as 10 per cent[17, 80]. Cornblath and Hartmann[23], observing that most cases occurred in infants less than 2 months old, have postulated that the pH of more than 4 in their gastric contents permits the growth of bacteria which can reduce nitrate to nitrite. Additional factors, however, may also contribute to the increased susceptibility of infants. Although not sufficient to cause visible cyanosis, the concentration of methemoglobin in the erythrocytes of newborn infants and, especially, of premature infants is significantly higher than that in the erythrocytes of children older than one year and adults[77]. The spontaneous oxidation of hemoglobin to methemoglobin is about twice as rapid in intact cord blood erythrocytes as it is in the erythrocytes of adults when glycolysis is inhibited by fluoride or iodoacetate[79]. Although purified oxyhemoglobin F is no more susceptible to spontaneous oxidation than is oxyhemoglobin A, the rate at which nitrite oxidizes fetal oxyhemoglobin is twice as rapid as the rate with adult oxyhemoglobin[8]. The capacity of the erythrocytes of newborn infants to reduce methemoglobin to hemoglobin appears to be less than that of the erythrocytes of adults[78]. This decrease is probably due to a transient deficiency in the acitivity of DPNH-methemoglobin reductase[87, 96]. Thus, the metabolic differences of the erythrocytes of the neonatal period may predispose to the development of methemoglobinemia.

Many drugs probably induce the oxidation of hemoglobin after being converted to intermediate forms which are either direct oxidants or which participate in coupled oxidation with hemoglobin and atmospheric oxygen. The nature of these intermediate compounds is, for the most part, unknown. Nitrosobenzene (C_6H_5NO) can be reduced to phenylhydroxylamine (C_6H_5NHOH), a potent methemoglobin-former, by TPNH and the methemoglobin reductase system isolated from mammalian erythrocytes by Kiese[72]. The interaction of phenylhydroxylamine, oxygen and hemoglobin results in the formation of nitrosobenzene and methemoglobin. A metabolic cycle which permits the formation of much more than a stoichiometric amount of methemoglobin by phenylhydroxylamine thus exists within erythrocytes. Exposure of glucose-6-P dehydrogenase deficient erythrocytes, which have a decreased capacity to generate TPNH, to nitrosobenzene in the presence of glucose results in the formation of much less methemoglobin than does similar treatment of normal cells[86]. Phenylhydroxylamine may be the active intermediate in the oxidation of hemoglobin by aniline dyes, nitrosobenzene, nitrobenzene, acetanilide, acetophenetidine and related compounds[13, 15, 71]. As with nitrite or nitrate intoxication, the effect of the potential methemoglobin-forming agents is more pronounced in infants and young children than in adults.

The degree of methemoglobinemia which these chemicals produce is dependent upon several factors: 1) the extent and rate of entry of the compound into the individual's circulation and into the erythrocytes, 2) the rate of metabolism and excretion of the compound, 3) the rate and extent to which the compound is converted to intermediates with either increased or decreased oxidizing capacities, and 4) the rate at which erythrocytes can reduce methemoglobin to hemoglobin. Additional deleterious effects on essential constituents of erythrocytes, especially their membranes, may result from the action of these compounds or their metabolites. As stated before, the question of the relationship between the formation of methemoglobin and the hemolysis of erythrocytes *in vivo* remains unanswered. Primaquine causes methemoglobinemia without hemolysis in normal subjects and produces extensive hemolysis with little methemoglobinemia in individuals whose erythrocytes are deficient in glucose-6-P dehydrogenase activity. This observation may be explained by the rapid removal from the circulation of those enzyme-deficient cells which are damaged most severely and which also contain the most methemoglobin[14].

B. *Hereditary Methemoglobinemia Associated with an Abnormality in the Metabolism of the Erythrocyte*

Since 1844, over 200 cases of probable hereditary methemoglobinemia have been recorded. Unfortunately, it is not possible to determine accurately how many are the result of a deficiency in DPNH-methemoglobin reductase activity and how many are due to the recently reported variants described below (Table I) or to hemoglobin M. It is not unreasonable, however, to assume that those patients in whom complete biochemical studies were not performed, but whose methemoglobinemia responded to the administration of methylene blue or ascorbic acid, did have an abnormality in erythrocyte metabolism. The majority of these cases are probably the result of a deficiency in DPNH-methemoglobin reductase activity. Thus, about 150 examples of presumed DPNH-methemoglobin reductase deficiency can be collected.

Although most instances of this disorder have been described in individuals of European origin, over 20 Alaskan Eskimos and Indians with hereditary methemoglobinemia have been reported[100]. Two Puerto Rican[58, 93], two Hindu[95], one Chinese[19] and one Cuban[33] subject with this abnormality have been described. There are at least 37 families where more than one member was affected or where the results of biochemical studies have been compatible with a hereditary disorder[4, 18, 25, 40, 62, 100, 109]. There does not appear to be

TABLE I.—*Characteristics of Variants of Hereditary Methemoglobinemia Associated with an Abnormality in the Metabolism of the Erythrocyte*

Reported metabolic abnormality	Reduction of nitrite-induced methemoglobin upon incubation with		Mode of Inheritance	Remarks
	Glucose	Lactate		
Deficient DPNH-methemoglobin reductase activity	Markedly decreased	Markedly decreased	Recessive, autosomal, but ? of exceptions	Probably most common form of hereditary methemoglobinemia; may be associated with severe mental retardation.
Decreased erythrocyte GSH; ? impaired glyceraldehyde-3-P dehydrogenase activity	Markedly decreased	Normal	Dominant, autosomal	One patient reported[118, 119], but another possible case has been described[30].
Deficient TPNH-methemoglobin reductase activity (?)	Markedly decreased	Normal	Recessive	One patient reported[91].

a sex predilection. Three cases[27, 58, 93] have been diagnosed initially during pregnancy, and in two[27, 58] the cyanosis appeared to become more pronounced during each gestation. Deleterious effects on these pregnancies or the newborn infants have not been noted. Life expectancy is not affected adversely; patients aged 60 to 80 have been reported[122]. Thus, the disorder appears to be widespread and to be benign.

Blood from patients with hereditary methemoglobinemia is unusually dark, contains 20 to 45 per cent methemoglobin, and the color does not change even after remaining at room temperature for several days[27, 84, 109]. Incubation of nitrite-treated erythrocytes from such blood samples with compounds which are metabolized and which promote the reduction of methemoglobin in normal nitrite-treated cells fails to result in the reduction of a significant amount of methemoglobin[39, 58] (Figure 3). The erythrocytes of 35 patients have been found to be deficient in DPNH-methemoglobin reductase activity[18, 59, 63, 81, 93, 100, 112]. In 12 patients, the concentration of ascorbic acid in the blood has been less than 1 mg per 100 ml[20, 25, 30, 39, 74, 95, 102, 109, 120]. It is of interest that patients with scurvy do not appear to have methemoglobinemia. One patient whose erythrocytes contained a decreased concentration of GSH has been reported[30], but normal concentrations have been found in other instances[63, 74, 102]. It is conceivable that the decreased concentrations of ascorbic acid and of GSH are the result of their being utilized in the reduction of methemoglobin by compensatory mechanisms.

Extensive investigations of erythrocytes from patients with hereditary met-

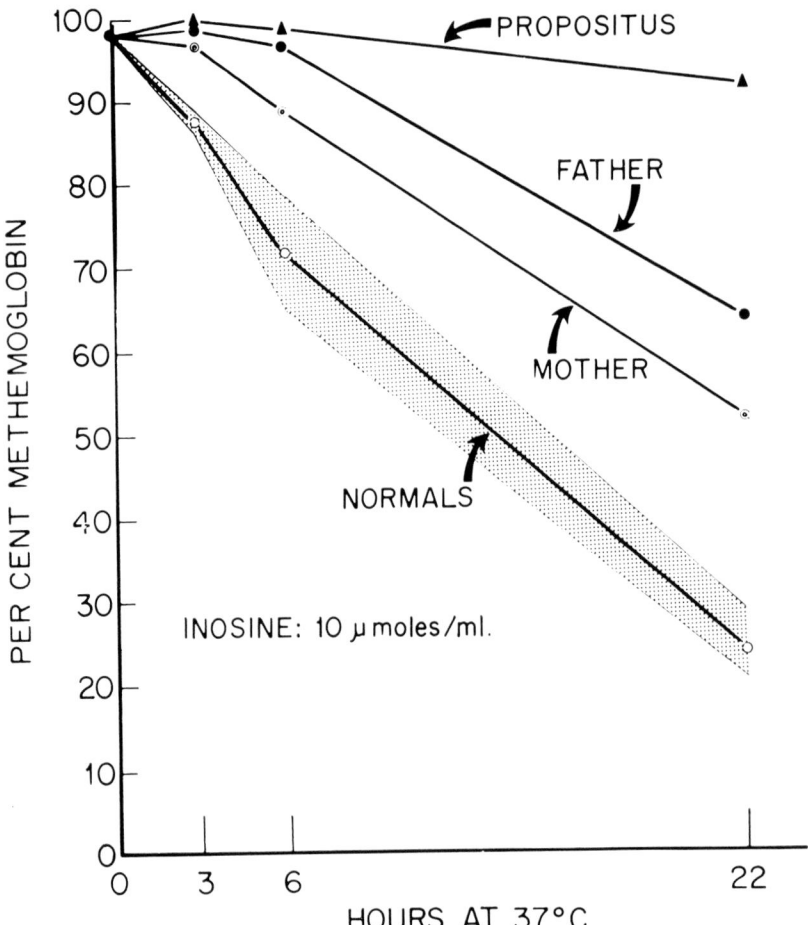

Fig. 3.—Reduction of methemoglobin to hemoglobin during incubation of nitrite-treated erythrocytes. The propositus is a child with hereditary methemoglobinemia associated with severe deficiency in erythrocyte DPNH-methemoglobin reductase activity; the parents' erythrocytes have intermediate levels of DPNH-methemoglobin reductase activity. Normal values are shown for comparison (shaded area indicates the variation in 10 experiments)[63]. Under these experimental conditions, reduction of methemoglobin in suspensions incubated without added substrate does not occur.

hemoglobinemia with proven or presumed DPNH-methemoglobin reductase deficiency have failed to reveal other abnormalities. The rate of spontaneous oxidation of hemoglobin in hemolysates of such cells is not increased[121]. Plasma factors which can enhance the oxidation of hemoglobin or which inhibit the normal reduction of methemoglobin have been excluded[74, 84, 109]. Electrophoresis has revealed only normal hemoglobin A[58, 93, 100]. The ability of erythrocytes deficient in DPNH-methemoglobin reductase activity to metabolize glucose, ribose and purine nucleosides is normal[58]. When nitrite-treated deficient cells are incubated with glucose, less pyruvate[38] and slightly more lactate[58] are produced than when normal erythrocytes are treated similarly. Presumably, more DPNH is available for lactate dehydrogenase activity in cells which are unable to utilize DPNH for the reduction of methemoglobin. The activities of various enzymes of the Embden-Meyerhof and hexose monophosphate shunt pathways and of catalase in these erythrocytes are normal[30, 63, 121]. The concentrations of organic phosphate esters, including pyridine nucleotides, do not differ from those in normal erythrocytes[30, 102, 121]. Ascorbic acid promotes the reduction of methemoglobin in such cells *in vitro*[58, 84]. Incubation of nitrite-treated erythrocytes with methylene blue plus glucose or a purine nucleoside which can be metabolized results in normal reduction of methemoglobin[38, 58]. This latter observation, as well as the results of direct assay for TPNH-methemoglobin reductase activity[59, 93], indicate that the TPNH-methemoglobin reductase system is normal.

The findings of most family studies are compatible with a recessive, autosomal mode of inheritance of hereditary methemoglobinemia due to DPNH-methemoglobin reductase deficiency[9, 18, 62, 100, 112]. Affected individuals are homozygotes and their erythrocytes contain low or absent DPNH-methemoglobin reductase activity. Intermediate levels of enzyme activity have been demonstrated in the erythrocytes of parents of affected children and of children of an affected parent. The erythrocytes of heterozygous subjects contain normal[62, 100, 112] or nearly normal[18] concentrations of methemoglobin. Impaired ability of nitrite-treated erythrocytes of heterozygous subjects to reduce methemoglobin can be demonstrated *in vitro* (Figure 3)[9, 62]. This decreased capacity to reduce methemoglobin in heterozygotes might contribute to variability in susceptibility to toxic methemoglobinemia. Codounis[20] has interpreted his family sudies as indicating a dominant mode of inheritance. Scott[101] has examined one affected member of each of the four families described by Codounis. DPNH-methemoglobin reductase activity is deficient and only normal hemoglobin A is present in their erythrocytes. The absence of close linkage of methemoglobinemia and blood group loci has been reported recently[104]. Additional investigations will be required to resolve the contradictory conclusions about the inheritance of this disorder.

B. 1. *Hereditary Methemoglobinemia Associated with Mental Retardation*

At least nineteen patients have been reported in whom methemoglobinemia has been associated with various degrees of mental retardation[28, 41, 43, 63, 81, 82, 122]. The most severely affected children have, in addition, strabismus, hyporeflexia and frequent vomiting, and they die in infancy or childhood. Treatment with methylene blue and ascorbic acid has failed to alter this course, although the methemoglobinemia has been alleviated. Less severe central nervous system involvement occurs in other affected individuals. The erythrocytes of four patients have been found to be severely deficient in DPNH-methemoglobin reductase activity[63, 81, 112]. The erythrocytes of other subjects are presumed to have had the same metabolic abnormality. The possibility that the association of the two disorders is due to coincidence has been inferred from the findings in one of five families[41]. Cerebral anoxia, secondary to intrauterine methemoglobinemia, has been suggested as the cause of the neurological disability[28, 81]. Since the majority of patients with hereditary methemoglobinemia are neurologically and mentally normal, this expla-

nation appears to be inadequate. There is, at present, no satisfactory explanation for the simultaneous occurrence of DPNH-methemoglobin reductase
deficiency and severe neurological impairment.

B. 2. *Hereditary Methemoglobinemia Associated with an Abnormality in
Erythrocyte Metabolism, but not DPNH-Methemoglobin Reductase
Deficiency*

An unusual variant of hereditary methemoglobinemia has been described
by Townes and his associates[118, 119]. Nitrite-treated erythrocytes from their
patient reduce methemoglobin upon incubation with lactate, but not with
glucose (Table I). Production of lactate from glucose is decreased. DPNH-
and TPNH-methemoglobin reductase activities are normal, and the
methemoglobinemia responds to methylene blue and ascorbic acid. The erythrocytes contain a decreased concentration of GSH, but it is stable upon incubation with acetylphenylhydrazine. Townes and Lovell have postulated that
inadequate synthesis of GSH results in impaired glyceraldehyde-3-P dehydrogenase activity which leads to insufficient generation of DPNH. A dominant
mode of inheritance has been inferred from the family history. It is conceivable that the patient with hereditary methemoglobinemia whose erythrocytes contained a similarly decreased concentration of GSH[30] is also an
example of this variant, but lactate production from glucose is stated to have
been normal.

A patient in whom methemoglobinemia has been attributed to a hereditary
deficiency in TPNH-methemoglobin reductase activity has been reported[91].
The erythrocytes of this patient contain a normal concentration of GSH. His
cells are able to reduce nitrite-induced methemoglobin upon incubation with
lactate, but not with glucose (Table I). Erythrocytes obtained from two
brothers of this patient appear to have the same metabolic abnormality, but
contain normal concentrations of methemoglobin. A recessive mode of inheritance is suggested by the authors. The patient's methemoglobinemia responds dramatically to the administration of methylene blue. If TPNH-
methemoglobin reductase activity is required for the therapeutic effect of this
dye, the existence of a deficiency in this methemoglobin reductase does not
appear to have been established.

C. Hereditary Methemoglobinemia Due to Hemoglobin M

In 1948, Hörlein and Weber[53] described a family with hereditary methemoglobinemia in which this disorder was dominantly transmitted through four
generations. The absorption spectrum of acid methemoglobin prepared from the
erythrocytes of three affected subjects differed from that of normal methemoglobin. This abnormal spectrum could be reproduced by the recombination of
normal heme and globin obtained from the patients' hemolysates, but not by
the reciprocal arrangement. Seven years later, Singer[110] recognized that these
simple heme-globin exchange experiments had established this type of hereditary
methemoglobinemia as a hemoglobinopathy. He suggested, therefore, that the
abnormal hemoglobin underlying this abnormality be designated as hemoglobin
M.

Subsequently, individuals with this abnormal hemoglobin have been detected in various parts of the world[5, 7, 34, 35, 37, 51, 66, 94, 105, 107] and some of these methemoglobins have been found to have different absorption spectra. This heterogeneity has been shown to be due to different single amino acid substitutions in the α or β polypeptide chain of hemoglobin[36, 65, 89] (Table II). On the basis of such differences, hemoglobins M_{Boston} (M_B)[34-36], $M_{Saskatoon}$ (M_S)[35-37], $M_{Milwaukee-1}$ (M_{M-1})[36, 94, 111] and M_{Iwate} (M_I)[65, 89, 107] are well established as separate entities. Several other described variants, hemoglobin $M_{Milwaukee-2}$ (M_{M-2})[36, 94, 111], $M_{Leipzig}$ (M_L)[5, 7], $M_{Chicago}$ (M_{Ch})[66]*, $M_{Freiburg}$[6], $M_{Hamburg}$[6] have not yet been fully characterized by amino acid analysis, but have certain other distinctive properties (vide infra). Others, first described as distinct variants, e.g., hemoglobins $M_{Kankakee}$[51], M_{Kurume}[106], etc., have later been found to be identical with previously reported variants (Table II).

Hemoglobin M is transmitted as a co-dominant characteristic. Hemoglobin A is the other major component in all cases with one exception, hemoglobin M_{M-2}, which has been found to be associated with hemoglobin E[36, 94, 111]. The homozygous state probably is incompatible with life. In several reported families, the disorder has not been present in the parents and known ancestors of the probands, but the children are affected[6, 51, 66]. In these families the disorder might have originated by recent mutation.

Hemoglobin M disease has not been observed in Negroes, but the reason for this apparent absence might be the fact that the cyanosis is masked by the skin pigment. Moreover, electrophoresis for screening purposes is usually performed at alkaline pH which does not permit clear separation of the M fraction.

A lower rate of synthesis of the abnormal hemoglobin may be inferred from the observation that in most affected individuals only 25–30 per cent of the total hemoglobin is in the oxidized state. Hemoglobin M is likely to be present in all erythrocytes of affected subjects, as suggested by the results of a recently described elution test for methemoglobin[76]. This test, performed with blood samples containing hemoglobin M_I (obtained from affected individuals living near Kankakee, Illinois), revealed methemoglobin in all cells, but equal distribution could not be determined with certainty.

The cyanosis of affected individuals is not altered by the administration of methylene blue or ascorbic acid. The presence of hemoglobin M usually is not associated with disability, but a mild secondary erythrocytosis has been observed in one of the individuals with hemoglobin M_I[51]. The erythrocytes of the individual with hemoglobin M_{M-2}[36, 94] who is a double heterozygote for hemoglobin M and E have a diminished survival time. The child with hemoglobin M_{Ch}[66] and the patient with hemoglobin $M_{Freiburg}$[6] have an unexplained hemolytic anemia of fluctuating severity.

The absorption spectra of the methemoglobin M variants are characteristically different from those of normal acid methemoglobin. The normal absorption maxima at 502 and 632 mμ are displaced towards a lower wave length (Figure

* Recent studies[51a] of hemoglobin M_{Ch} (hybridization with canine hemoglobin, "fingerprint" of tryptic digests, amino acid analysis of the abnormal peptide) have shown that this abnormal hemoglobin has the same structural abnormality ($\alpha_2^A \beta_2^{63Tyr}$) as that reported for hemoglobin M_S.[36] (See Table II.)

TABLE II.—*Characteristics of Various Hemoglobin M Variants*

Variant	Spectroscopic maxima of acid methgb† in 480–630 mμ range (Normal: 502,632)	Velocity of cyanide reactivity and cyanmethgb spectrum	Electrophoresis of oxidized hemolysate pH 7.1	Molecular formula	Remarks
M_{Boston} [34-36]	495,600	Slow and incomplete Spectrum abnormal	More anodic than A	α_2^{58} Tyr β_2^A	Also found in Sweden[35] and Germany[5]
$M_{Saskatoon}$ [35-37]	490,602	Fast‡ Spectrum normal	As M_B	$\alpha_2^A \beta_2^{63}$ Tyr	Identical with hgbs M_{Emory}[36], M_{Kurume}[106], $M_{Chicago}$[51a, 66], probably also with $M_{Leipzig}$[5,7] and Hörlein and Weber's hemoglobin.[5,53] The individual with M_{Ch} has hemolytic anemia.
$M_{Milwaukee\ 1}$ [36, 94]	500,622	Fast? Spectrum normal	As M_B	$\alpha_2^A \beta_2^{67}$ Glu	Small spectral differences from hgb A make recognition in whole hemolysate difficult
$M_{Milwaukee\ 2}$ [36, 94, 111]	490,588	?	?	?	Probably β chain abnormality because of observed pseudo-allelism with hgb E
M_{Iwate} [51, 65, 89, 107]	490,610	Fast Spectrum abnormal	More anodic than M_B	α_2^{87} Tyr β_2^A	Identical with hgb $M_{Kankakee}$*. Perhaps most frequent variant. Other families in Chicago[22] Israel[105], Germany[6]
$M_{Freiburg}$ [6]	500,630 Atypical maxima at 530 and 560	Fast Spectrum normal	Not separable (separable as cyanmethgb at alkaline pH)	?	Associated with hemolytic process

* The identity was established by two separate studies of Hgb M_I and M_K, in Dr. Shibata's and the laboratory of one of the authors (P.H.).

† Methgb = Methemoglobin, hgb = hemoglobin.

‡ Quantitative measurements of cyanide reactivity according to the technic of Betke[7] are not available for M_S, but have been performed with $M_{Leipzig}$ and M_{Ch}.[5,66] Their reactivity is slower than that of methemoglobin A.

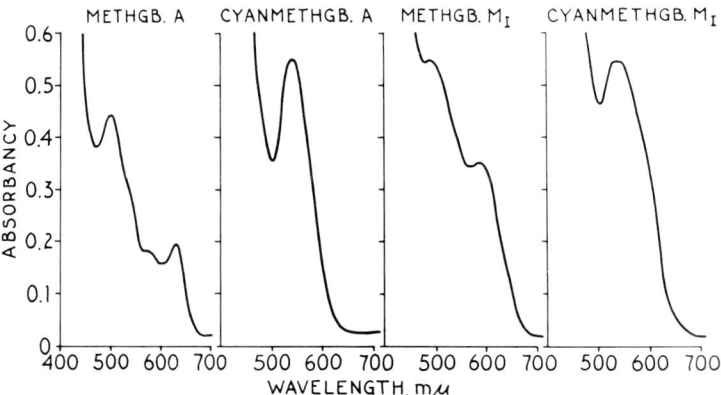

Fig. 4.—Absorption spectra (0.1 M phosphate buffer, pH 6.5, 0.65 mg methemoglobin per ml) of methemoglobins A and M_{Iwate} (obtained from affected family in Kankakee, Illinois) before and after mixing with excess potassium cyanide[51, 107].

4, Table II). This shift of the 632 mμ peak is smallest in hemoglobin M_{M-1} (622 mμ) and greatest in hemoglobin M_{M-2} (588 mμ). There are also alterations in the spectrum between 500 and 600 mμ which are distinctive for some of the variants. The shifts of the absorption maxima provide a simple method for detecting hemoglobin M in whole hemolysates. The ratio of the absorbancies at 500 and 600 mμ, determined in oxidized normal hemolysates at pH7, is approximately 2.8, and at pH 6.5 it is approximately 3.2; in hemolysates containing hemoglobin M these ratios are less. The spectral characteristics can also be utilized for a quantitative determination of the amount of methemoglobin M in hemolysates, if the absorption coefficients are known. Quantification of hemoglobin M, however, is best accomplished by electrophoresis. Gerald[34, 35] has shown that separation of the M fraction from hemoglobin A is most distinct after the hemolysate is oxidized by potassium ferricyanide and electrophoresis is performed at neutral pH. Under these circumstances, methemoglobin M is less positively charged than methemoglobin A. For still unknown reasons, hemoglobin $M_{Freiburg}$ separates more distinctly after conversion to cyanmethemoglobin[6].

Normal methemoglobin forms complexes with certain anions (e.g., cyanide, fluoride, azide) which replace water in the sixth coordination position of iron. These complexes have characteristic absorption spectra. The reaction of methemoglobin A with excess potassium cyanide is practically instantaneous and complete. If oxidized hemolysates containing hemoglobin M are mixed with this ligand, the reaction rate is usually measurably slower and the resulting spectrum may or may not be identical with that of cyanmethemoglobin A. This behavior has become another distinguishing criterion for the hemoglobin M variants[5]. For example, methemoglobins M_S and M_{M-1} react rapidly and the resulting absorption spectra do not differ from cyanmethemoglobin A. Methemoglobin M_B reacts very slowly and the reaction is incomplete, resulting in an abnormal absorption spectrum[34]. Cyanmethemoglobin M_I also has an abnormal spectrum, but the reaction rate is only slightly slower than normal[51, 107]. Characteristic differences among the variants of hemoglobin M also exist for the rate of oxidation by hydrogen peroxide and reduction with sodium dithionite.

For the study of the structural abnormalities of hemoglobin M, the same technics have been used which have proved valuable for the characterization of other abnormal hemoglobins. Hybridization experiments have aided in determining which of the two pairs of polypeptide chains has the abnormality. In the case of hemoglobin M_I, the hybrid between the human α chain and the canine β chain $(\alpha_2^M\beta_2^{Can})$ has been found to have the grey-greenish color of methemoglobin M_I and the spectrum of this hybrid resembles that of the abnormal hemoglobin[51]. The presence of an α chain abnormality can also be recognized from the color of the minor hemoglobin fraction, A_2 $(\alpha_2^M\delta_2^{A2})$[105]. A clinical clue to the chain abnormality in hemoglobin M is the presence of cyanosis at birth in the case of abnormal α chains. With the anomaly in the β chains, cyanosis develops only with the progressively increasing postnatal synthesis of these chains at the expense of the γ chains of fetal hemoglobin.

Electrophoretic and chromatographic analysis of tryptic digests of the M fraction and amino acid analysis of the abnormal peptides have resulted in the elucidation of the structural abnormality of several variants of hemoglobin M (Table II)[36, 65, 89]. In hemoglobin M_B, the histidine residue in position 58 of the α chain is replaced by tyrosine and the molecular formula is written as α_2^{58Tyr}-β_2^A. In hemoglobin M_S, an analogous substitution has occurred in the β chain $(\alpha_2^A\beta_2^{63Tyr})$, in M_{M-1} glutamic acid is present in position 67β instead of valine $(\alpha_2^A\beta_2^{67Glu})$, and M_I is characterized by the substitution of histidine by tyrosine in 87 α.

The accumulation of abnormal amounts of methemoglobin in the erythrocytes can be causally related to these amino acid substitutions. Under normal conditions *in vivo*, some oxidation of hemoglobin to methemoglobin occurs, but the reducing system of the normal erythrocyte keeps the concentration at about one per cent. The enzyme system for reducing methemoglobin functions normally in erythrocytes of individuals with hemoglobin M[35, 51, 66], but it is unable to reduce methemoglobin M to hemoglobin M. A possible reason for this inability to reduce methemoglobin M has been suggested by Gerald and George[35, 37]. Impressed by the similarity of the acid methemoglobin spectrum of hemoglobin M_B and M_S to that of certain methemoglobin complexes (fluoride methemoglobin A) and also phenol metmyoglobin[111], these investigators have developed the following hypothesis: In methemoglobin M, ferric iron forms a complex with an "internal ligand" in a manner analogous to the reaction of normal methemoglobin with fluoride, cyanide and azide. This internal ligand is furnished by a reactive side chain of an amino acid of the polypeptide chain, e.g., the phenolic group of tyrosine, provided it is in a sterically suitable position near iron (Figure 5). As soon as methemoglobin M forms as the result of the normal oxidative processes in the erythrocyte, the trivalent iron reacts with the internal ligand and the resulting internal complex is an unsuitable substrate for enzymatic reduction. Thus, the abnormal methemoglobin accumulates, apparently limited only by the number of abnormal hemoglobin molecules in each erythrocyte. This hypothesis satisfactorily explains the charge difference enabling electrophoretic separation of methemoglobin M from methemoglobin A at neutral pH: one of the three positive charges of ferric iron is not externally manifest because of the internal ionic bond. The occupation of the sixth coordination position of iron by the

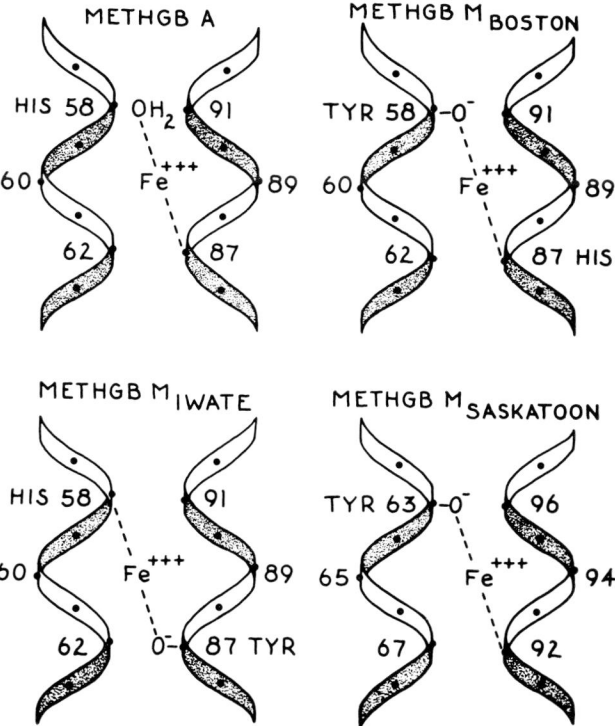

FIG. 5.—Schematic representation of internal-complex-hypothesis and its adaptation to hemoglobin M_{Iwate}. Only the portions of the polypeptide chains around residues 58 and 87 of the α chain (A, M_B, M_I) and residues 63 and 92 of the β chain (M_S) are shown. Only the fifth and sixth coordination positions of iron are indicated and the protoporphyrin part of heme is omitted.

internal ligand also explains the usually diminished reaction velocity of methemoglobin M variants with external ligands, such as cyanide. Depending on the altered steric configuration and the strength of the internal bond, the sixth coordination position of iron is less accessible to the external ligand than normally. It is of interest that in the known β chain variants of hemoglobin M the ligand reactivity appears to be less impaired than in α chain variants.

The internal-complex-hypothesis has received additional support from the rapidly evolving concept of the primary, secondary, tertiary and quaternary structure of the hemoglobin molecule that has developed from the studies of Kendrew, Perutz, Braunitzer, Schroeder, Hill and Königsberg, and others (summarized in references[3, 13a, 56, 99a]. In this molecular model, the heme of the normal α chain is bound to histidine in position 87 via the fifth coordination position of iron, while the sixth coordination position which is reversibly occupied by oxygen is opposite histidine 58. In the β chain, the analogous positions are 92 histidine and 63 histidine, respectively (Figure 5). The amino acid substitutions in hemoglobin M_B (tyrosine in 58 α) and hemoglobin M_S (tyrosine in 63 β) appear to meet the requirements for the formation of internal complexes according to this hypothesis (Figure 5). Because of the helical arrangement of the polypeptide chains, the amino acid in position 67 of the β chain is also sufficiently close to the heme iron (Figure 5) to permit internal complex formation, if endowed with a reactive group. This appears to be the case in hemoglobin M_{M-1} ($\alpha_2{}^A\beta_2{}^{67Glu}$). Certain conceptual difficulties in the application of the internal complex hypothesis to hemoglobin M_1 arise. In this hemoglobin, tyrosine replaces histidine in position 87 α, normally the site of the covalent bond with the fifth coordination position of the heme iron (Figure 5). It seems unlikely that tyrosine in this position could do two things: form a bond with the fifth and interfere with the reversible oxygenation of the sixth coordination position of iron. It appears more likely that histidine 58 has assumed the function of forming the covalent bond with heme iron, thus enabling tyrosine in position 87 to form a stable internal complex with ferric iron.

The differences between the physical and chemical characteristics of the α- and β-chain variants of hemoglobin M will, undoubtedly, receive more intensive attention in the future because they may help to explain the mechanism of heme-heme interaction. Similar reactivity of hemoglobin M_B and hemoglobin M_S with oxygen and ligands might have been expected. In these hemoglobins, the distal histidine in the α-chain (hemoglobin M_B) or the β-chain (hemoglobin M_S) is replaced by tyrosine. There are, however, considerable differences between these two altered hemoglobins in their absorption spectra (Table II: acid methemoglobin, cyanmethemoglobin), in the rate of ligand combination and in the reduction with dithionite.[5] These observations are in keeping with the x-ray crystallographic findings of conformational differences between the α- and β-chains during oxygenation[90] and with certain characteristics of hemoglobin $H^{4a, 93a}$ which consists of four β-chains. Thus, it is likely that the study of hemoglobin M will enhance the understanding of the apparent need for two unequal pairs of polypeptide chains for human hemoglobin to function normally.

Therapy of Methemoglobinemia

Treatment of toxic methemoglobinemia is relatively simple. Concentrations of 20 to 30 per cent methemoglobin do not require specific therapy. They will decrease spontaneously to normal levels in 24 to 72 hours after exposure to the offending agent is discontinued[13, 32]. When unconsciousness or semi-stupor is present or when the concentration of methemoglobin exceeds 40 per cent, more active treatment is indicated. Hemodialysis to remove the toxic agent or its metabolites may be extremely helpful. Methylene blue, 1 to 2 mg per kg intravenously, will often correct the methemoglobinemia within 30 to 60 minutes[13]. Repeated doses may be given, if the initial response has been incomplete. Toxicity from methylene blue with the recommended doses probably does not occur, but excessively large doses (over 15 mg per kg) may cause hemolytic anemia in infants[42]. Although no examples have been reported, it is possible that individuals whose erythrocytes are deficient in glucose-6-P dehydrogenase activity might respond suboptimally to the administration of this dye. The capacity of ascorbic acid to promote the reduction of methemoglobin is so much smaller than that of the normal intrinsic mechanism for the reduction of methemoglobin that it has no place in the therapy of toxic methemoglobinemia.

Hereditary methemoglobinemia associated with a metabolic abnormality in the erythrocytes does not require treatment, except for cosmetic and psychological reasons. Methylene blue, intravenously or orally, will reduce the methemoglobinemia whenever the degree of cyanosis becomes distressing. The rationale for the use of methylene blue is based upon the observation that the capacity of this dye to activate the reserve TPNH-methemoglobin reductase system, in the presence of glucose, greatly exceeds its tendency to oxidize hemoglobin. Menadione sodium bisulfite (vitamin K_3) can accelerate the reduction of methemoglobin *in vitro*[47] and can enhance slightly the oxidation of TPNH by isolated TPNH-methemoglobin reductase[99]. The administration of vitamin K_3 to a patient whose erythrocytes are deficient in DPNH-methemoglobin reductase activity results in the reduction of methemoglobin, but its effect is only about 20 per cent of that of an equimolar amount of methylene blue[61]. Ascorbic acid, 500 mg per day orally for adults, will reduce the methemoglobinemia slowly and will maintain the concentration at between 5 and 13 per cent[13, 58, 74].

The methemoglobinemic cyanosis due to methemoglobin M does not respond to methylene blue or ascorbic acid. Since the causal abnormality resides in the structure of the hemoglobin, the usual treatment for methemoglobinemia is not indicated and no other effective form of therapy has been reported.

REFERENCES

1. Aebi, H., Heiniger, J. P., and Suter, H.: Some properties of red cells and other tissues from normal and acatalatic humans. Biochem. J. 89: 63P, 1963.
2. Allen, D. W., and Jandl, J. H.: Oxidative hemolysis and precipitation of hemoglobin. II. Role of thiols in oxidant drug action. J. Clin. Invest. 40: 454–475, 1961.
3. Baglioni, C.: Correlation between genetics and chemistry of human hemoglobins. *In* Taylor, J. H. (Ed.): Molecular Genetics. Part I. New York and London, Academic Press, 1963, pp. 405–475.
4. Baikie, A. G., and Valtis, D. J.: Gas transport function of the blood in congenital familial methaemoglobinaemia. Brit. Med. J. 2: 73–76, 1954.
4a. Benesch, R. E., Ranney, H. M., Benesch, R., and Smith, G. M.: The chemistry of the Bohr effect. II. Some properties of hemoglobin H. J. Biol. Chem. 236: 2926–2929, 1961.
5. Betke, K.: Hämoglobin M: Typen und ihre Differenzierung (Übersicht). *In* Lehmann, H. and Betke, K. (Eds.): Haemoglobin-Colloquium. Stuttgart, Georg Thieme, 1962, pp. 39–47.
6. Betke, K.: Personal communciation.
7. Betke, K., Gröschner, E., and Bock, K.: Properties of a further variant of haemoglobin M. Nature (London) 188: 864–865, 1960.
8. Betke, K., Kleihauer, E., and Lipps, M.: Vergleichende Untersuchungen über die Spontanoxydation von Nabelschnur- und Erwachsenenhämoglobin. Z. Kinderheilk. 77: 549–553, 1956.
9. Betke, K., Steim, H., and Tönz, O.: Untersuchung einer Familie mit kongenitaler Methämoglobinämie durch Reduktaseinsuffizienz. Deutsch. Med. Wschr. 87: 65–68, 1962.
10. Beutler, E.: The effect of methemoglobin formation in sickle cell disease. J. Clin. Invest. 40: 1856–1871, 1961.
11. Beutler, E., and Baluda, M. C.: The role of methemoglobin in oxidative degradation of hemoglobin. Acta Haemat. (Basel) 27: 321–333, 1962.
12. Beutler, E., and Baluda, M. C.: Methemoglobin reduction. Studies of the interaction between cell populations and of the role of methylene blue. Blood 22: 323–333, 1963.
13. Bodansky, O.: Methemoglobinemia and methemoglobin-producing compounds. Pharmacol. Rev. 3: 144–196, 1951.
13a. Braunitzer, G., and Rudloff, V.: Die Haemoglobine. Deutsch. Med. Wschr. 87: 959–968, 1962.
14. Brewer, G. J., Tarlov, A. R., Kellermeyer, R. W., and Alving, A. S.: The hemolytic effect of primaquine. XV. Role of methemoglobin. J. Lab. Clin. Med. 59: 905–917, 1962.
15. Brodie, B. B., and Axelrod, J.: The fate of acetanilide in man. J. Pharmacol. Exp. Ther. 94: 29–38, 1948.
16. Brooks, J.: The oxidation of haemoglobin to methaemoglobin by oxygen. J. Physiol. (London) 107: 332–335, 1948.

17. Bucklin, R., and Myint, M. K.: Fatal methemoglobinemia due to well water nitrates. Ann. Intern. Med. 52: 703–705, 1960.
18. Cawein, M., Behlen, C. H., II, Lappat, E. J., and Cohn, J. E.: Hereditary diaphorase deficiency and methemoglobinemia. Arch. Intern. Med. (Chicago) 113: 578–585, 1964.
19. Chang, H., and Wu, S.: Congenital methemoglobinemia. Report of a case. Chin. Med. J. 72: 153–157, 1954.
20. Codounis, A.: A genetic study on the "hereditary methaemoglobinaemic cyanosis" (H. M. C.). Acta Genet. (Basel) 7: 131–140, 1957.
21. Cohen, G., and Hochstein, P.: Glutathione peroxidase: The primary agent for the elimination of hydrogen peroxide in erythrocytes. Biochemistry (Wash) 2: 1420–1428, 1963.
22. Coleman, R. D., and Heller, P.: Unpublished observations.
23. Cornblath, M., and Hartmann, A. F.: Methemoglobinemia in young infants. J. Pediat. 33: 421–425, 1948.
24. Darling, R. C., and Roughton, F. J. W.: Effect of methemoglobin on equilibrium between oxygen and hemoglobin. Amer. J. Physiol. 137: 56–68, 1942.
25. DePree, H. E., and Hickman, M. J.: Familial congenital methemoglobinemia: Report of a case and family study. Ann. Intern. Med. 51: 1078–1084, 1959.
26. Desforges, J. F.: Glutathione instability in normal blood. Blood 20: 186–195, 1962.
27. Dieckmann, W. J.: Methemoglobinemia. Arch. Intern. Med. (Chicago) 50: 574–578, 1932.
28. Dine, M. S.: Congenital methemoglobinemia in the newborn period. Amer. J. Dis. Child. 92: 15–19, 1956.
29. Ebaugh, F. G., Jr., Samuels, A. J., Dobrowolski, P., and Heisterkamp, D.: The site of the $CrO_4^=$—hemoglobin bond as determined by starch electrophoresis and chromatography. Fed. Proc. 20: 70, 1961.
30. Eder, H. A., Finch, C., and McKee, R. W.: Congenital methemoglobinemia. A clinical and biochemical study of a case. J. Clin. Invest. 28: 265–272, 1949.
31. Evelyn, K. A., and Malloy, H. T.: Microdetermination of oxyhemoglobin, methemoglobin, and sulfhemoglobin in a single sample of blood. J. Biol. Chem. 126: 655–662, 1938.
32. Finch, C. A.: Methemoblobinemia and sulfhemoglobinemia. New Eng. J. Med. 239: 470–478, 1948.
33. Gasul, B. M., Fell, E. H., Casas, R., and Pereiras, R.: Congenital methemoglobinemia simulating tricuspid atresia. J.A.M.A. 149: 258–260, 1952.
34. Gerald, P. S.: The electrophoretic and spectroscopic characterization of hgb M. Blood 13: 936–949, 1958.
35. Gerald, P. S.: The hereditary methemoglobinemias. In Stanbury, J. B., Wyngaarden, J. B., and Fredrickson, D. S. (Eds.): The Metabolic Basis of Inherited Disease. New York, McGraw-Hill Book Company, 1960, pp. 1068–1085.
36. Gerald, P. S., and Efron, M. L.: Chemical studies of several varieties of Hb M. Proc. Nat. Acad. Sci. U.S.A. 47: 1758–1767, 1961.
37. Gerald, P. S., and George, P.: Second spectroscopically abnormal methemoglobin associated with hereditary cyanosis. Science 129: 393–394, 1959.
38. Gibson, Q. H.: The reduction of methaemoglobin in red blood cells and studies on the cause of idiopathic methaemoglobinaemia. Biochem. J. 42: 13–23, 1948.
39. Gibson, Q. H.: Methaemoglobin and sulphaemoglobin. In Williams, R. T. (Ed.): The Chemical Pathology of Animal Pigments. Biochem. Soc. Sympos. No. 12. London and New York, Cambridge University Press, 1954, pp. 55–70.
40. Gibson, Q. H., and Harrison, D. C.: Familial idiopathic methaemoglobinaemia. Five cases in one family. Lancet 2: 941–943, 1947.
41. Gibson, R.: Familial idiopathic methaemoglobinaemia associated with oligophrenia. Amer. J. Ment. Defic. 61: 207–209, 1956.
42. Goluboff, N., and Wheaton, R.: Methylene blue induced cyanosis and acute hemolytic anemia complicating the treatment of methemoglobinemia. J. Pediat. 58: 86–89, 1961.
43. Graybiel, A., Lilienthal, J. L., Jr., and Riley, R. L.: The report of a case of idiopathic congenital (and probably familial) methemoglobinemia. Bull. Hopkins Hosp. 76: 155–162, 1945.
44. Greenberg, M., Birnkrant, W. B., and Schiftner, J. J.: Outbreak of sodium nitrite poisoning. Amer. J. Public Health 35: 1217–1220, 1945.
45. Harley, J. D., and Mauer, A. M.: Studies on the formation of Heinz bodies. II. The nature and significance of Heinz bodies. Blood 17: 418–433, 1961.
46. Harley, J. D., and Robin, H.: The effect of the nitrite ion on intact human erythrocytes. Blood 20: 710–721, 1962.
47. Harley, J. D., and Robin, H.: The effect of menadione on the reduction of methaemoglobin. Aust. J. Exp. Biol. Med. Sci. 40: 473–483, 1962.
48. Harley, J. D., and Robin, H.: Adaptive mechanisms in erythrocytes exposed to naphthoquinones. Aust. J. Exp. Biol. Med. Sci. 41: 281–292, 1963.
49. Harris, J. W.: The Red Cell. Production, Metabolism, Destruction: Normal and Abnormal. Cambridge, Harvard University Press, 1963, p. 229.

50. Heiniger, J. P., and Aebi, H.: Methämoglobinbildung durch Röntgen-Bestrahlung in Hämolysat und intakten Erythrocyten von verschiedenem Katalasegehalt. Helv. Chim. Acta 46: 255–268, 1963.
51. Heller, P., Weinstein, H. G., Yakulis, V. J., and Rosenthal, I. M.: Hemoglobin M$_{Kankakee}$, a new variant of hemoglobin M. Blood 20: 287–301, 1962.
51a. Heller, P., Coleman, R. D., Yakulis, V. J., and Josephson, A. M.: The molecular abnormality of hemoglobin M$_{Chicago}$. To be published.
52. Hill, A. S., Jr., Haut, A., Cartwright, G. E., and Wintrobe, M. M.: The role of nonhemoglobin proteins and reduced glutathione in the protection of hemoglobin from oxidation in vitro. J. Clin. Invest. 43: 17–26, 1964.
53. Hörlein, H., and Weber, G.: Über chronische familiäre Methämoglobinämie und eine neue Modifikation des Methämoglobins. Deutsch. Med. Wschr. 73: 476–478, 1948.
54. Holmquist, W. R., and Vinograd, J. R.: Reduction of human ferrihemoglobin A in the presence of cysteine and the effect of carbon monoxide. Biochim. Biophys. Acta 69: 337–354, 1963.
55. Huennekens, F. M., Caffrey, R. W., and Gabrio, B. W.: The electron transport sequence of methemoglobin reductase. Ann. N.Y. Acad. Sci. 75: 167–174, 1958.
56. Ingram, V. M.: The Hemoglobins in Genetics and Evolution. New York, Columbia University Press, 1963, pp. 16–36.
57. Itano, H. A., and Robinson, E.: Electrophoretic separation of intermediate compounds in two reactions of ferrihemoglobin. Biochim. Biophys. Acta 29: 545–555, 1958.
58. Jaffé, E. R.: The reduction of methemoglobin in human erythrocytes incubated with purine nucleosides. J. Clin. Invest. 38: 1555–1563, 1959.
59. Jaffé, E. R.: The reduction of methemoglobin in erythrocytes of a patient with congenital methemoglobinemia, subjects with erythrocyte glucose-6-phosphate dehydrogenase deficiency, and normal individuals. Blood 21: 561–572, 1963.
60. Jaffé, E. R.: Metabolic processes involved in the formation and reduction of methemoglobin in human erythrocytes. In Bishop, C., and Surgenor, D. M. (Eds.): Red Blood Cells. New York and London, Academic Press, 1964, pp. 397–422.
61. Jaffé, E. R., and Neumann, G.: A comparison of the effect of menadione, methylene blue and ascorbic acid on the reduction of methaemoglobin in vivo. Nature (London) 202: 607–608, 1964.
62. Jaffé, E. R., and Neumann, G.: DPNH-methemoglobin reductase activity and the reduction of methemoglobin in human erythrocytes. Fed. Proc. 23: 470, 1964.
63. Jaffé, E. R., Neumann, G., Rothberg, H., Wilson, F. T., and Webster, R. M.: Hereditary methemoglobinemia associated with severe mental retardation. Clin. Res. 12: 216, 1964.
64. Jandl, J. H., Engle, L. K., and Allen, D. W.: Oxidative hemolysis and precipitation of hemoglobin. I. Heinz body anemias as an acceleration of red cell aging. J. Clin. Invest. 39: 1818–1836, 1960.
65. Jones, R. T., Coleman, R. D., and Heller, P.: The chemical structure of Hgb M$_{Iwate}$ (M$_{Kankakee}$). Fed. Proc. 23: 173, 1964.
66. Josephson, A. M., Weinstein, H. G., Yakulis, V. J., Singer, L., and Heller, P.: A new variant of hemoglobin M disease: Hemoglobin M$_{Chicago}$. J. Lab. Clin. Med. 59: 918–925, 1962.
67. Jung, F.: Methämoglobinbildung und Blutkörperchenresistenz. Klin. Wschr. 19: 1016–1017, 1940.
68. Keilin, D.: Reactions of haemoproteins with hydrogen peroxide and the supposed formation of hydrogen peroxide during the autoxidation of haemoglobin. Nature (London) 191: 769–770, 1961.
69. Keilin, D., and Hartree, E. F.: Properties of catalase. Catalysis of coupled oxidation of alcohols. Biochem. J. 39: 293–301, 1945.
70. Kiese, M.: Die Reduktion des Hämiglobins. Biochem. Z. 316: 264–294, 1944.
71. Kiese, M., and Waller, H. -D.: Kinetik der Hämiglobinbildung: VII. Die Stoffwechselvorgänge in roten Zellen bei der Hämiglobinbildung durch den Kreisprocess Phenylhydroxylamin-Nitrosobenzol. Naunyn Schmiedeberg Arch. Exp. Path. 211: 345–361, 1950.
72. Kiese, M., Resag, K., and Schneider, Cl.: Reduktion von Nitrosobenzol durch Hämiglobinreduktase und durch altes gelbes Ferment. Naunyn Schmiedeberg Arch. Exp. Path. 231: 170–175, 1957.
73. Kiese, M., Schneider, Cl., and Waller, H. -D.: Hämiglobinreduktase. Naunyn Schmiedeberg Arch. Exp. Path. 231: 158–169, 1957.
74. King, E. J., White, J. C., and Gilchrist, M.: A case of idiopathic methaemoglobinaemia treated by ascorbic acid and methylene blue. J. Path. Bact. 59: 181–188, 1947.
75. Klebanoff, S. J.: An ergothioneine-dependent oxidation of reduced pyridine nucleotides by methemoglobin and metmyoglobin. Stimulation by thyroxine. Biochim. Biophys. Acta 64: 554–556, 1962.
76. Kleihauer, E., and Betke, K.: Elution procedure for the demonstration of methaemoglobin in red cells of human blood smears. Nature (London) 199: 1196–1197, 1963.
77. Kravitz, H., Elegant, L. D., Kaiser, E., and Kagan, B. M.: Methemoglobin values in premature and mature infants and children. Amer. J. Dis. Child. 91: 1–5, 1956.

78. Künzer, W., and Schneider, D.: Zur Aktivität der reduzierenden Fermentsysteme in den Erythrozyten junger Säuglinge. Acta Haemat. (Basel) 9: 346–353, 1953.
79. Künzer, W., Schütz, A., and Schütz, E.: Vergleichende Untersuchung der Spontanoxydation der Blutfarbstoffes in Nabelschnur- und Erwachsenen-erythrocyten nach Glykolysehemmung. Acta Haemat. (Basel) 16: 137–146, 1956.
80. Lachhein, L., Thal, W., and Harnack, O.: Methämoglobinämien durch Brunnenwasser bei Säuglingen. Deutsch. Geshundh. 15: 2291–2303, 1960.
81. Lamy, M., Frézal, J., Jammet, M. -L., and Josso, N.: La méthémoglobinémie congénitale récessive. Nouv. Rev. Franc. Hemat. 3: 105–120, 1963.
82. Lees, M. H., and Jolly, H.: Severe congenital methaemoglobinaemia in an infant. Lancet 2: 1147–1150, 1957.
83. Lemberg, R., and Legge, J. W.: Hematin Compounds and Bile Pigments. New York, Wiley (Interscience) 1949, pp. 218–222, 389–396, 515–532.
84. Lian, C., Frumusan, P., and Sassier, R.: Méthémoglobinémie congénitale et familiale. Action favorable de l'acide ascorbique. Bull. Soc. Med. Hop. Paris 55: 1194–1203, 1939.
85. Litarczek, G., Aubert, H., Cosmulesco, I., Comanesco, V., and Litarczek, S.: Sur un cas de cyanose auto-toxique par méthémoglobinémie intra-globulaire. Le Sang 4: 188–202, 1930.
86. Löhr, G. W., and Waller, H. D.: Biochemie und Pathogenese der enzymopenischen hämolytischen Anämien. Deutsch. Med. Wsch. 86: 27–29, 87–93, 1961.
87. McDonald, C. D., Jr., and Huisman, T. H. J.: A comparative study of enzymic activities in normal adult and cord blood erythrocytes as related to the reduction of methemoglobin. Clin. Chim. Acta 7: 555–559, 1962.
88. Mills, G. C.: The purification and properties of glutathione peroxidase of erythrocytes. J. Biol. Chem. 234: 502–506, 1959.
89. Miyaji, T., Ueda, S., Shibata, S., Tamura, A., and Sasaki, H.: Further studies on the fingerprint of Hb M_{Iwate}. Acta Haemat. Jap. 25: 169–175, 1962.
90. Muirhead, H., and Perutz, M. F.: Structure of haemoglobin. Nature (London) 199: 633–638, 1963.
91. Müller, J., Murawski, K., Szymanowska, Z., Koziorowski, A., and Radwan, L.: Hereditary deficiency of $NADPH_2$-methaemoglobin reductase. Acta Med. Scand. 173: 243–247, 1963.
92. Neill, J. M., and Hastings, A. B.: The influence of the tension of molecular oxygen upon certain oxidations of hemoglobin. J. Biol. Chem. 63: 479–492, 1925.
93. Pepper, G., Weinstein, H. G., and Heller, P.: Congenital methemoglobinemia in pregnancy. J.A.M.A. 177: 328–330, 1961.
93a. Perutz, M. F., and Mazarella, L.: A preliminary x-ray analysis of hemoglobin H. Nature (London) 199: 639, 1963.
94. Pisciotta, A. V., Ebbe, S. N., and Hinz, J. E.: Clinical and laboratory features of two variants of methemoglobin M disease. J. Lab. Clin. Med. 54: 73–87, 1959.
95. Ray, R. N., Chatterjea, J. B., and Ghosh, S. K.: Hereditary methaemoglobinaemia. J. Indian Med. Ass. 33: 165–168, 1959.
96. Ross, J. D.: Deficient activity of DPNH-dependent methemoglobin diaphorase in cord blood erythrocytes. Blood 21: 51–62, 1963.
97. Rostorfer, H. H., and Cormier, M. J.: The formation of "hydrogen peroxide" in the reaction of oxyhemoglobin with methemoglobin-forming agents. Arch. Biochem. 71: 235–249, 1957.
98. Rubinstein, D., Ottolenghi, P., and Denstedt, O. F.: The metabolism of the erythrocyte. XIII. Enzyme activity in the reticulocyte. Canad. J. Biochem. Physiol. 34: 222–235, 1956.
99. Sass-Kortsak, A., Thalme, B., and Ernster, L.: Haemolytic activity of vitamin K_3: Evidence for a direct effect on cellular enzymes. Nature (London) 193: 480–481, 1962.
99a. Schroeder, W. A.: The hemoglobins. Ann. Rev. Biochem. 32: 301–320, 1963.
100. Scott, E. M.: The relation of diaphorase of human erythrocytes to inheritance of methemoglobinemia. J. Clin. Invest. 39: 1176–1179, 1960.
101. Scott, E. M.: Personal communication.
102. Scott, E. M., and Hoskins, D. D.: Hereditary methemoglobinemia in Alaskan Eskimos and Indians. Blood 13: 795–802, 1958.
103. Scott, E. M., and McGraw, J. C.: Purification and properties of diphosphopyridine nucleotide diaphorase of human erythrocytes. J. Biol. Chem. 237: 249–252, 1962.
104. Scott, E. M., Lewis, M., Kaita, H., Chown, B., and Giblett, E. R.: The absence of close linkage of methemoglobinemia and blood group loci. Amer. J. Hum. Genet. 15: 493–494, 1963.
105. Shechter-Mani, A., Kende, G., and Ramot, B.: Hemoglobin M disease. Harefuah 62: 195–198, 1962.
106. Shibata, S., Miyaji, T., Iuchi, I., Ueda, S., Takeda, I., Kimura, N., and Kodama, S.: Hemoglobin M_{Kurume}: Its identify with hemoglobin $M_{Saskatoon}$. Acta Haemat. Jap. 25: 690–694, 1962.
107. Shibata, S., Tamura, A. Iuchi, I., and Takahashi, H.: Hemoglobin M_I: Demonstration of a new abnormal hemoglobin in hereditary nigremia. Acta Haemat. Jap. 23: 96–105, 1960.

108. Shrago, E., and Falcone, A. B.: Human-erythrocyte reduced triphosphopyridine nucleo-
     tide oxidase. Biochim. Biophys. Acta 67: 147–149, 1963.
109. Sievers, R. F., and Ryon, J. B.: Congenital idiopathic methemoglobinemia. Favorable
     response to ascorbic acid therapy. Arch. Intern. Med. (Chicago) 76: 299–307, 1945.
110. Singer, K.: Hereditary hemolytic disorders associated with abnormal hemoglobins.
     Amer. J. Med. 18: 633–652, 1955.
111. Smith, M. H.: Spectral properties of the M haemoglobins. *In* Lehmann, H., and Betke,
     K. (Eds.): Haemoglobin-Colloquium. Stuttgart, Georg Thieme, 1962, pp. 49–53.
112. Sparkes, R. S., and Browder, A.: Personal communication.
113. Spicer, S. S., Wooley, J. G., and Kessler, V.: Ergothioneine depletion in rabbit erythro-
     cytes and its effect on methemoglobin formation and reversion. Proc. Soc. Exp. Biol.
     Med. 77: 418–420, 1951.
114. Strömme, J. H.: Methaemoglobin formation induced by thiols. Biochem. Pharmacol.
     12: 937–948, 1963.
115. Strömme, J. H., and Eldjarn, L.: The role of the pentose phosphate pathway in the
     reduction of methaemoglobin in human erythrocytes. Biochem. J. 84: 406–410, 1962.
116. Szeinberg, A., and Marks, P. A.: Substances stimulating glucose catabolism by the oxida-
     tive reactions of the pentose phosphate pathway in human erythrocytes. J. Clin. Invest.
     40: 914–924, 1961.
117. Touster, O., and Yarbro, M. C.: The ergothioneine content of human erythrocytes; the
     effect of age, race, malignancy, and pregnancy. J. Lab. Clin. Med. 39: 720–724, 1952.
118. Townes, P. L., and Lovell, G. R.: Hereditary methemoglobinemia: A new varient ex-
     hibiting dominant inheritance of methemoglobin A. Blood 18: 18–33, 1961.
119. Townes, P. L., and Morrison, M.: Investigation of the defect in a variant of hereditary
     methemoglobinemia. Blood 19: 60–74, 1962.
120. Waisman, H. A., Bain, J. A., Richmond, J. B., and Munsey, F. A.: Laboratory and
     clinical studies in congential methemoglobinemia. Pediatrics 10: 293–305, 1952.
121. Waller, H. D., and Löhr, G. W.: Beitrag zur idiopathischen Methämoglobinämie.
     Folia Haemat. (Leipzig) 78: 588–599, 1961–1962.
122. Worster-Drought, C., White, J. C., and Sargent, F.: Familial idiopathic methaemo-
     globinaemia, associated with mental deficiency and neurological abnormalities. Brit.
     Med. J. 2: 114–118, 1953.

Erythropoietin

—ROBERT D. LANGE and VERA PAVLOVIC-KENTERA—

THE existence of a humoral regulatory mechanism for erythropoiesis, as postulated first by Carnot and Deflandre[34, 35] and later verified by Reissmann,[182] Erslev[54] and Stohlman et al.,[207] is now generally accepted. The humoral substance, erythropoietin, which stimulates the formation of red blood cells has been the subject of numerous editorials,[55, 146, 147] reviews,[3-5, 23, 27, 36a, 44, 46, 56, 92, 95, 102, 107, 111, 112, 124, 129, 145, 163, 175, 177, 188, 208] sections of books,[189, 209, 231] and finally entire books.[113, 141, 186] The proceedings of a conference on erythropoiesis[113] were published in 1962. This paper reviews progress in this field during the past two years. The report has been divided into the following sections:

1. Erythropoietin Assays.
2. Immuno-Studies on Erythropoietin.
3. Site of Erythropoietin Production.
4. Chemistry of Erythropoietin.
5. Site of Action of Erythropoietin.
6. Clinical Studies.
7. Metabolic, Neurohumoral and Kinetic Studies.
8. Miscellaneous Investigations.

1. Assays for Erythropoietin

Erythropoietin has not yet been purified and an immuno-assay is not available, thus bioassays remain the mainstay for indirectly detecting erythropoietin in the body fluids and tissue extracts, and for studying the rate of production and utilization of the hormone as well. The numerous methods used to assay erythropoietin have been reviewed several times.[91, 92, 120] Most investigators now use either mice or rats (although guinea pigs have been found to respond to erythropoietin[81]) and measure the reticulocytosis or incorporation of radioiron into the red blood cells of the recipient animals as the method for assay. Mice have the advantage of requiring a much smaller amount of test substances. The assay animals are prepared to make them more sensitive than normal animals to the injection of test substances. Plethora induced by transfusions, exposure to lowered barometric pressures or starvation, all reduce erythropoiesis by suppression of endogenous erythropoietin and increase the sensitivity of the animals. DeGowin, Hofstra and Gurney[42] have shown that the transfused plethoric mouse is sensitive to 0.05 cobalt unit* of erythropoietin. A starved rat would be sensitive to approximately 10–20 times the same amount of erythropoietin. It is of interest that mice

From the Division of Hematology of the Department of Medicine, Medical College of Georgia, Augusta, Georgia.

This report was supported in part by a PHS research grant #AM-07705-01 AI from the National Institute of Arthritis and Metabolic Diseases, Public Health Service.

* A cobalt unit is defined as the response of fasted rats to 5 μ moles of $CoCl_3$.

and rats may be transfused intraperitoneally; in rats the blood is absorbed from the peritoneal cavity in ten hours.[84]

An economical method for producing hypoxia-induced polycythemic mice has been developed by DeGowin, Hofstra and Gurney[43] based on a method originally suggested by Cotes and Bangham,[39] and B. M. Wright[233] has developed an economical chamber for maintaining low atmospheric pressure for long periods. DeGowin et al.[43] produced polycythemia by keeping mice at one half atmosphere for three weeks. Discontinuous hypoxia of mice at 0.4 atmosphere was found by Weintraub and Gordon[228] to be more efficacious. In our laboratory both the transfused plethoric mouse and the mouse made polycythemic by hypoxia have proven to be very sensitive assay animals. Table I gives the values for saline injected control mice and polycythemic mice receiving 0.25 unit of sheep plasma erythropoietin and compares the two types of polycythemia.

Other investigators have utilized the incorporation of radioiron into heme[190] in the spleens of polycythemic animals injected with erythropoietin as a measure of erythropoietic activity. The Fe^{59} incorporation was found to be maximal in the spleen at 8 hrs. and in the red blood cells at 48 hrs.

The idea of utilizing an in vitro model for erythropoietin assay occurred quite early in the last decade. Although the morphological studies by Matoth,[148] Friederici,[75] Bernadelli[19, 20] and Rosse and Gurney[191] revealed an enhancing effect of anemic sera and concentrated erythropoietin on bone marrow cells in vitro, the methods were not commonly used. Matoth and his co-workers have introduced an improved method of rabbit and human bone marrow cultures in homologous plasma clots for the study of the effect of erythropoietin.[148] Colchicine was added to arrest mitosis and the number of mitoses at metaphase was counted at the end of a given period of incubation. This was used as an index of the number of cells which had entered mitosis during the incubation period. Erythroblasts exposed to erythropoietin in vivo or in vitro showed high mitotic rates when subsequently cultured in an erythropoietin poor medium.

The early in vitro methods utilizing Fe^{59} or C^{14} incorporation were very discouraging. Thus, Thomas et al.,[218] Alpen et al.,[1] and Erslev and Hughes[57] utilizing isotopic incorporation in vitro were unable to demonstrate any difference between bone marrow incubated with normal or anemic serum. In spite of the fact that Schroeder[202] had demonstrated a difference, the general impression remained that erythropoietin did not have an effect in vitro.

Powsner and Berman,[176] and Erslev[58] and Korst[126] have all reported that erythropoietin has a demonstrable effect on the metabolic functions of bone

TABLE I.—*Polycythemic Mouse Assay*

	Saline	0.25 u. Erythropoietin
Transfusion	0.23 ± 0.02 (21)	3.84 ± 0.97 (18)
Hypoxic	0.25 ± 0.02 (38)	3.73 ± 0.52 (20)

Values represent 48 hr. percentage of erythrocyte iron incorporation ± standard error of the mean. Number in parentheses is the number of animals. Each animal received 1 ml. of saline or 1 ml. of saline containing 0.25 unit of erythropoietin.

marrow in suspension culture. Recently Krantz, Gallien-Lartigue and Gold-wasser[128] have developed a rat bone marrow suspension culture in vitro and measured the amount of radioiron incorporated into heme. Their study demonstrated that the cells responded to added erythropoietin with a marked increase in heme synthesis and a definite dose-response relationship. Bone marrow cells from fasted rats were found to be more sensitive to added erythropoietin than were cells from normal rats. The increase in the C^{14} glycine incorporation caused by purified sheep plasma erythropoietin in human bone marrow suspension culture demonstrated by Powsner and Berman[176] was less pronounced but quite definite. When an ethanol extract of erythropoietically active urine was added in vitro, negative results were obtained and the authors postulated the existence of an inhibitory substance.

In our laboratory rabbit bone marrow suspension cultures have been used and the radioiron incorporation has been measured. The increase in Fe^{59} due to added sheep plasma erythropoietin was 22 to 142 per cent with a mean value of 70 per cent, compared to control samples without added erythropoietin. Approximately 50 per cent of the iron was incorporated into heme. Bone marrow from polycythemic animals was found to be the most sensitive, paralleling in vivo experience; the marrow of such animals offers a promising system for the study of erythropoietin effect in vitro. The same system was used to study urinary erythropoietin. Crude urinary extracts not only failed to cause an increase in Fe^{59} incorporation, but just as in Powsner's experience, some extracts inhibited the activity of the marrow. However, when the extracts were partially purified by column chromatography, an enhancing effect on Fe^{59} incorporation was evident.

Although erythropoietin stimulates heme synthesis in vitro, Dukes and Goldwasser[51] found no stimulating effect of 15 units of erythropoietin on the incorporation of labeled formate into nucleic acid bases in vitro.

2. *Immuno-Studies on Erythropoietin*

Erythropoietin has been characterized as a poor antigen.[89, 114, 143] However, recently antibodies to erythropoietin have been produced in two laboratories. Schooley and Garcia first described an antiserum to erythropoietically active human urinary concentrate.[199] The antisera neutralized the antigen in vivo and a significant depression in erythropoiesis was observed in normal mice after the injection of antisera. The production of antisera to concentrated sheep plasma erythropoietin has recently been reported from this laboratory;[135] in addition, antisera to human urinary material have been produced. These antisera have been found to inhibit the erythropoietin-induced in vitro incorporation of iron in rabbit bone marrow suspension cultures.[171] Garcia and Schooley have extended their work to show that the neutralizing antibodies cross reacted with erythropoietin produced in mice, rats, rabbits and sheep.[82] Their studies suggest that the erythropoietins of the various animal species studied are similar. Injections of normal mice with antisera resulted in a daily progressive decrease in the number of erythroid cells in the bone marrow and a decrease in radioiron incorporation.[200] Injections of the antisera into polycythemic mice 24 to 44 hours after initiating a wave of erythropoiesis had no effect on the erythropoietic response, although injections of antisera at the same time that exogenous erythropoietin was administered completely abolished the erythropoietic response.

The immunological studies hold great promise for the future. The use of these antisera may give rise to a long awaited immuno-assay and information regarding the cellular site of production of erythropoietin.

3. *Site of Production of Erythropoietin*

In 1957 Jacobson et al. postulated, on the basis of their extirpation experiments, that erythropoietin was either produced or activated in the kidney.[115] Experimental evidence from other laboratories has provided support for the belief that the kidney is responsible for the elaboration of erythropoietin. In 1962 Naets[160] published the results of experiments which showed that the kidney in dogs was the sole source of erythropoietin. The erythropoietic response of starved nephrectomized rats to sheep plasma erythropoietin and cobalt was studied by Sanzari and Fisher who demonstrated that nephrectomy reduced the response to cobalt but did not modify the response to erythropoietin.[197]

Other investigators, while confirming the importance of the kidney, have demonstrated that the kidney is not the sole source of erythropoietin in all species.[77, 192] Fischer and Friederici[65] examined the bone marrows of bilaterally nephrectomized rabbits daily for a period of ten days after the operation and found no significant difference in the percentage of erythroid cells of those rabbits as compared to unoperated control rabbits. In contrast to the experience in dogs, the production of erythroblasts increased after phlebotomy. Erythroid precursors remain plentiful in the bone marrow of human patients who have undergone bilateral nephrectomy.[165] Rosse and Waldmann, in an impressive series of experiments,[192, 221] used parabiotic rats in which one parabiont was either nephrectomized or underwent ureteral ligation; erythropoiesis was stimulated by hypoxia and radioiron incorporation into the red blood cells was measured (Figure 1). The radioiron incorporation was found to be less in pairs in which the nephrectomized partner was hypoxic than in pairs in which either the unoperated or ureter-ligated partner was hypoxic (Figure 2). These results suggested that the kidney was important in the stimulation of erythropoiesis in response to hypoxia. However, the radioiron incorporation was greater in pairs in which the nephrectomized partner was hypoxic than in those pairs in which one partner was nephrectomized, but neither was hypoxic. Tissues other than the kidney seemed to contribute to the erythropoietic response to hypoxia. From all of these observations it can be concluded that species differences exist regarding the production of erythropoietin; in some species other tissues in addition to the kidney can produce erythropoietin. These other sites have not yet been clearly delineated although Rambach, et al. found erythropoietic stimulating substances in extracts of many tissues.[180]

While extirpation experiments have indirectly linked the kidney to erythropoietin production, perfusion studies have provided further evidence for a renal source of erythropoietin. Kuratowska and her associates perfused isolated rabbit kidneys with anoxic blood and Tyrode's solution; the perfusate

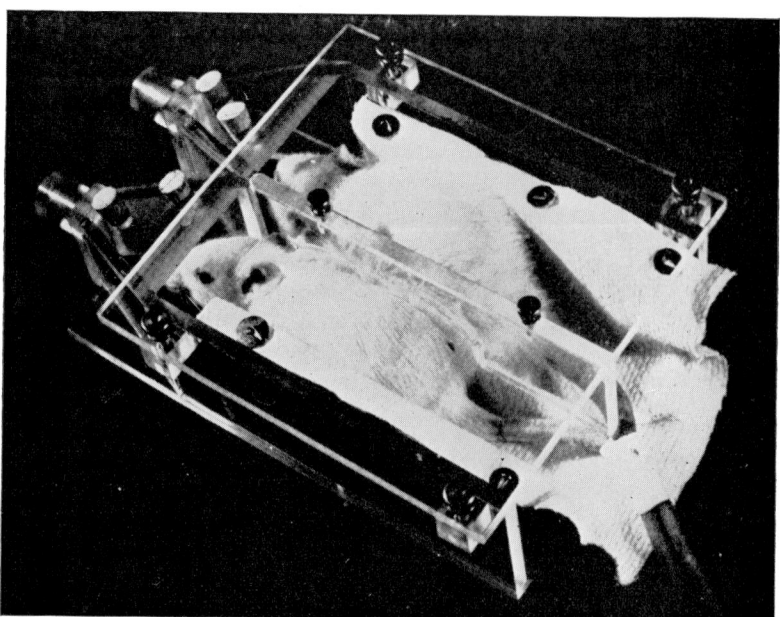

Fig. 1.—Parabiotic rats placed in a divided chamber. (Reprinted by permission of Rosse, et al. Blood 19: 75–81, 1962.)

contained erythropoietic activity.[130, 131] Nakao has reported an increase in erythropoietin in rabbit kidney perfusates when the blood flow was impaired.[164] Reissmann and Nomura demonstrated that perfusion of isolated rabbit kidneys by fully oxygenated blood did not influence erythropoietin production, while perfusion with extremely hypoxic blood caused the production of erythropoietin.[183] Using cobalt as a stimulus, Fisher, et al. found erythropoietic stimulating activity in the perfusate from dog kidneys in situ.[66] The isolated dog kidney was also used by Zangheri and his co-workers; they perfused the kidneys with anoxic blood and found significant erythropoietic stimulating activity in the perfusate.[235] When anemic, but fully oxygenated blood was used for perfusion no erythropoietic stimulating effect was found. Kentera, Hall and Lange used venous blood to perfuse dog kidneys in situ.[171a] The unilateral perfusion was carried out at normal flow rates and the dogs were artificially ventilated to maintain constant oxygen saturation. Increased erythropoietin levels were found in the renal vein blood of the perfused kidney when the perfusion was continued for periods of more than three hours. Similar results with perfusion of isolated calf kidneys have also been reported by Warter, Mantz, and Hammann.[226]

Although the kidney is considered to be the main source of erythropoietin, the cellular site of production is not known. The renal cortex,[206] the renal medulla,[183] both the cortex and medulla,[157] the kidney tubules[67] or renal vasculature[132] have been implicated as a specific site of production of erythropoietin or perhaps as responding to a messenger substance from another site such as the juxtaglomerular cells. The juxtaglomerular cells were first suggested as a site of erythropoietin production by Osnes in 1960.[170] This view has

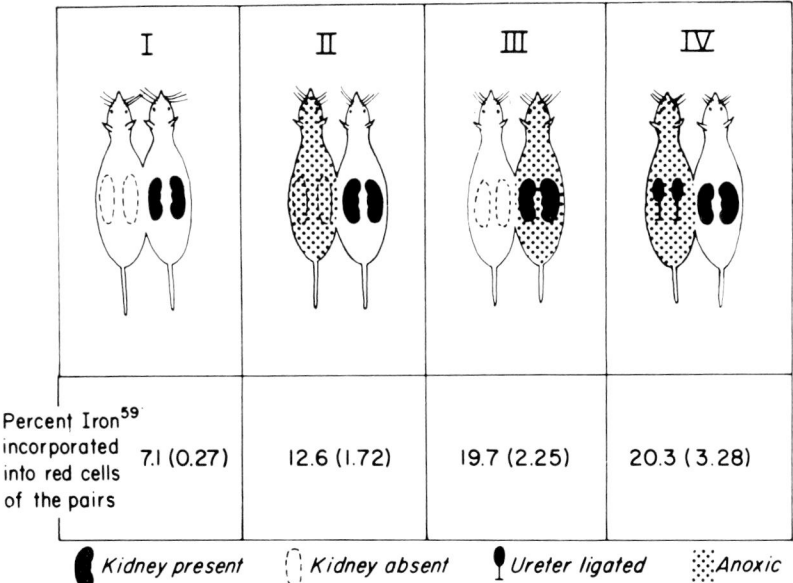

FIG. 2.—Studies on the effect of nephrectomy or ureter ligation on the erythropoietic response to anoxia in parabiotic rats. The standard error of the mean is shown in parenthesis. (Reprinted by permission of Waldmann, et al. *Erythropoiesis*, Grune & Stratton, 1962.)

been championed by Takaku, Hirashima[106, 216] and Nakao[164]; they used rats in which a Goldblatt kidney had been produced. The parallel association of erythropoietin production and granularity of the juxtaglomerular cells led these workers to suggest that the juxtaglomerular cells may secrete erythropoietin. In human cirrhotic and non-cirrhotic patients Reeves, et al. found that hemoglobin values and the juxtaglomerular cell counts correlated only in the non-cirrhotic patients with recent hemorrhage.[181] They suggested that the hypervolemia of cirrhotic patients inhibited erythropoietin production.

However, contradictory results have been obtained by other investigators. Neither Mitus[156] nor Cooper and Nocenti[38] were able to increase erythropoietin production by clamping the renal artery of experimental animals. Goldfarb and Tobian have also investigated juxtaglomerular granularity under different physiological conditions and were unable to record any differences between normal, hypoxic or hyperoxic animals.[86, 88] The same authors measured the erythropoietic activity of saline extracts of kidneys with varying degrees of juxtaglomerular granularity. Their results did not conclusively prove nor disprove that the juxtaglomerular apparatus secretes erythropoietin.[87]

Many other investigators have studied the erythropoietic activity of tissue extracts. The results, while interesting, have been somewhat contradictory as have so many studies in the field of erythropoietin. Thus, normal and anemic kidney extracts have been found to exert an erythropoietic effect,[83, 155, 161, 174, 236] while as previously mentioned, Rambach, Alt and Cooper[180] found activity in the homogenates of many tissues. Further experiments are obviously needed to bring some uniformity to the methods of extraction and assay in order to obtain meaningful results.

4. Chemistry of Erythropoietin

Erythropoietin has not been crystallized. As a consequence any discussion of chemistry is somewhat premature. Berry, Rambach and Alt[21] performed DEAE cellulose column chromatography on plasma filtrates from normal rabbits and on filtrates obtained from rabbits stimulated by bleeding, hypoxia, treatment with phenylhydrazine or cobalt; all of the effluent diagrams were found to be of similar shape. They suggested that erythropoietin may be either a small glycoprotein or may be carried by a glycoprotein. The concept that erythropoietin may exist in a free and bound form has been proposed by other investigators.[89]

Evidence for the presence of at least two humoral erythropoietic factors has been presented by Linman.[142] He found a thermolabile factor that was erythropoietically inactive orally and a thermostable factor which was active orally. This investigator originally suggested that batyl alcohol had some erythropoiesis stimulating properties.[140] However, Bassi and Dunjic[17] have shown that neither batyl nor salachyl alcohol given during the first three days following irradiation changes the effect of radiation, nor do they modify the evolution of erythropoietic activity between the third through the twelfth day after exposure to x-ray.

Khalifa and Keller have described another method of alcohol fractionation and purification of erythropoietin.[123] In column chromatography, Lowy and Keighley found that the recovery of erythropoietin was enhanced when they used 0.1% phenol in all equilibrations and in the elution buffers.[144] Rosse and his co-workers by x-ray defraction have estimated the molecular weight of a crude urinary erythropoietin to be approximately 28,000.[194] Studies of erythropoietically active material from extracts obtained from renal tumors and cerebellar hemangioblastomas suggested that the biologically active molecule from those sources was nearly the same weight. Other investigators have found molecular weights of 40,000[230] and 10,000[179] for erythropoietin; it is entirely possible, however, that carrier proteins are being measured and that active erythropoietin may be a relatively small polypeptide. Erythropoietin has been characterized as being non-dialyzable, but other evidence has shown that under certain circumstances erythropoietically active material can be dialyzed.[139, 174, 220]

A description of active erythropoietic stimulating material has been published by Goldwasser, White and Taylor.[90] They used ion exchange chromatography, ammonium sulfate precipitation and batch gel adsorption in their method of partial purification. The most active fraction obtained had an activity of 450 units/mg. protein and represented a purification of about 64,000-fold. This fraction was found to have an adsorption maximum of 270 mμ with A $_{280 \, m\mu}^{1\%, 1cm}$ of 10.0. The protein content was 80.8 per cent as measured by Lowry method and 68.1 per cent by the Westly method. Carbohydrates made up 29.2 per cent of the material; the hexosamine and sialic acid contents were 17.5 and 13 per cent, respectively. These chemical characteristics are those of a glycoprotein.

5. *Mode of Action of Erythropoietin*

Rats and mice have been given exogenous erythropoietin for periods of from 40 to over 200 days by Keighley, Hammond and Lowy.[122] Increased erythropoiesis persisted as long as erythropoietin was given; when the injections were stopped, erythropoiesis returned to pretreatment level.

Impressive evidence from a number of laboratories has shown that erythropoietin exerts an influence at the stem cell level to initiate changes causing the differentiation of these cells into erythrocytic elements.[2, 59, 63, 134, 210] More recent studies that have supported this belief include Schooley and Garcia's results[200] from injection of antiserum to erythropoietin into polycythemic mice which had been pretreated with erythropoietin. Bernardelli, using an in vitro hanging drop culture[19] and Matoth using a plasma clot,[148] have interpreted their results as showing a stem cell effect. Kinetic studies by Kurtides, et al., using tritiated thymidine, showed that erythropoietin administration led to increased mitotic activity in the stem cell compartment.[133] In addition, Gurney, Lajtha and Oliver[97] have presented results which support the former evidence that erythropoietin does not shorten the intermitotic time and infer, therefore, a stem cell action.

Although erythropoietin exerts an effect on stem cells, this is not the only action since erythropoietin has further effects on erythroid proliferation, maturation and release of cells from the bone marrow. In this regard, Linman[142] has again postulated the existence of two erythropoietins, one affecting the rate of erythrocyte differentation and the other said to determine the number of mitoses which erythrocyte precursors undergo during maturation. The thermostable factor he isolated led to the production of microcytes. These observations have not been confirmed. Brecher, Stohlman, and Moores have found that defective, short-lived macrocytes were produced in rats in response to severe anemia caused by bleeding or severe iron deficiency.[28, 158, 211] Strzhizhovskii also has noted an increase in mean cell size after hemorrhage, but, in addition, he has noted a diminished hemoglobin content.[214]

More direct evidence for other actions of erythropoietin has been obtained by Gordon and his co-workers in rats[93] and by Fisher, et al. in dogs.[70] Both of these groups found that purified sheep plasma erythropoietin effected a prompt release of reticulocytes from the marrow of isolated perfused femurs. Similar results were obtained in intact starved rats[76] by Fruhman and Fischer, who concluded that erythropoietin has some action on nucleated erythrocytes in the bone marrow well beyond the stem cell stage. Further evidence for this effect was presented by Gallagher and Lange.[78] When polycythemia in rats was sustained for two or more weeks, increases in red blood cell radioiron incorporation and reticulocytosis resulting from stimulation by erythropoietin did not occur until at least 24 hours had elapsed following injection (Figure 3 ✕3). In rats that were polycythemic for only one day prior to the injection of erythropoietin, an increase in reticulocytes and iron incorporation was seen within the first 24 hours (Figure 3 ✕4). In extention of these studies[79] control

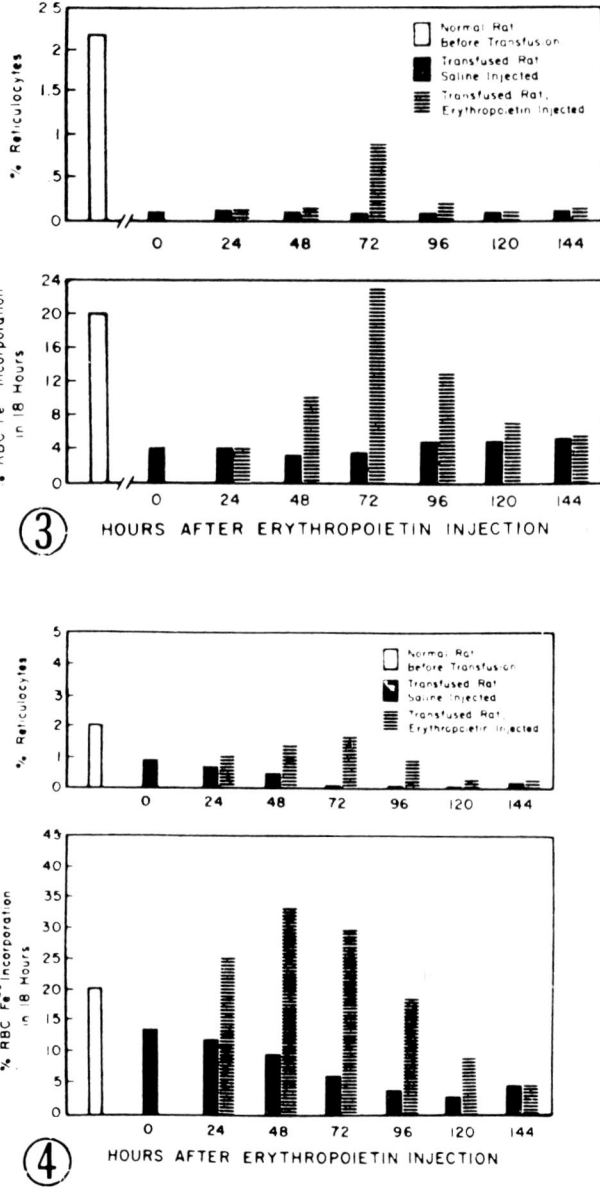

Fig. 3. No. 3.—Response of polycythemic rats to human urinary erythropoietin. These rats were transfused once weekly and the polycythemic state was maintained for thirty days prior to injection of 2 ml. of urine concentrate on the 31st day.

No. 4.—Response of polycythemic rats to human urinary erythropoietin. These rats were given a single transfusion and on the following day 2 ml. of urine concentrate were injected. (Reprinted by permission of Gallagher, et al., Proc. Soc. Exp. Biol. Med. 110: 422, 1962.)

hypertransfused rats injected with saline, and test animals injected with erythropoietin were bled for a determination of reticulocyte counts and radio-iron incorporation at 24, 48, 72, 96, 120, and 144 hours after erythropoietin injection. Several rats in each group were given a second injection of erythropoietin 24 hours prior to bleeding. Response to a single injection began after 24 hours and was maximal between 72 and 96 hours. Second injections at increasing intervals after the first caused a prompt additive effect during each 24 hour interval. It was concluded that erythropoietin influences erythropoiesis by more than one mechanism. Bruce and McCulloch, studying the effect of erythropoietin on the hematopoietic colony forming cells in mice, concluded that the primitive erythroid precursor that is sensitive to erythropoietin is not the colony forming cell.[31]

6. *Clinical Studies*

The plasma and urine erythropoietin titers from patients with diverse types of anemia have been measured. In general, elevated levels have been found in post-hemorrhagic, vitamin deficiency, hemolytic and refractory anemias.[24, 25, 74, 84, 109, 110, 118, 162, 167, 203] Three observers have found low erythropoietin titers in iron deficiency anemia; titers then rose after iron therapy.[109, 110, 203] Naets[162] found increased erythropoietin levels in 47 per cent of anemic patients with normal renal function; in 39 anemic uremic patients, elevated erythropoietin levels were found in only a single case. Similar results were reported by Dolder,[48] who found that the serum of 2 of 7 patients with renal disease, when incubated with erythropoietically active serum, decreased the activity of the latter serum. However, other investigators found a slight increase in erythropoietin in approximately one-half of the patients with chronic renal disease.[24, 25, 74, 109]

The recent investigations of Halvorsen are most fascinating. In his first study, in collaboration with Finne,[100] he reported that high levels of erythropoietin were found in the amniotic fluid of mothers of severely anemic infants. Since the anemia was caused by Rh immunization, it was suggested that an estimation of erythropoietin levels in the amniotic fluid might aid in the prenatal diagnosis of erythroblastosis. In another study, slightly elevated erythropoietin levels were found at birth in the cord plasma obtained from non-hypoxic infants who were not anemic; high erythropoietin levels were found in infants with severe anemia or hypoxia. During the first few weeks of life the erythropoietin levels in the non-hypoxic, non-anemic infants decreased to normal levels. The author concluded that the erythropoietin regulating mechanism was present during the last part of intrauterine life and in the neonatal period.

The association of erythrocytosis and erythropoietin levels has been frequently studied. There is still no agreement regarding the role of erythropoietin in the production of the erythrocytosis of polycythemia vera. Normal erythropoietin levels in seven cases of polycythemia vera were obtained by Noyes and his co-workers.[167] They found elevated levels in hypoxic polycythemia only if the patient had been phlebotomized in the previous six weeks. Van Dyke[220a] also found this to be true, but contradictory results have been reported. Moderate increases in erythropoietin levels were obtained in 4 of 8 cases of polycythemia vera studied by Boivin et al.,[24] and Gráf[94] reported that the serum of 10 patients with polycythemia caused a reticulocyte response in his assay animals. Increased levels of erythropoietin were found by Freedman and Penington[72] in 7 of 8 patients with pulmonary insufficiency and Strausz[212] has reported elevated plasma erythropoietin levels in 28 of 30 patients with right sided congenital cardiac defects.

The relationship of the kidney and erythrocytosis has been pointed out once more by Donati, Lange and Gallagher[50] who reported seven patients with nephrogenic erythrocytosis. The plasma erythropoietin level of four patients was increased and the erythropoietin content of the cyst fluid in a fifth patient was elevated. The results of erythropoietin assay of the cyst fluid of nine patients with renal cystic disease have been reported by Rosse et al.[193] In three of the six patients with polycythemia, the erythropoietin level was elevated. Erythropoietic stimulating activity was also found in the cyst fluid of patients with normal hemoglobin and hematocrit levels. Erythrocytosis has been described in a case of hydronephrosis[116] and one case of nephrosis,[52] but erythropoietin levels were not reported. The erythrocytosis in the former case was relieved by decompression and cured by nephrectomy.

The association of erythrocythemia and malignancies has been reviewed by Donati et al.[49] Tables II and III are taken from his article. Table II lists

TABLE II.—*Cases with Assay for Erythropoietic Activity*†

	Hb	Hema-tocrit	RBC	Red Cell Mass	WBC	Platelets	Remis-sion	Erythropoietic Activity	
								Plasma	Tumor Extract
	g/100 ml.	%	10⁶/mm³	ml/kg	/mm³	/mm³	Months		
Renal carcinoma									
*Barnard (15)	(33%)	65	6.6		5,000	120,000	12	—	
Gurney (98)	20.8	68	7.5				2	—	+
*Hewlett, et al. (105)	20.0	62	6.0	51	7,900	400,000	6		+
Korst, et al. (125)								+(Preop)	+
								−(Postop)	
*Conley, et al. (37)	21.5	70.8	8.64		9,200	280,000	None	—	
Donati, et al. (50)									
I.	20.7	70			8,700	184,000		+	
II.	19.4	64			8,250	240,000		+	
III.	23.0	60			8,200	138,000		+	
Cerebellar hemangioblas-toma									
Brody & Rodriguez (29)	20.0	69			5,100	210,000	None	—	
Waldmann, et al. (224)	17.3	58	6.1	44	7,500	254,000		−‡	+§
Pheochromocytoma									
*Bradley, et al. (26)	21.0	65	8.3	40	8,000	745,000	12	+	+
Hepatocellular carcinoma									
Kan, et al. (119)									
Pt. 12	14.4	50		46.1				—	
Pt. 13	16.2	56		46.5				—	
Pt. 16	20.7	69		75.0				—	
Pt. 17	21.3	70		70.5					

* Cases also recorded in Table 3.

† Adapted from Donati, et al, Ann. Int. Med., 58: 47, 1963.

‡ Urine and cerebrospinal fluid also not erythropoietically active.

§ Tumor cyst fluid.

TABLE III.—*Cases With Apparent Relationship Between Tumor and Erythrocythemia*†

	Hb*	Hematocrit	RBC	Red Cell Mass	WBC	Platelets	Remission
	g/100 ml	%	10⁶/mm³	ml/kg	/mm³	/mm³	months
Uterine myomata							
Thomson & Marson (219)	(148%)	72	7.77	111	6700	161,000	22
Horwitz & McKelway (108)	(141%)		10.4		12,000		96
Engel & Singer (53)	21.4	61	6.8	52	7000	300,000	6
Fleming & Markley (70a)	19.1	64	7.5	Inc.	9850	230,000	15
Babuna, et al. (12)	20.2	62	6.17		6400		7
Zilliacus (237)	17.1		5.3		13,100	275,000	24
Laurin, et al. (136)	19.5	78	8.1	Inc.			26
Menzies (153)	20		6.5		Normal		25
Cerebellar hemangioblastoma							
Woolsey (232)	21.1	69	7.89		6850	645,000	22
Ward, et al. (225)	19.4	63	7.95	Inc.	13,900	272,000	12
Schmid & French (201)	21.0	65	6.6		8600	200,000	36
Carpenter, et al. (33)	23	68	7.13	73.2	6600		13
	20		6.5		9150	295,000	7
Stroebel & Fowler (213)	21.5	76	7.28	89	4800		22
Renal carcinoma							
Ways (227)	21.5	69	8.6		6050	Normal	12
Frey (73)	22.2	63	6.5	63	4600		20
Omland (169)	(135%)		7.3		7100		108
DeWeerd & Hagedorn (47)	20.7	66	6.63		7400		24
	19.4	71	8.32	64	6400	174,000	66
	19.8	71	6.86	81	6000	235,000	20
	21.3	70	6.27	76	7300	108,000	9
Damon, et al. (41)	20		8.2		9050	202,000	132
‡Barnard (15)	(133%)	65	6.6		5000	120,000	12
Messmer (154)	22.9	69		51	17,000	170,000	12
Conley, et al. (37)	19.6	68	7.03		13,000	280,000	12
Campbell, et al. (32)	23	76	7.7			750,000	
Forssell (71)			8.3		Normal	673,000	14
‡Hewlett, et al. (105)	20	62	6.0	51	7900	400,000	6
Renal adenoma							
DeMarsh & Warmington (45)	20.5	72	9.2		6500		36
Pheochromocytoma							
‡Bradley, et al. (26)	21	65	8.3	40		745,000	12

* Percent as indicated.

† Adapted from Donati, et al. Ann. Int. Med., 58: 47, 1963.

‡ With erythropoietin assay see Table 2.

cases in which an assay for erythropoietin has been carried out; Table III records the cases with an apparent relationship between the tumors and erythrocythemia. The criteria for selection were: (1) a histologic diagnosis; (2) remission for 6 months or more following surgical or radiologic extirpation of the tumor without use of myelosuppressive therapy; and (3) absence of the characteristics of polycythemia vera. Since hepatic carcinoma cannot be definitively excised, these criteria could not be applied to those reports; thus, they are not included in the table. Among the tumors with erythrocythemia recently reported have been two cases with uterine myomas but no erythropoietin assays were made.[36, 166] Both patients responded to the removal of the tumor. Waldmann and Bradley found elevated erythropoietin levels in the serum of a patient with pheochromocytoma and polycythemia.[223] Saline extracts of the tumor tissue stimulated erythropoiesis in the assay animals.

Absolute polycythemia has been described in approximately 10 per cent of 145 cases of hepatic carcinoma reported by Kan and his co-workers.[119] Lehman et al.[138] added another case; however, no erythropoietic activity was found in the patients' serum or hepatic tumor. Other instances have been described by other authors.[18, 60, 117, 198] Polycythemia is found in 9 to 20 per cent of cases of cerebellar hemangioblastoma; at least 40 cases have been described. In one patient reported by Waldmann, Levin and Baldwin[224] fluid aspirated from the cystic cerebellar tumor was shown to contain erythropoietic stimulating activity. Increased activity was not detected in the patients' urine, plasma or spinal fluid. The authors suggested that the patient's polycythemia may have been caused by increased marrow erythroid activity in response to an erythropoietic stimulating factor produced by the tumor.

7. Metabolic, Neurohumoral and Kinetic Studies

Many other substances have been found to have an effect on erythropoiesis. The glycoprotein apoceruloplasmin has an erythropoietic stimulating activity[103, 234] not found in the copper containing ceruloplasmin.[204]

Endocrine preparations have been extensively studied. Fisher[68] has found that adrenalectomy decreases the response to erythropoietin, but such animals have a reduced rate of inactivation of erythropoietin. Together with Crook,[69] he found that many pituitary, thyroid and adrenal hormones induced a moderate to marked erythropoietic stimulation in hypophysectomized rats. They also found that angiotensin, indirectly a product of the juxtaglomerular cells, had erythropoietic stimulating ability. However, Bilsel and his co-workers were unable to confirm this observation.[22] Waldmann, Weissman and Levin[222] administered 7.5 gms. of thyroid to dogs over a long period and found a consistant elevation in the peripheral hematocrit and rate of red cell synthesis. The elevated parameters returned to normal when the treatment was discontinued. Extirpation studies by Shirakura[205] showed a reduction in erythropoiesis after adrenalectomy, thyroidectomy and gonadectomy; however, the animals were still able to be stimulated by bleeding or cobalt injections. He also observed that ACTH stimulated erythropoiesis in hypophysectomized-adrenalectomized rats. However, bilaterally nephrectomized animals were unable to respond to corticotropin whereas animals with ureteral ligation responded to this stimulus. Most observers think that the endocrine effects exerted on the hematopoietic organs are secondary to their influence on metabolic reactions.

Piliero, Medici and Orr measured erythrocytic parameters in rats having meticulously placed tissue defects in the hypothalamus.[173] No significant change occurred following bilateral lesions in the anterior, middle or posterior hypothalamic regions, although these animals still demonstrated an erythropoietic response to lowered barometric pressure. Baciu,[14] using a technique which permitted separation of the circulation of the head and trunk of dogs followed by compression of the carotid arteries, concluded that hypoxia acts through the central nervous system by means of two mechanisms. One mechanism was thought to be reflex in origin and to be triggered in the sinocarotid chemoreceptors; the other was thought to be neurohumoral and associated with the production of erythropoietin. The effect of bilateral section of the splanchnic nerves on erythropoietin production in rats was reported by Takaku, et al.[217] After section, the elevation of erythropoietin levels following hemorrhage was markedly inhibited presumably because of a reduction in renal blood flow.

Sanchez-Medal found in dogs that recovery from post hemorrhagic anemia was quicker if products of hemolysis were injected.[196] That observation was of interest since Brown and his fellow workers have shown that lysed mammalian red blood cells have erythropoietic stimulating activity.[30] This property was found to reside in the heme portion of the cell, particularly in compounds containing the 4 pyrrole ring configuration. Somewhat contradictory findings were obtained by Hellens, et al.;[104] they subjected intact and partially hemolyzed cells to a low atmospheric pressure and found that an active erythropoietic stimulating agent was lost from the blood during hemolysis.

Several investigations relating to hypoxia were carried out during the past two years. Grant and Smith[96] compared histologic appearance with oxygen content of 29 sternal marrow aspirates in patients with normal, hypoplastic and hyperplastic bone marrows. The studies confirmed the fact that bone marrow is not stimulated to greater activity by marrow anoxia and that the increased metabolic requirements of a stimulated marrow can be met by increased arterial perfusion. In pulmonary insufficiency, a nearly normal marrow oxygen tension was found despite arterial anoxia. Naets[159] observed that both hypophysectomy and starvation reduced the marrow response to hypoxia; the diminished response was not as striking when cobalt was used as a stimulant. The effect of hypocapnia and hypoxia in the production of erythropoietin was studied by Bartlett and Phillips[16] who found that the addition of CO_2 to a hypoxic atmosphere prevented the erythropoietic effect of hypoxia. In a most interesting study, Rosse, Waldmann and Hull[195] investigated the factors stimulating erythropoiesis in frogs. Sublethal levels of hypoxia and cobalt did not stimulate erythropoiesis in frogs as measured by the incorporation of thymidine-2-C^{14} into peripheral erythrocytes. Bleeding of approximately one third of the blood volume increased erythropoiesis 70-fold, and the serum of bled animals increased thymidine uptake in recipient frogs, but not in polycythemic mice. Conversely, serum of an anemic patient, which contained large amounts of erythropoietin, as measured in polycythemic mice, did not stimulate erythropoiesis in the frog. It must be concluded that erythropoiesis in the frog is regulated by a different mechanism than in mammals.

Several workers have continued studies of the kinetics of erythropoietin production and inactivation. Prentice and Mirand produced anemia in rabbits by bleeding and phenylhydrazine administration.[178] Erythropoietin did not appear in the plasma or urine of bled rabbits until the hematocrit was lowered to 15 per cent. The urine showed one-sixth the activity of the plasma. With the use of phenylhydrazine, higher titers of erythropoietin were found. The authors stated that it is not known whether erythropoietin in the plasma and urine is one substance and speculated as to the role of the liver in inactivating erythropoietin. Fischer and Roheim,[64] however, perfused rat livers with concentrated sheep plasma erythropoietin by the method of Miller. No difference was found in the erythropoietin activities between samples obtained after perfusion and control samples incubated with Ringer's solution. Also of interest are the studies of Krzymowski and Krzymowska who found a thermolabile plasma factor in polycythemic plasma filtrates which inhibited erythropoiesis in normal rabbits.[127]

The half-time clearance of erythropoietin has been reinvestigated by Weintraub and co-workers.[229] In the dog, two components were found, an initial rapid phase in the range of 25 to 40 minutes and a slower component of 9 to 10.5 hours. Although 70 per cent of the administered erythropoietin was lost from the plasma compartment, recovery in the urine was low. Clearance studies showed a low renal clearance, with values ranging from 0.2 to 0.6 ml. per minute. These results would indicate that renal excretion in the active form does not represent a major pathway for the elimination of exogenous erythropoietin.

The limitations of space do not permit a discussion of the theories of regulation based on (1) feed-back mechanisms,[56] (2) the effect of oxygen supply and demand,[112] (3) ineffective erythropoiesis,[208] or (4) products of red cell destruction[208] although they are most important.

8. *Miscellaneous*

A number of interesting studies have been conducted that are difficult to classify. McCall and his fellow workers[149] administered cobalt to growing rats maintained on a synthetic diet supplemented with varying amounts of iron. The addition of 3 to 10 mg./kg. of cobalt caused an erythremia in the rat; the duration and degree appeared to depend upon both the size of the Co supplement and the quantity of Fe in the diet. Aschkenasy[7-11] has published five papers on the relationship of proteins to erythropoiesis or erythropoietin. During the first week of a protein deficient diet, he found that erythropoiesis was inhibited and the lack of a single essential amino acid could cause similar changes. However, early in starvation, animals injected with erythropoietin responded by increasing mitosis of the erythroid elements. During the second week of protein deprivation erythropoietin was much less effective. This investigator produced a chronic protein deficiency and found that animals given proteins for 5 days after a 50 day deprivation are deficient in erythropoietin. Earlier studies by McCarthy, et al.[150] had shown that acutely starved animals could be stimulated to form erythropoietin. These results have been confirmed by Reissmann in well planned studies.[184] This investigator found that the decrease in the red cell mass during protein deficiency could be prevented by erythropoietin injections. After further studies, the author concluded that protein deficiency does not affect cytoplasmic protein synthesis in erythroid precursors directly; instead, the depression of erythropoiesis is attributed to a diminished formation of erythropoietin.[185]

Reynafarje and Ramos found that plasma filtrates from rabbits exposed to a simulated altitude of 22,000 feet increased the intestinal absorption of ferrous iron in rats.[187] The subject of erythropoietin and iron absorption has been thoroughly reviewed by Mendel[152] who found that the augmentation of iron absorption from the gastro-intestinal tract produced by hypoxia can occur independently of acceleration of erythropoiesis. Erythropoietin also enhanced iron absorption but this was found to be indirect and dependent on acceleration of erythropoiesis. The presence of erythropoietic stimulating factors in gastric juice has been found by Fedorov and his fellow workers.[61, 62] The results remain to be confirmed by more commonly used assay techniques.

The erythropoietic responses of normal mice and mice with a genetically transmitted anemia to exogenous erythropoietin and oxygen deprivation have been measured by Keighley, Russell and Lowy.[121] The anemic adult WWv mice failed to respond to injections of erythropoietin, but did respond to hypoxia. Normal mice responded to both stimuli. The authors considered that the contrasting reactions of normal and anemic WWv mice to the two different hematopoietic stimuli demonstrated that there is more than one fundamental stimulus to erythropoiesis.

A possible source of large quantities of erythropoietin was suggested by Swanson, et al.,[215] who found that plasma of anemic cattle is active in the frozen state for at least a year. Hammond has reported erythropoietic activity to be preserved by storage at $-4°C$ for periods as long as 18 months.[102a]

The plasma from anemic rabbits has been used by Cumming and Khoyi to alter beneficially the effect of post-irradiation anemia in mice.[40] In dogs, Pesic, Radotic and Hajdukovic[172] found irradiated animals were capable of producing erythropoietin in response to bleeding and it was thought that early and sustained stimulus to erythropoiesis could favorably influence the recovery of bone marrow following a 300 rad exposure to irradiation.

The anemia of infection remains an enigma. Gutnisky and Van Dyke have shown, however, that rats made mildly anemic by production of a turpentine abscess had an erythropoietic response comparable to normal controls following treatment with exogenous erythropoietin or exposure to hypoxia.[99] Since the rats having a turpentine abscess are capable of producing erythropoietin and the marrow is capable of responding when stimulated, it was suggested that the mild anemia which accompanies a turpentine abscess does not serve as an adequate stimulus for increased red cell production. Medici, Piliero and Hurst[151] found that in rats, splenectomy seemed to prevent erythropoietin from exhibiting its maximum effect in untreated as well as in rats with bone marrow supression caused by busulfan.

In a most provocative paper, Leaders, Dixon, Osborne and Long[137] presented evidence that the action of erythropoietin may not be entirely specific. These investigators studied the effect of four experimental procedures on the growth of Novikoff hepatomas in rats. Two erythropoietin preparations, partial hepatectomy and cobalt all were found to be capable of stimulating the growth of Novikoff hepatoma.

In summary, we would like to present Figure 4 as a diagramatic representation of our thinking regarding the production, mechanism of action and

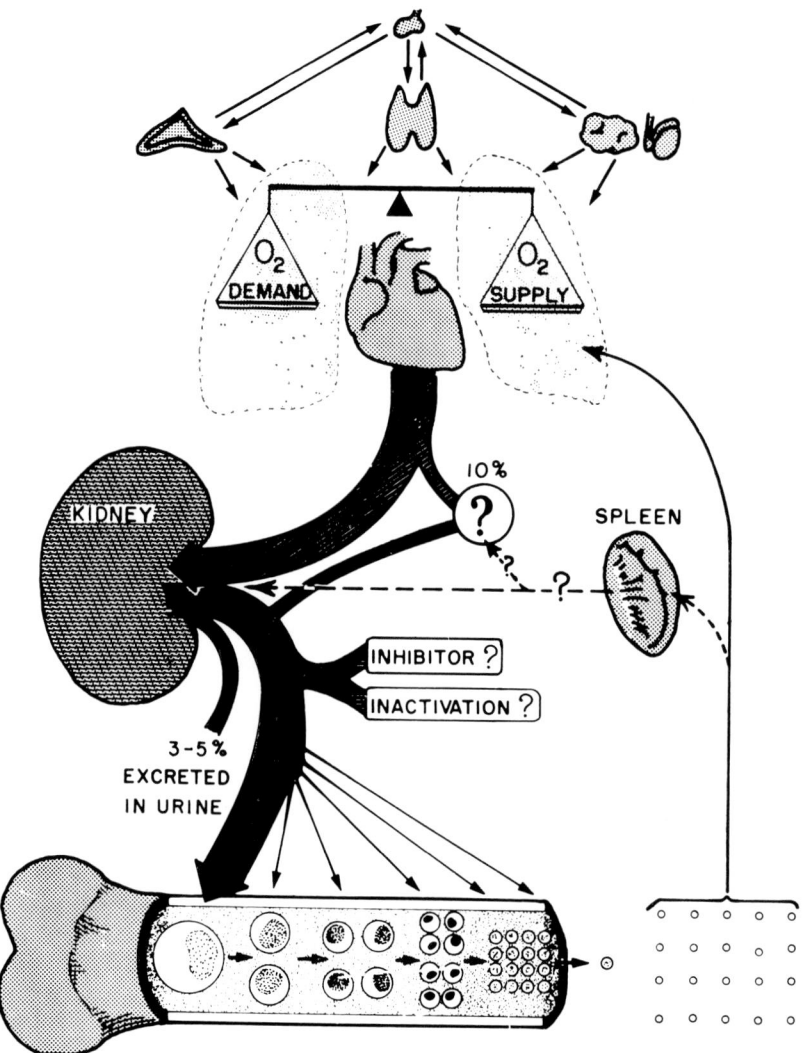

FIG. 4.—Schematic representation of erythropoietin production and action. Erythropoietin production is depicted as occurring mainly in the kidney with 10% from other sources. Production is thought to be regulated in part by a balance of oxygen supply and demand with the endocrine glands exerting their action as a secondary influence on metabolic reactions. A small amount of the erythropoietin is excreted in the urine; probably some is inactivated and inhibited. The main action of erythropoietin is on the stem cells of the bone marrow, but more peripheral actions including reticulocyte release are known. The developed red blood cells contribute to a feed-back through their influence on oxygen supply; perhaps the destruction of the red blood cells represents another controlling mechanism.

metabolism of erythropoietin. We can all look forward to the removal of the question marks as new experiments continue to shed further light on this subject.

ACKNOWLEDGMENT

The authors gratefully acknowledge the advice of Drs. T. Findley, E. Gardner, and N. I. Gallagher together with the assistance of Mr. L. Ruby and Mrs. Mary Jane Lange. We appreciate the co-operation of Miss Octavia Garlington, of the Department of Medical Illustration of the Medical College of Georgia, who drew Figure 4. Miss Elinore Pollock and Mrs. Patricia Strickland gave valuable stenographic assistance.

REFERENCES

1. Alpen, E. L., Lajtha, L. G., and Van Dyke, D. C.: Lack of direct effect of erythropoietin on human erythroid cells in vitro. Nature, London 184(Suppl. 16): 1228–1229, 1959.
2. Alpen, E. L., and Cranmore, D.: Observations on regulation of erythropoiesis and on cellular dynamics by Fe 59 autoradiography. In Stohlman, F., Jr. (Ed.): The Kinetics of Cellular Proliferation. New York, Grune & Stratton, 290–300, 1959.
3. Althoff, H.: Zur Bedeutung des Erythropoietins für die klinische Hämatologie. Ärztl. Forsch. 16: I/484–487, 1962.
4. Althoff, H.: Die Regulation des Erythrocytenbestandes durch das Erythropoetin. Mschr. Kinderheilkunde. 110: 413–417, 1962.
5. Amick, A. F.: The kidney and erythropoiesis with special consideration of the anemia of chronic renal disease. J. Lancet 82: 314–319, 1962.
6. Aschkenasy, A.: L'anemic experimentale par carence en proteines: Etat actuel de la question. Rev. Franc. Etud. Clin. Biol. 8: 435–438, 1963.
7. Aschkenasy A.: Reactivation par l'érythropoietine des mitoses erythroblastique inhibees par la privation de proteines alimentaires. C. R. Soc. Biol. 157: 275–280, 1963.
8. Aschkenasy, A.: Inhibition précoce de l'érythropoiese aprés privation de divers acides aminés essentiels chez la rat mâle. C. R. Soc. Biol. 156: 1971–1976, 1962.
9. Aschkenasy, A.: Le contenu d'erythropoiétine du plasma chez le ratiqui se manque de proteinés. J. Physiol. 54: 279, 1962.
10. Aschkenasy, A.: Nouvelles recherches sur la tarissement de la production d'érythro-poiétine au cours de l'inanition protidique du rat. C. R. Soc. Biol. 156: 1599–1605, 1962.
11. Aschkenasy, A.: Teneurs en érythropoiétine du plasmia sanguin de rats, au cours de la carence protidigue et de sa réparation. C. R. Soc. Biol. 156: 226–232, 1962.
12. Babuna, C., Gardner, G. H., and Green, R. R.: Erythrocytosis associated with a myomatous uterus. Amer. J. Obstet. Gynec. 77: 424–429, 1959.
13. Baciu, I.: Fractiuni electroforetice biologic active in plasma sanguina. Stud. Cercet. Med. Intern 3: 441–449, 1962.
14. Baciu, J.: La régulation nerveuse et humorale de l'érythropoïése. J. Physiol. (Paris) 54: 431–458, 1962.
15. Barnard, H. F.: Polycythemia and renal carcinoma. Brit. Med. J. 1: 1214–1215, 1961.
16. Bartlett, R. G., Jr. and Phillips, N. E.: Hypocapnia and erythropoiesis. Aerospace Med. 33: 831–833, 1962.
17. Bassi, P. and Dunjic, A.: L'exploration de la fanction érythropoïétique à l'aide du fer rodioaetif chez le rat irradié et traité par l'alcool batylique ou sélachylique. Rev. Franc. Etud. Clin. Biol. 7: 187–191, 1962.
18. Becker, F.: Extremitätennekrose bei Polycythaemia vera. Klin. Wchnschr. 11: 1260–1262, 1932.
19. Bernardelli, E.: Mécanisme d'action de l'érythropoïétine. Schweiz. Med. Wchnschr. 92: 1329–1331, 1962.
20. Bernardelli, E.: Mecanisme d'action de l'érythropoïétine recherches in vitro. Boll. Soc. Ital. Biol. Sper. 38: 979–982, 1962.
21. Berry, E. R., Rambach, W. A., and Alt, H. L.: Ion-exchange chromatography of erythro-poietically active plasma filtrates. Quart. Bull. Northwest. Univ. Med. Sch. 36: 285–289, 1962.
22. Bilsel, Y. C., Wood, J. E., and Lange, R. D.: Angiotensin II and erythropoiesis. Proc. Soc. Exper. Biol. & Med. 114: 475–479, 1963.
23. Boivin, P.: L'activité erythropoïétique du plasma. Stud. Cercet. Med. Intern 4: 135–143, 1963.
24. Boivin, P., Lagrue, G., and Fauvert, R.: L'activite erythropoietique du plasma humain au cours de quelques affections hematologigues et autres. Nouv. Rev. Fr. d'Hematologie. 3: 35–50, 1963.
25. Boulet, P., Mirouze, J., and Barjon, P.: Le facteur érythropoïétique plasmatique dans l'anémie des néphropathies chroniques urémiques. J. Urol. Nephrol. 67: 416–424, 1961.
26. Bradley, J. E., Young, J. D., and Lentz, G.: Polycythemia secondary to pheochromocytoma. J. Urol. 86: 1–6, 1961.
27. Brecher, G. and Stohlman, F. Jr.: Humoral factors in erythropoiesis. In Tocantins, L. M. (Ed.): Progress in Hematology II. New York, Grune & Stratton, 110–132, 1959.
28. Brecher, G. and Stohlman, F. Jr.: Reticulocyte size and erythropoietin stimulation. Proc. Soc. Exp. Biol. & Med. 107: 887–891, 1961.
29. Brody, J. I. and Rodriguez, F.: Cerebellar hemagioblastoma and polycythemia (erythrocythemia). Amer. J. Med. Sci. 242: 579–584, 1961.
30. Brown, J. R., Altschuler, N., and Cooper, J. A.: Erythropoietic effect of red blood cell components and heme-related compounds. Proc. Soc. Exp. Biol. & Med. 112: 840–843, 1963.

31. Bruce, W. R. and McCulloch, E. A.: The effect of erythropoietic stimulation on the hemopoietic colony-forming cells of mice. Blood. 23: 216–232, 1964.
32. Campbell, J. H., Pasquier, C. M., St. Martin, E. C., and Worley, P. C.: Hypernephroma associated with polycythemia and eczematoid dermatitis. J. Urol. 79: 12–15, 1958.
33. Carpenter, G., Schwartz, H., and Walker, A. E.: Neurogenic polycythemia. Ann. Intern. Med. 19: 470–481, 1943.
34. Carnot, P. and Deflandre, C.: Sur l'activité hémopoiétique du sérum au cours de la régénération du sang. Compt. rend. Acad. Sc. 143: 384–386, 1906.
35. Carnot, P. and Deflandre, C.: Sur l'activité hémopoiétique des differents organes au cours de la régénération du sang. Compl. rend. Acad. Sc. 143: 432–435, 1906.
36. Cohen, M. and Rothenberg, S. P.: Erythrocytosis associated with uterine fibromyomas. Report of a case. Obstet. Gynec. (N.Y.). 19: 96–100, 1962.
37. Conley, C. L., Kowal, J., and D'Antonio, J.: Polycythemia associated with renal tumors. Bull. Johns Hopkins Hosp. 101: 63–73, 1957.
38. Cooper, G. W. and Nocenti, M. R.: Unilateral renal ischemia and erythropoietin. Proc. Soc. Exp. Biol. & Med. 108: 546–549, 1961.
39. Cotes, P. M. and Bangham, D. R.: Bio-assay of erythropoietin in mice made polycythemic by exposure to air at a reduced pressure. Nature, London. 191: 1065–1067, 1961.
40. Cumming, J. D. and Khoyi, M. A.: Effect of plasma from anaemic rabbits on the postirradiation anaemia of mice. Nature, London. 193: 1196–1198, 1962.
41. Damon, A., Holub, D. A., Melicow, M. M., and Uson, A. C.: Polycythemia and renal carcinoma. Report of ten new cases, two with long hematologic remission following nephrectomy. Amer. J. Med. 25: 182–197, 1958.
42. DeGowin, R. L., Hofstra, D., and Gurney, C. W.: A comparison of erythropoietin bioassays. Proc. Soc. Exp. Biol. & Med. 110: 48–51, 1962.
43. DeGowin, R. L., Hofstra, D., and Gurney, C. W.: The mouse with hypoxia-induced erythremia, an erythropoietin bioassay animal. J. Lab. & Clin. Med. 60: 846–852, 1962.
44. De La Torre Fernandez, J. M.: Conceptos actuales sobre la eritropoyesis. Rev. Esp. Enferm. Apar. Dig. 21: 1509–1516, 1962.
45. DeMarsh, Q. B. and Warmington, W. J.: Polycythemia associated with renal tumor. Northwest Med. 54: 976–979, 1955.
46. DeRitis, G.: Le eritropoietine. Ann. Ist. Forlanini. 22: 99–105, 1962.
47. De Weerd, J. H. and Hagedorn, A. B.: Hypernephroma associated with polycythemia. J. Urol. 82: 29–35, 1959.
48. Dolder, G. von: Humorale aspecten vande erythropëse. Nederl. T. Geneesk. 107: 312–316, 1963.
49. Donati, R. M., McCarthy, J. M., Lange, R. D., and Gallagher, N. I.: Erythrocythemia and Neoplastic Tumors. Ann. Int. Med. 58: 47–55, 1963.
50. Donati, R. M., Lange, R. D., and Gallagher, N. I.: Nephrogenic erythrocytosis. Arch. Intern. Med. 112: 960–965, 1963.
51. Dukes, P. P. and Goldwasser, E.: Lack of effect of plasma erythropoietin on formate incorporation into nucleic acids in vitro. Nature, London. 195: 1222, 1962.
52. Emanuel, D. A. and Wenzel, F. J.: Erythrocytosis associated with the nephrotic syndrome. J. A. M. A. 181: 788–790, 1962.
53. Engel, H. W. and Singer, K.: Polycythemia with fibroids. J. A. M. A. 159: 190–191, 1955.
54. Erslev, A.: Humoral regulation of red cell production. Blood 8: 349–357, 1953.
55. Erslev, A. J.: Le contrôl de l'erythropoïèse. Rev. France Etud. Clin. Biol. 8: 225–228, 1963.
56. Erslev, A.: Hematology: Control of red cell production. In Rytand, D. A. and Creger, W. P. (Eds.): Annual Review of Medicine 11. Palo Alto, California. Annual Reviews, Inc. 315–332, 1960.
57. Erslev, A. J. and Hughes, J. R.: The influence of environment on iron incorporation and mitotic division in a suspension of normal bone marrow. Brit. J. Hemat. 6: 414–432, 1960.
58. Erslev, A. J.: Effect of erythropoietin on the uptake and utilization of iron by bone marrow cells in vitro. Proc. Soc. Exp. Biol. & Med. 110: 615–620, 1962.
59. Erslev, A. J.: Control of the proliferative steady state. In Stohlman, F. Jr. (Ed.): The Kinetics of Cellular Proliferation. New York, Grune & Stratton, 313–317, 1959.
60. Escobar, M. A. and Trobaugh, F. E., Jr.: Erythrocythemia in primary carcinoma of the liver. A case report. Arch. Int. Med. 110: 339–344, 1962.
61. Fedorov, N. A., Kakhetelidze, M. G. and Namiatysheva, A. M.: Quantitative hemopoietin changes in the gastric juice following repeated bloodletting and blood transfusion in the dog. Biull. Eksp. Biol. Med. 53: 28–32, 1962.
62. Fedorov, N. A. and Kakhetelidze, M. G.: On the relation between the intrinsic factor of the stomach and hemopoietins. Probl. Gemat. 7: 3–7, 1962.
63. Filmanowicz, E. and Gurney, C. W.: Studies on erythropoiesis. XVI. Response to a single dose of erythropoietin in polycythemic mouse. J. Lab. & Clin. Med. 57: 65–72, 1961.
64. Fischer, S. and Roheim, P. S.: Role of the liver in the inactivation of erythropoietin. Nature 200: 899–900, 1963.

65. Fischer, J. and Friederici, L.: Erythropoese bei bilateral nephrektomierten kaninchen. Experienta. 17: 318–319, 1961.
66. Fisher, J. W. and Birdwell, B. J.: The production of an erythropoietic factor by the in situ perfused kidney. Acta Haemat. 26: 224–232, 1961.
67. Fisher, J. W., Knight, D. B., and Couch, C.: The influence of several diuretic drugs on erythropoietin formation. J. Pharmacol. Exp. Ther. 141: 113–121, 1963.
68. Fisher, J. W.: Effect of adrenalectomy on the erythropoietic response to sheep erythropoietin and cobalt. Endocrinology. 70: 243–248, 1962.
69. Fisher, J. W. and Crook, J. J.: Influence of several hormones on erythropoiesis and oxygen consumption in the hypophysectomized rat. Blood 19: 557–565, 1962.
70. Fisher, J. W., Roh, B. L., Couch, C., and Nightingale, W. O.: Influence of cobalt, sheep erythropoietin and several hormones on erythropoiesis in bone marrows of isolated perfused hind limbs of dogs. Blood 23: 87–98, 1964.
70a. Fleming, A. R., Markley, J. C.: Polycythemia associated with uterine myomas. Amer. J. Obstet. Gynec. 74: 677, 1957.
71. Forssell, J.: Polycythemia in patient with hypernephroma. Nord. Med. 30: 1415–1418, 1946.
72. Freedman, B. J. and Penington, D. G.: Erythrocytosis in emphysema. Brit. J. of Hemat. 9: 425–430, 1963.
73. Frey, W. G., III: Polycythemia and hypernephroma: Review and report of a case with apparent surgical cure. New England J. Med. 258: 842–844, 1958.
74. Friederici, L. and Fischer, J.: Die Erythropoese bei Nierenerkrankungen unter besonderer Berüchsichtigung der Erythropoetin aktivitat des Blutes. Folia. Haemat. 8: 398–404, 1963.
75. Friederici, L.: Über den Nachweis des Erythropoetins in der Gewebekultur. Klin. Wchnschr. 36: 132–134, 1958.
76. Fruhman, G. J. and Fischer, S.: The short term effects of a single dose of erythropoietin upon reticulocytes in starved rats. Experientia. 18: 462–464, 1962.
77. Gallagher, N. I., McCarthy, J. M., and Lange, R. D.: Erythropoietin production in uremic rabbits. J. Lab. & Clin. Med. 57: 281–289, 1961.
78. Gallagher, N. I. and Lange, R. D.: Response to erythropoietin. Proc. Soc. Exp. Biol. & Med. 110: 422–426, 1962.
79. Gallagher, N. I., Seifert, G. L., Callinan, J. L., Maes, A. A., and Lange, R. D.: Influence of erythropoietin on erythropoiesis in polycythemic rats. J. Lab. & Clin. Med. 61: 258–265, 1963.
80. Gallagher, N. I., McCarthy, J. M., and Lange, R. D.: Observations on erythropoietic stimulating factor (ESF) in the plasma of uremic and nonuremic anemic patients. Ann. Int. Med. 52: 1201–1212, 1960.
81. Garcia, J. F. and Schooley, J. C.: Erythropoietic stimulation in the hypertransfused guinea pig following injections of human urinary erythropoietin. Nature, London. 196: 279–280, 1962.
82. Garcia, J. F. and Schooley, J. C.: Immunological neutralization of various erythropoietins. Proc. Soc. Exp. Biol. & Med. 112: 712–714, 1963.
83. Giono, H., Manoussos, G., Dormard, Y., and Thuillier, Y.: Etude chez le rat de l'activité érythropoiétique d'un extrait rénal. Thérapie. 17: 349–354, 1962.
84. Goetze, E., Buhler, H., and Petermann, R.: Erythro-und Leukopoese bei experimenteller Polyzythämie von Ratten. Folia Haemat. Leipzig 80: 1–8, 1963.
85. Goltner, E. and Friederici, L.: Die erythropoetische Aktivität des blutserums nach Blutverlusten bei Karzinomen ohne und mit Urämie. Med. Welt. 11: 586–589, 1962.
86. Goldfarb, B. and Tobian, L.: Effect of high oxygen concentrations on erythropoietin and the renal juxtaglomerular cell. Proc. Soc. Exper. Biol. & Med. 113: 35–36, 1963.
87. Goldfarb, B. and Tobian, L.: Relationship of erythropoietin to renal juxtaglomerular cells. Proc. Soc. Exp. Biol. & Med. 112: 65–69, 1963.
88. Goldfarb, B. and Tobian, L.: The interrelationship of hypoxia, erythropoietin and the renal juxtaglomerular cell. Proc. Soc. Exp. Biol. & Med. 111: 510–511, 1962.
89. Goldwasser, E., White, W. F., and Taylor, K. B.: On the purification of sheep plasma erythropoietin. In Jacobson, L. O. and Doyle, M. (Eds.): Erythropoiesis. New York, Grune & Stratton, 43–49, 1962.
90. Goldwasser, E., White, W. F., and Taylor, K. B.: Further purification of sheep plasma erythropoietin. Biochem. Biophys. Acta 64: 487–496, 1962.
91. Gordon, A. S. and Weintraub, A. H.: Assay of erythropoietic stimulating factor (ESF). In Jacobson, L. O. and Doyle, M. (Eds.): Erythropoiesis. New York, Grune & Stratton, 1–16, 1962.
92. Gordon, A. S.: Hemopoietine. Physiol. Rev. 39: 1–40, 1959.
93. Gordon, A. S., LoBue, J., Dornfest, B. S., and Cooper, G. W.: Reticulocyte and leukocyte release from isolated perfused rat legs and femurs. In Jacobson, L. O. and Doyle, M. (Eds.): Erythropoiesis. New York, Grune & Stratton, 321–327, 1962.
94. Gráf, F. and Takácsi-Nagy, L.: Die neurohumorale Regulation der Erythropoese. Folia Haemat. (Leipzig) 80: 129–137, 1963.
95. Grant, W. C. and Root, W. S.: Fundamental stimulus for erythropoiesis. Physiol. Rev. 32: 449–498, 1952.

96. Grant, J. L. and Smith, B.: Bone marrow gas tensions, bone marrow blood flow, and erythropoiesis in man. Ann. Int. Med. 58: 801–809, 1963.
97. Gurney, C. W., Lajtha, L. G., and Oliver, R.: A method for investigation of stem cell kinetics. Brit. J. Haemaet. 8: 461–466, 1962.
98. Gurney, C. W.: Erythremia in renal disease. Trans. Ass. Amer. Physicians. 73: 103–112, 1960.
99. Gutnisky, A. and Van Dyke, D.: Normal response to erythropoietin or hypoxia in rats made anemic with turpentine abscess. Proc. Soc. Exp. Biol. & Med. 112: 75–78, 1963.
100. Halvorsen, S. and Finne, P. H.: Transfer of erythropoietin to amniotic fluid in Rh immunized pregnant women. Brit. Med. J. 5338: 1132–1134, 1963.
101. Halvorsen, S.: Plasma erythropoietin levels in cord blood and in blood during the first weeks of life. Acta Paediatrica. 52: 425–435, 1963.
102. Hammond, D.: Humoral hematopoietic factors in the control of erythrocyte production. Pediat. Clin. N. Amer. 9: 549–557, 1962.
102a. Hammond, D. G.: In Jacobson, L. O. and Doyle, M. (Eds.): Erythropoiesis. New York, Grune & Stratton, 31, 1962.
103. Hatta, Y., Maruyama, Y., Tsuruoka, N., Yamaguchi, A., Kukita, M., Sho, C. T., Sugata, F., and Shimizu, M.: Studies on the erythropoietic stimulating factor apoceruloplasmin. Acta. Haemat. Jap. 25: 682–689, 1962.
104. Hellens, Y. von, Hirsjarvi, E., and Nikiforow, R.: Erythropoietic activity of saline washings of blood cells subjected to low atmospheric pressure in vitro II. Effect of partial hemolysis of the blood. Acta Physiol. Scand. 56: 381–384, 1962.
105. Hewlett, J. S., Hoffman, G. C., Senhauser, D. A., and Battle, J. D., Jr.: Hypernephroma with erythrocythemia: Report of a case and assay of the tumor for an erythropoietic-stimulating substance. New England J. Med. 262: 1058–1062, 1960.
106. Hirashima, K. and Takaku, F.: Experimental studies on erythropoietin. II. The relationship between juxtaglomerular cells and erythropoietin. Blood. 20: 1–8, 1962.
107. Hodgson, G.: Control de la eritropoyesis. Rev. Med. Chile 90: 817–825, 1962.
108. Horwitz, A., and McKelway, W. P.: Polycythemia associated with uterine myomas. J. A. M. A. 158: 1360–1361, 1955.
109. Iaroshevskii, A. I.: Plasma and serum erythropoietins in internal diseases. Ter. Arkh. 33: 3–17, 1961.
110. Idel'son, L. I.: Erythropoietic activity of the urine in erythraemia and anaemia. Prob. Gemat. 6: 810–817, 1961.
111. Jacobson, L. O.: Erythropoietin and the regulation of red blood cell formation. Physiol. Physicians. 1: 1–6, 1963.
112. Jacobson, L. O., Gurney, C. W., and Goldwasser, E.: The control of erythropoiesis. In Dock, W. and Snapper, I. (Eds.): Advances in Internal Medicine. The Year Book Publishers. 10: 297–327, 1960.
113. Jacobson, L. O. and Doyle, M. (Eds.): Erythropoiesis. New York, Grune & Stratton, 1962.
114. Jacobson, L. O., Goldwasser, E., and Gurney, C. W.: Control of red cell formation. In Stohlman, F., Jr., (Ed.): The Kinetics of Cellular Proliferation. New York, Grune & Stratton, 344–356, 1959.
115. Jacobson, L. O., Goldwasser, E., Fried, W., and Plzak, L.: Role of the kidney in erythropoiesis. Nature, London. 179: 633–634, 1957.
116. Jaworski, Z. F. and Wolan, C. T.: Hydronephrosis and polycythemia. A case of erythrocytosis relieved by decompression of unilateral hydronephrosis and cured by nephrectomy. Am. J. Med. 34: 523–534, 1963.
117. Josephs, B. N., Robbins, G., and Levine, A.: Polycythemia secondary to hamartoma of the liver. J. A. M. A. 179: 867–870, 1962.
118. Kakhetelidze, M. G. and Makorova, E. M.: Modified hemopoietin content of the blood serum following blood loss. Prob. Gemat. 7: 50–53, 1962.
119. Kan, Y. W., McFadzean, A. J. S., Todd, D., and Tso, S. C.: Further observations on polycythemia in hepatocellular carcinoma. Blood. 18: 592–598, 1961.
120. Keighley, G., Lowy, P. H., Borsook, H., Goldwasser, E., Gordon, A. S., Prentice, T. C., Rambach, W. A., Stohlman, F. Jr., and Van Dyke, D. C.: A cooperative assay of a sample with erythropoietic stimulating activity. Blood. 16: 1424–1432, 1960.
121. Keighley, G., Russell, E. S., and Lowy, P. H.: Response of normal and genetically anemic mice to erythropoietic stimuli. Brit. J. Haemat. 8: 429–441, 1962.
122. Keighley, G., Hammond, D., and Lowy, P. H.: The sustained action of erythropoietin injected repeatedly into rats and mice. Blood. 23: 99–107, 1964.
123. Khalifa, K. and Keller, H. M.: Study of erythropoietin production in sheep after repeated bleedings and phenylhydrazine. Acta. Hemat. 29: 242–248, 1963.
124. Kienel, G.: Erythropoietin ein humoraler Faktor für die Kontrolle der Blutbildung. Med. Mschr. 16: 310–313, 1962.
125. Korst, D. R., Whalley, B. E., and Bethell, F. H.: Erythropoietic activity of plasma in polycythemia. J. Lab. & Clin. Med. 54: 916, 1959. (Abstract)
126. Korst, D. R., Frenkel, E. P., and Wilhelm, J. E.: Studies utilizing short-term marrow culture. I. Ferrokinetics and erythropoietin. In Jacobson, L. O. and Doyle, M. (Eds.): Erythropoiesis. New York, Grune & Stratton, 310–320, 1962.

127. Krzymowski, T. and Krzymowska, H.: Studies on the erythropoiesis inhibiting factor in the plasma of animals with transfusion polycythemia. Blood. 19: 38–44, 1962.
128. Krantz, S. B., Gallien-Lartigue, O., and Goldwasser, E.: The effect of erythropoietin upon heme synthesis by marrow cells in vitro. J. Biol. Chem. 238: 4085–4090, 1963.
129. Kuratowska, Z.: Erythropoetyna postepy badan nad humoralna regulacja erytropoezy. Postepy. Hig. Med. Dosw. 16: 373–400, 1962.
130. Kuratowska, Z., Lewartowski, B., and Michalak, E.: Studies on the production of erythropoietin by isolated perfused organs. Blood 18: 527–534, 1961.
131. Kuratowska, Z. and Lewartowski, B.: Studies on the active principle released by the hypoxic kidney into Tyrode's solution. In Jacobson, L. O. and Doyle, M. (Eds.): Erythropoiesis. New York, Grune & Stratton, 101, 1962.
132. Kuratowska, Z., Lewartowski, B., and Michalak, E.: Studies on production of erythropoietin by the isolated hypoxic kidney. Bull. Acad. Pol. Sci. (Serie Biol.) 8: 77–80, 1960. Cited in Waldmann, T. A. and Rosse, W. F.: Sites of Formation of Erythropoietin. In Jacobson, L. O. and Doyle, M. (Eds.): Erythropoiesis. New York, Grune & Stratton, 1962.
133. Kurtides, E. S., Rambach, W. A., Alt, H. L., and Wurster, J. C.: Effect of erythropoietin on tritiated thymidine incorporation by the rat spleen. J. Lab. & Clin. Med. 61: 23–33, 1963.
134. Lajtha, L. G. and Oliver, R.: Studies of the kinetics of erythropoiesis a model of the erythron. In Wolstenholme, G. E. W. and O'Conner, M. (Eds.): Ciba Foundation Symposium on Haemopoiesis. London. J. & A. Churchill Ltd. 289–314, 1960.
135. Lange, R. D., Gardner, E., Wright, C-S., and Gallagher, N. I.: Neutralization of the biological activity of erythropoietin by immune sera. Brit. J. Hemat. 10: 69–74, 1964.
136. Laurin, J. G., Girard, Y., Gauthier, G., and Leduc, P. E.: Polycythaemia and fibromyoma of the uterus. Canad. Med. Ass. J. 83: 318–319, 1960.
137. Leaders, F. E., Dixon, R. L., Osborne, J. W., and Long, J. P.: Erythropoietic stimulating factor (ESF) as a stimulant of tumor growth. Proc. Soc. Exp. Biol. & Med. 110: 436–440, 1962.
138. Lehman, C. J., Erslev, A. J., and Myerson, R. M.: Erythrocytosis associated with hepatocellular carcinoma. Am. J. Med. 35: 439–442, 1963.
139. Lewis, J. P., Gallagher, N. I., Carmody, S., and Lange, R. D.: Erythropoietic activity in human urine concentrates. In preparation.
140. Linman, J. W., Long, M. J., Korst, D. R., and Bethell, F. H.: Studies on the stimulation of hemopoiesis by batyl alcohol. J. Lab. & Clin. Med. 54: 335–343, 1959.
141. Linman, J. W. and Bethell, F. H.: Factors Controlling Erythropoiesis. Springfield, Illinois. Charles C. Thomas, 1960.
142. Linman, J. W.: Factors controlling hemopoiesis: Erythropoietic effects of "anemic" plasma. J. Lab. & Clin. Med. 59: 249–261, 1962.
143. Lowy, P. H., Keighley, G., Borsook, H., and Graybiel, A.: On the erythropoietic principle in the blood of rabbits made severely anemic with phenylhydrazine. Blood. 14: 262–273, 1959.
144. Lowy, P. H. and Keighley, G.: Use of phenol in the isolation of erythropoietic glycoprotein. Nature, London. 192: 75, 1961.
145. Marinescu, S. and Bălăceapu, M.: Eritropoetina. Med. Intern. (Bucur) 13: 1351–1353, 1961.
146. Marinone, G.: Luci ed ombre sul problema dei fattori umorali di regolozione dell'emopoiesi. È possibile prospettare una patogenesi umorale di alcuni stati iperplastici ed aplastici midollari? Riv Emater Immunoemat. 8: 13–29, 1961.
147. Masson, M.: Le facteur érythropoiétique produit par le rein. Presse Med. 69: 2139–2140, 1961.
148. Matoth, Y. and Kaufmann, L.: Mitotic activity in vitro of erythroblasts previously exposed to erythropoietin. Blood. 20: 165–172, 1962.
149. McCall, M. G., Newman, G. E., O'brien, J. R., and Witts, L. J.: Studies in iron metabolism. 3. Cobalt and erythropoiesis in the growing rat. Brit. J. Nutr. 16: 325–332, 1962.
150. McCarthy, J. M., Gallagher, N. I., and Lange, R. D.: Fasting and the erythropoietic-stimulating factor. Metabolism. 8: 429–431, 1959.
151. Medici, P. T., Piliero, S. J., and Hurst, J.: Protective effect of sheep plasma erythropoietin against the hemato-depressent action of myleran in intact and splenemectomized rats. Blood 20: 783–784, 1962. (Abstract)
152. Mendel, G. A.: Studies on iron absorption. I. The relationships between the rate of erythropoiesis, hypoxia and iron absorption. Blood. 18: 727–736, 1961.
153. Menzies, D. N.: Ribromyomata and polycythaemia. J. Obstet. Gynaec. Brit. Comm. 68: 505–509, 1961.
154. Messmer, B. A.: Renal polycythaemia: A report of three cases, with discussion. Med. J. Aust. 48(2): 14–18, 1961.
155. Milliez, P., Lagrue, G., Tcherdakoff, P., and Boivin, P.: Reins et érythropoiése. Infom. Med. Paramed. 14: 1–9, 1962.
156. Mitus, W. J., Galbraith, P., and Gollerkeri, M.: Experimental renal erythrocytosis in Proc. IX Congress of the International Society of Hematology. (Abstract)

157. Muirhead, E. E., Kosinski, M., Jones, F., and Reno, E.: Erythropoietin and the state of renal tissue. Blood. 20: 782, 1962. (Abstract)
158. Moores, R. R., Stohlman, F., Jr., and Brecher, G.: Humoral regulation of erythropoiesis. XI. The pattern of response to specific therapy in iron deficiency anemia. Blood. 22: 286–294, 1963.
159. Naets, J. P.: Relation between erythropoietin plasma level and oxygen requirements. Proc. Soc. Exp. Biol. & Med. 112: 832–836, 1963.
160. Naets, J. P. and Heuse, A. F.: Effect of anaemic anoxia on erythropoiesis of nephrectomized dog. Nature (London) 195: 190, 1962.
161. Naets, J. P.: Erythropoietic factor in kidney tissue of anemic dogs. Proc. Soc. Exp. Biol. & Med. 103: 129–132, 1960.
162. Naets, J. P. and Heuse, A. F.: Measurement of erythropoietic stimulating factor in anemic patients with or without renal disease. J. Lab. & Clin. Med. 60: 365–374, 1962.
163. Najean, Y. and Bernard, J.: L'aspect quantitatif de l'érythropoiése et sa régulation humorale. Rev. Prat. 12: 2361–2367, 1962.
164. Nakao, K.: Studies on erythropoietin. Acta. Haem. Jap. 25: 253–279, 1962.
165. Nathan, D. G., Schupak, E., and Merrill, J. P.: Erythrokinetics in anephric man. Blood. 22: 811–812, 1963. (Abstract)
166. Nedwich, A., Frumin, A., and Meranze, D. R.: Erythrocytosis associated with uterine myomas. Amer. J. Obstet. Gynec. 84: 174–178, 1962.
167. Noyes, W. D., Domm, B. M., and Willis, L. C.: Regulation of erythropoiesis. I. Erythropoietin assay as a clinical tool. Blood. 20: 9–18, 1962.
168. Olesen, H.: Erythropoietin. Nord. Med. 68: 883–888, 1962.
169. Omland, G.: Polycythemia in renal carcinoma. Acta Med. Scand. 164: 451–454, 1959.
170. Osnes, S.: Influence of the pituitary on the erythropoietic principle produced in the kidney. Brit. Med. J. 1: 1153–1157, 1960.
171. Pavlovic-Kentera, V., Gardner, E., Jr., and Lange, R. D.: Effect of antisera to erythropoietin on the in vitro Fe[59] incorporation by rabbit bone marrow cells. Blood. 22: 809, 1963. (Abstract)
171a. Pavlovic-Kentera, V., Hall, D. P., and Lange, R. D.: Unilateral renal hypoxia and production of erythropoietin. In preparation.
172. Pesic, N., Radotic, M., and Hajdukovic, S.: Erythropoietin production following gamma irradiation and hemorrhage in dogs. Science. 143: 49–50, 1964.
173. Piliero, S. J., Medici, P. T., and Orr, A.: Influence of hypoxic stimuli upon erythropoiesis in hypothalamic lesioned animals. Acta Haemat. (Basel) 28: 101–112, 1962.
174. Piha, R. S.: Demonstration of erythropoietic activity in body fluids, organs and tissues. Ann. Acad. Sci. Fenn. 98: 1–40, 1962.
175. Plachecka-Gutowska, M.: Humoralna regulacja erytropoezy. Pol. Arch. Med. Wewnet. 32: 249–258, 1962.
176. Powsner, E. R. and Berman, L.: Effect of erythropoietin in vitro. J. Mich. Med. Soc. 62: 670–673, 1963.
177. Prankerd, T. A. J.: Current views on erythropoiesis. Practitioner. 188: 173–178, 1962.
178. Prentice, T. C. and Mirand, E. A.: Some aspects of the relationship between plasma and urine erythropoietin. Proc. Soc. Exp. Biol. Med. 109: 414–417, 1962.
179. Rambach, W. A., Cooper, J. A. D., and Alt, H. L.: Purification of erythropoietin by ion-exchange chromatography. Proc. Soc. Exp. Biol. & Med. 98: 602–604, 1958.
180. Rambach, W. A., Alt, H. L., and Cooper, J. A. D.: Erythropoietic activity of tissue homogenates. Proc. Soc. Exp. Biol. & Med. 108: 793–796, 1961.
181. Reeves, G., Lowenstein, L., and Sommers, S. C.: A suggested mechanism of erythropoietic control by juxtaglomerular cells. Am. J. Med. Sci. 245: 184–188, 1963.
182. Reissmann, K. R.: Studies on the mechanism of erythropoietic stimulation in parabiotic rats during hypoxia. Blood. 5: 372–380, 1950.
183. Reissmann, K. R. and Nomura, T.: Erythropoietin formation in isolated kidneys and liver. In Jacobson, L. O. and Doyle, M. (Eds.): Erythropoiesis. New York, Grune & Stratton, 71–77, 1962.
184. Reissmann, K.: Protein metabolism and erythropoiesis. I. The anemia of protein deprivation. Blood. 23: 137–145, 1964.
185. Reissmann, K.: Protein metabolism and erythropoiesis. II. Erythropoietin formation and erythroid responsiveness in protein deprived rats. Blood. 23: 146–153, 1964.
186. Remmele, Wolfgang: Die Humorale Steuerung der Erythropoiese. Berlin: Springer Verlag. 1963.
187. Reynafarje, C. and Ramos, J.: Influence of plasma filtrate containing erythropoietic factor on intestinal iron absorption in rats. Proc. Soc. Exp. Biol. & Med. 109: 868–869, 1962.
188. Riabov, S. I.: On hormonal regulation of hematopoiesis. Usp. Sovr. Biol. 52: 225–240, 1961.
189. Root, W. S. (Ed.): Hemopoietic mechanisms. Ann. of N. Y. Acad. of Science. 77: 407–820, 1959.
190. Rosse, W. F., Waldmann, T. A., and Houston, D. E.: Erythropoietin assays using iron 59 incorporation into blood and spleen of the polycythemic mouse. Proc. Soc. Exp. Biol. & Med. 109: 836–839, 1962.

191. Rosse, W. F. and Gurney, C. W.: Studies on erythropoiesis. X. The use of bone marrow tissue culture in demonstrating erythropoietin. J. Lab. & Clin. Med. 53: 446–456, 1959.
192. Rosse, W. F. and Waldmann, T. A.: The role of the kidney in the erythropoietic response to hypoxia in parabiotic rats. Blood. 19: 75–81, 1962.
193. Rosse, W. F., Waldmann, T. A., and Cohen, P.: Renal cysts, erythropoietin and polycythemia. Am. J. Med. 34: 76–81, 1963.
194. Rosse, W. F., Berry, R. J., and Waldmann, T. A.: Some molecular characteristics of erythropoietin from different sources determined by inactivation ionizing radiation. J. Clin. Inv. 42: 124–129, 1963.
195. Rosse, W. F., Waldmann, T., and Hull, E.: Factors stimulating erythropoiesis in frogs. Blood. 22: 66–72, 1963.
196. Sanchez-Medal, L.: Hemolysis y activadad eritropoyética. Rev. Invest. Clin. 14: 199–209, 1962.
197. Sanzari, N. P. and Fisher, J. W.: The influence of cobalt and sheep erythropoietin on radioactive iron incorporation in RBC of starved intact and nephrectomized rats. Blood. 21: 729–738, 1963.
198. Schonfeld, A., Babbott, D., and Gundersen, K.: Hypoglycemia and polycythemia associated with primary hepatoma. New England J. Med. 265: 231–233, 1961.
199. Schooley, J. C. and Garcia, J. F.: Immunochemical studies of human urinary erythropoietin. Proc. Soc. Exp. Biol. & Med. 109: 325–328, 1962.
200. Schooley, J. C. and Garcia, J. F.: Immunologic studies on the mechanism of action of erythropoietin. Proc. Soc. Exp. Biol. & Med. 110: 636–641, 1962.
201. Schmid, R. and French, L. A.: Cerebellares Hämangioblastom mit Polycythämie. Schweiz. Med. Wschr. 85: 1274–1277, 1955.
202. Schroeder, L. R., Gurney, C. W., and Wackman, N.: Assay of erythropoietin in bone marrow suspensions. Nature, London. 181: 1537–1538, 1958.
203. Shekhter, S. Y.: Erythropoietic properties of the sera from patients with gastroenterogenous iron-deficiency anemia. Prob. Gemat. 6: 817–823, 1961.
204. Shimizu, M.: Hematopoietic hormone. J. Showa Med. Ass. 21: 765–768, 1962.
205. Shirakura, T.: Experimental studies on the relationship between erythropoiesis and endocrine organs. Acta Haemat. Jap. 24: 536–544, 1961.
206. Sokabe, H., and Grollman, A.: Localization of blood pressure regulating and erythropoietic functions in rat kidney. Amer. J. Physiol. 203: 991–994, 1962.
207. Stohlman, F., Jr., Rath, C. E., and Rose, J. C.: Evidence for a humoral regulation of erythropoiesis: Studies on a patient with polycythemia secondary to regional hypoxia. Blood. 9: 721–733, 1954.
208. Stohlman, F., Jr.: Erythropoiesis. New England J. Med. 267: 342–348, 392–399, 1962.
209. Stohlman, F., Jr: (Ed.): The Kinetics of Cellular Proliferation. New York, Grune & Stratton, 1959.
210. Stohlman, F., Jr.: Humoral regulation of erythropoiesis. VI. Mechanism of action of erythropoietine in the irradiated animal. Proc. Soc. Exp. Biol. & Med. 107: 751–754, 1961.
211. Stohlman, F., Jr.: Humoral regulation of erythropoiesis. VII. Shortened survival of erythrocytes produced by erythropoietine or severe anemia. Proc. Soc. Exp. Biol. & Med. 107: 884–887, 1961.
212. Strausz, I., Kekes, E., Janikovsky, B., and Molnar, A.: Erythropoietic effect of the blood serum of patients with cardiac decompensation. Kiserl Orvostud. 15: 29–32, 1962.
213. Stroebel, C. F. and Fowler, W. S.: Secondary polycythemia. Med. Clin. N. Amer. 40: 1061–1076, 1956.
214. Strzhizhovskii, A. D.: On some kinetic mechanisms of erythropoiesis. Bull. Eksp. Biol. Med. 54: 102–105, 1962.
215. Swanson, R. N., Underbjerg, G. K., and Fryer, H. C.: Evaluation of an erythropoietic factor in the blood of anemic cattle using iron-59. Am. J. Vet. Res. 24: 307–312, 1963.
216. Takaku, F., Hirashima, K., and Nakao, K.: Studies on the mechanism of erythropoietin production. I. Effect of unilateral constriction of the renal artery. J. Lab. & Clin. Med. 59: 815–820, 1962.
217. Takaku, F., Hirashima, K., and Okinaka, S.: Studies on the mechanism of erythropoietin production. II. Effect of bilateral section of the splanchnic nerves. J. Lab. & Clin. Med. 59: 821–825, 1962.
218. Thomas, E. D., Lochte, H. L., Jr., and Stohlman, F., Jr.: Attempts to develop an in vitro system for the assay of erythropoietin. J. Lab. & Clin. Med. 55: 311–318, 1960.
219. Thomson, A. P. and Marson, F. G. W.: Polycythemia with fibroids. Lancet 2: 759–760, 1953.
220. Tohá, J., Eskuche, I., Abarca, F., Salávtore, F., and Hodgson, G.: Chemical properties of a plasma factor accelerating haemoglobin recovery in bled rabbits. Nature, London 175: 167–168, 1955.
220a. Van Dyke, D., Lawrence, J. H., and Siri, W. E.: Erythropoietin as an etiologic factor in blood dyscrasias. Acta Isotopica 1: 217–225, 1961.
221. Waldmann, T. A. and Rosse, W. F.: Sites of formation of erythropoietin. In Jacobson,

L. O. and Doyle, M. (Eds.): Erythropoiesis. New York, Grune & Stratton, 87–92, 1962.

222. Waldmann, T. A., Weissman, S. M., and Levin, E. H.: Effect of thyroid administration on erythropoiesis in the dog. J. Lab. & Clin. Med. 59: 926–931, 1962.

223. Waldmann, T. A., Bradley, J. E.: Polycythemia secondary to a pheochromocytoma with production of an erythropoiesis stimulating factor by the tumor. Proc. Soc. Exp. Biol. Med. 108: 425–427, 1961.

224. Waldmann, T. A., Levin, E. H., and Baldwin, M.: The association of polycythemia with a cerebellar hemangioblastoma. The production of an erythropoiesis stimulating factor by the tumor. Am. J. Med. 31: 318–324, 1961.

225. Ward, A. A., Foltz, E. L., and Knopp, L. M.: Polycythemia associated with cerebellar hemangioblastoma. J. Neurosurg. 13: 248–259, 1956.

226. Warter, J., Mantz, J., and Hammann, B.: Research on hemopoietin (erythropoietin) I. Erythropoietic potency of the wash liquid from the isolated and hypoxic calf kidney. C. R. Soc. Biol. 156: 897–900, 1962.

227. Ways, P., Huff, J. W., Kosmaler, C. H., and Young, L. E.: Polycythemia and histologically proven renal disease. A. M. A. Arch. Intern. Med. 107: 154–162, 1961.

228. Weintraub, A. H., Gordon, A. S., and Camiscoli, J. F.: Use of the hypoxia induced polycythemic mouse in the assay and standardization of erythropoietin. J. Lab. & Clin. Med. 62: 743–752, 1963.

229. Weintraub, A. H., Gordon, A. S., Becker, E. L., Camiscoli, J. F., and Contrera, J.: Studies on the bioassay and metabolism of erythropoietin. Blood. 22: 808–809, 1963. (Abstract)

230. White, W. F., Gurney, C. W., Goldwasser, E., and Jacobson, L. O.: Studies on erythropoietin. Recent Progr. Hormone Res. 16: 219–262, 1960.

231. Wolstenholme, G. E. W. and O'Conner, M. (Eds.): Haemopoesis Cell Production and its Regulation. Boston, Mass. Little Brown & Co. 1960.

232. Woolsey, R. D.: Hemangioblastoma of cerebellum with polycythemia. J. Neurosurg. 8: 447–450, 1951.

233. Wright, B. M.: Apparatus for exposing animals to reduced atmospheric pressure for long periods. Brit. J. Hemat. 10: 75–77, 1964.

234. Yamaguchi, A., Tsuruoka, N., Maruyama, Y., Yamamoto, M., Ando, M., Ueno, T., Hatta, Y., and Shimizu, M.: Studies on erythropoietic stimulating substance, apoceruloplasmin. II. Effects of apoceruloplasmin on peripheral blood picture, iron and copper metabolism. Acta Haemata. Jap. 25: 773–780, 1962.

235. Zangheri, E. O., Campana, H., Ponce, F., Silva, J. C., Fernández, F. O., and Suárez, J. R.: Production of erythropoietin by anoxic perfusion of the isolated kidney of a dog. Nature. 199: 572–573, 1963.

236. Zangheri, E. O., Suárez, J. R., Fernández, F. O., Campana, H., Silva, J. C., and Ponce, F. E.: Erythropoietic action of tissue extracts. Nature (London) 194: 938–939, 1962.

237. Zilliacus, H.: Polycythaemia associated with uterine fibromyoma. Acta Obstet. Gynec. Scand. 38: 737–741, 1959.

Chemistry of the ABH Blood Group Substances

—GERALD SCHIFFMAN and DONALD M. MARCUS—

INTRODUCTION

THERE is great interest in the blood group antigens not only because of the primary role they play in transfusion reactions but also because they are very useful in the study of many aspects of immunochemistry, genetics and biosynthetic mechanisms. This review will attempt to present the newer knowledge of the structures of the antigenic determinants of the ABH blood group system. Problems involved in the correlation of structure with biological activities are presented in the first section. The recently acquired information about the ABH blood group substances from secretions and from erythrocytes is presented in the second and third sections respectively. The last section discusses the Watkins-Morgan-Ceppellini scheme for biosynthesis of the blood group mucopolysaccharides.

I. THE ASSAY OF BLOOD GROUP SUBSTANCES

Before reviewing recent data on the structure of ABH substances it is essential to consider some complexities and limitations of the assay systems in common use. The factors which give rise to difficulties include heterogeneity in the serological behavior and specificity of isoagglutinins, differences in the nature of the hemagglutination and precipitin assay techniques, and the role of the physical state of the antigen in modifying its immunological activity.

Serological properties of isoagglutinins

ABH isoantibodies are inhomogeneous, differing in serological properties such as agglutinating activity in saline vs. colloid media, enhancement of titer by use of enzyme-treated erythrocytes or indirect antiglobulin (Coombs') tests, ease of neutralization by soluble blood group substances, and hemolytic activity (reviewed in 1, chap. 9). These observations have led to the arbitrary classification of isoantibodies as "natural" or "immune" in origin. The properties attributed to "immune" antibodies include resistance to neutralization by soluble blood group substances, hemolytic activity, and enhancement of agglutinating activity in colloid media[1, p. 261]. It is now clear that these diverse serological activities reflect the physical and immunochemical heterogeneity of the antibody globulins (immunoglobulins).

Three major classes of serum immunoglobulins are recognized at present[2-8]: $7S\gamma_2$-globulins; $19S\gamma$-macroglobulins $(\gamma_{1M}; \beta_{2M})$; and $\beta_{2A}(\gamma_{1A})$-globulins which have sedimentation rates varying from 7S to $15S^9$. Studies of the pri-

From the John Herr Musser Department of Research Medicine, University of Pennsylvania, Philadelphia, Pa. and the Department of Medicine, Albert Einstein College of Medicine, Yeshiva University, New York.

mary antibody response to a variety of antigens in man and animals have revealed that the first antibody to appear is a 19Sγ-macroglobulin[10-19]. In response to most antigens, 7S antibodies then appear and become preponderant, or entirely replace the 19S antibodies[12-19]. Even with repeated immunization, however, the response to some antigens consists mostly of macroglobulin antibodies[13-15, 19].

The anti-A and anti-B isoagglutinins of both $7S\gamma_2$ and 19Sγ varieties have been identified by many workers[20-28]. Many human sera contain both types of isoagglutinin, though preponderantly the latter, but sera containing only 19S, or, more rarely, only $7S\gamma_2$ antibodies have been described[22]. Individuals of blood group O appear to have more 7S isohemagglutinin than do those of the other ABO phenotypes[22-25, 26, 29, 30].

Rockey and Kunkel[31] found isoagglutinins which sedimented at a rate intermediate between 7S and 19S. These isoagglutinins were eluted from DEAE-cellulose columns between the 7S and 19S isoagglutinin peaks, and their serological activity was abolished by mercaptoethanol. Kunkel and Rockey[32] reported subsequently that the proteins which sedimented at an intermediate rate reacted with individual sera monspecific for β_{2A} and $7S\gamma_2$-globulins. It is not known whether the proteins with the antigenic characteristics of $7S\gamma_2$-globulins were complexed to the β_{2A}-globulins, or if they were in polymeric form. These authors established the existence of β_{2A} isoagglutinins in the following manner. Anti-A agglutinins were precipitated with blood group A substance, and the precipitates were dissolved in excess antigen or in an acid buffer. The dissolved material was then allowed to react in agar gel plates with antisera monospecific for $7S\gamma_2$,β_{2A} , and 19Sγ-globulins. β_{2A} proteins were detected in most of the dissolved precipitates.

The presence of an intermediate isoagglutinin fraction obtained by DEAE-cellulose chromatography has been reported by several groups[21, 26, 30, 33]. The antibody activity found by these authors to be present in the intermediate area represented, however, a small fraction of the total serum activity, and it is not clear if any of these fractions corresponded to the material studied by Rockey and Kunkel.

Sera containing isoagglutinins were fractionated by gel filtration on Sephadex G-200 columns by Killander and Högman[28]. They detected isoagglutinin activity in the area between the peaks containing the serum macroglobulins and the 7Sγ globulins, and suggested that it might correspond to the agglutinins with intermediate sedimentation rates found by Rockey and Kunkel.

Although the isoagglutinins have not been completely purified, some of the serologic properties discussed above can be assigned tentatively to different classes of isoagglutinins[cf. 30]: the activity of the $7S\gamma_2$ antibodies, but not the 19S, is enhanced by colloid media or antiglobulin tests[21, 27-30]; both types of antibody may be hemolytic[21, 23, 30]; 19S antibodies are more readily neutralized by soluble blood group substances[21, 30].

The isoagglutinins which appear in an intermediate area on DEAE-cellulose chromatography have many serological properties in common with the 19S agglutinins[21, 30]. However, Abelson and Rawson's intermediate fractions were not hemolytic[23]. Purified β_{2A} isohemagglutinins were devoid of hemolytic activity[23a].

Immunization, whether by transfusion of incompatible blood, by administration of soluble blood group substances, or by a hetero-specific pregnancy, generally produces a rise in titer of all isoagglutinin fractions[29, 30]. This finding is in accord with previous work on the increase of the so-called "natural" and "immune" antibodies following immunization[34, 35], and it would be reasonable to discard these terms.

The Origin and Specificity of Isoagglutinins

To account for the regular occurrence of ABH isoagglutinins in the absence of known antigenic stimulation two hypotheses have been proposed. One hypothesis invokes a genetically directed synthesis of antibody in the absence of an external stimulus, and the other postulates immunization by cross-reacting exogenous material[reviewed in 1, p. 260; 36, 37]. A considerable body of evidence may now be adduced in favor of the latter hypothesis.

The presence of material with ABH blood group activity in animals, plants, and bacteria has been amply documented[1, chap. 3; 38-44]. The prevalence of blood group-active material is attested to by the finding of Springer et al. of blood group activity in approximately half of 282 strains of aerobic Gram-negative bacteria[40]. It is significant that naturally-occurring isoantibodies rarely are found in the Rh blood group system, and none of the 70 strains of bacteria tested possessed Rh activity. Springer et al. have also shown that the anti-human blood group B agglutinins found in the majority of ordinary White Leghorn chicks were absent from the sera of germ-free chicks, but that they could be induced in the latter by feeding blood group B-active E. coli O_{86} or human meconium[37]. Bacterial products may be found in the serum[45] or on the erythrocytes[46] of infants with enteritis, which indicates that humans may be immunized in the same manner.

One manifestation of the heterogeneity of human isoagglutinins not discussed above is their variable degree of cross-reactivity with erythrocytes and soluble blood group substances of other animal origin[36]. This variability is due probably to differences in antibody specificity, arising from immunization by exogenous materials, as well as to differences in sizes of combining sites and/or affinity of the antibody for antigen.

The various observations cited above indicate that immunization with exogenous antigens having blood group activity could account for the presence of naturally-occurring isoagglutinins. There is no evidence for the elaboration of isoagglutinins under genetic control in the absence of antigenic stimulation, but this possibility has not been excluded.

Plant Lectins and Heterologous Sera

The infrequent occurrence of human isoantibodies of certain specificities has led to the use of plant lectins and of heterologous sera for blood typing and in immunological research. Although valuable information has been acquired through the use of these reagents, they may differ in specificity from each other and from human isoantibodies. For example, several groups have reported differences in specificity among anti-H reagents in common use[47-51]. Two anti-N reagents—*Vicia graminea* and rabbit anti-N have also been found to differ in specificity[52, 53].

Some Problems in the Assay of Blood Group Substances

Substances of low molecular weight are generally assayed for blood group activity by measuring their ability to inhibit precipitation, hemolysis or hemagglutination. The isoagglutinins in human sera vary considerably in the extent to which they are inhibited by small oligosaccharides, and some sera are not measurably inhibited by monosaccharides or disaccharides of known activity[54]. Some light may be thrown on this phenomenon by the work on inhibition of human antidextran antibodies by isomaltose oligosaccharides of varying chain length[54, 55, p. 242-246]. Schlossman and Kabat have shown that an individual human antiserum to dextran may be separated, by hapten dissociation of antibody bound to Sephadex, into a fraction which is almost completely inhibited by small oligosaccharides, and a fraction requiring larger oligosaccharides for appreciable inhibition[56]. This heterogeneity has been attributed to differences in the size of the specific antibody combining sites, but the possible contribution of other factors has not been excluded. Whatever the underlying mechanism(s) may be, it should be appreciated that appropriate sera must be selected for inhibition studies with small haptens.

Another important consideration is the fact that it requires much less hapten to inhibit precipitation than it does to inhibit hemagglutination, even though much larger amounts of serum may be employed in the precipitin reaction[57, 58]. There is no ready explanation for this phenomenon.

Macromolecular blood group substances may be assayed by their ability to precipitate isoagglutinins or to inhibit hemagglutination. The two types of assay may give strikingly divergent results at times. Blood group substances which were altered by enzymatic treatment[59-61], or ultrasonic disintegration[62] appeared to be totally inactive in inhibiting hemagglutination, but were capable of precipitating substantial amounts of isoagglutinin. This apparent discrepancy reflects a basic difference in the two assays. In the hemagglutination inhibition test, the antigen must compete with the erythrocyte determinant for the antibody; and, if the antigen is partially degraded, it will compete less effectively. In the precipitin test, only antigen and antibody are present, and even a weak bond between the two may lead to the formation of insoluble complexes. To some extent these two types of assays complement each other; the hemagglutination inhibition technique is more likely to detect a partial loss of antigenic activity, but a weak cross-reaction would be more readily detected by the precipitin reaction. The exclusive use of either system to assay an antigen for blood group activity provides limited, and possibly misleading, information.

ABH Substances Derived From Erythrocytes

Substances with considerable ABH activity may be extracted from erythrocyte stroma in the form of glycolipids (reviewed in section III). Compounds of this type form micelles in aqueous solution[63-66] and the characteristics of the micelle are critical in determining immunological reactivity. In the course of purification of the glycolipid, a large loss of activity occurs, which is recovered by combining the active or "essential" lipid with an inactive or "auxiliary" fraction[67-69]. The auxiliary lipid is totally inactive alone and can be obtained from stroma of any ABO type; simple lipids, such as lecithin or sphingomyelin, also provide some reactivation[68]. Similar findings have been reported in the purification of Forssman hapten from sheep erythrocytes[70] and in the isolation of cytolipin H from human tissues[71]. Rapport has reviewed the specificity of lipid haptens[72] and lipid-lipid interactions[69]. The precise role of the auxiliary lipid is not clear. The carbohydrate determinant groups on the surface of the micelle may differ in orientation and spacing from their native configuration on the erythrocyte membrane, and their full immunological potential may not be measured in the usual assay system. The comparison of the specific activity of a glycolipid with a water-soluble "standard" substance derived from secretions is therefore of limited utility. In view of the large number of blood group-active materials encountered in nature, it is probable that each individual receives a unique series of antigenic stimuli, and, strictly speaking, there is no single "standard" substance. Koscielak and Zakrzewski noted that their glycolipid preparation was less active than a "standard A substance" in inhibiting most anti-A sera, but the reverse situation obtained with some sera[73].

II. Blood Group Mucopolysaccharides

Substances with blood group activity can be isolated from most secretions, e.g., saliva, meconium, urine, etc.[1, chap. 3]. The richest source of such material is fluid from ovarian pseudomucinous cysts[74] and hence this material has been studied most extensively. The chemical composition, molecular size and shape, as well as the structures involved in antigenic specificity have been investigated for many years. Reviews of the results obtained are available[1, 62, 75-81] and a complete recapitulation at this time is unnecessary. A brief resumé would seem to be useful, however, before considering recent advances in knowledge of the structure of the antigenic determinants.

Chemical Composition

Ovarian blood group substances are composed of 75–80% carbohydrate and 20–25% amino acids. The carbohydrate moiety consists of L-fucose, D-galactose, N-acetyl-D-galactosamine and N-acetyl-D-glucosamine. Table 1 shows the composition of several blood group substances. Small quantities of sialic acid are usually observed in preparations of ovarian blood group substances[80, 82]. Dische has found that there is an inverse relationship between the sialic acid and fucose content of many glycoproteins. A review of these observations and a discussion of their possible meaning has been presented recently[83]. Pusztai and Morgan[84] isolated an interesting blood group mucopolysaccharide from ovarian cyst fluid, the composition of which reflects the inverse relationship between fucose and sialic acid noted by Dische. The mucopolysaccharide, which contained 18% sialic acid and 7% fucose, had two biological specificities: the ability to inhibit viral hemagglutination and Le[a] activity. Each activity

TABLE 1.—*Blood Group Substances*

Preparation used	Blood group activity	Source	N	Galac- tose	Hexosa- mine	Fucose	References
			%	%	%	%	
Hog mucin Fr. 2	A + H	Hog gastric mucin	6	20	33	9	(85)
McDon	A	Human ovarian cyst fluid	5.2	21	33	20	(86)
MSS 10%	A	Human *serous* ovarian cyst fluid	7	18	30	16	(87)
MSM 10%	A	Human *mucinous* ovarian cyst fluid	5	19	32	15	(87)
Beach φH insol	B	Human ovarian cyst fluid	5.2	26	25	21	(88, 89)
J.S.	H	Human ovarian cyst fluid	4	19	25	23	(87)

was independent and could be destroyed enzymatically without affecting the other.

The amino acids of blood group substances have an unusual distribution. Serine, threonine and proline account for about half of the total, although some 12 or 14 amino acids are present[80, 85]. A similar pattern of amino acids has been reported to be present in bovine submaxillary mucin and in an erythrocyte mucoprotein which inhibits viral hemagglutination[91, 92]. The possibility that serine and/or threonine might be involved in a carbohydrate-amino acid linkage is suggested by two observations: 1) blood group substances extracted from erythrocytes do not contain amino acids and are stable in the presence of alkali[73, 93], in contrast to the alkaline lability of blood group mucopolysaccharides derived from secretions[1, p. 229; 87, 94-97]; and 2) a sugar component of chondroitin sulfate is eliminated by alkaline treatment which results in the disappearance of serine alone among the amino acids, probably by a β-carbonyl elimination of an alkoxide from O-substituted serine[98].

Size and Shape of the Blood Group Molecule

Estimates of the molecular weight (MW) of blood group substances range from 250,000 to 1,000,000 or more[1, p. 154]. A MW of 300,000 is usually assumed for the purposes of calculations. Diffusion and viscosity measurements[62] as well as periodate oxidation studies[89] have been interpreted to indicate that blood group substances are highly branched asymmetric molecules containing a periodate resistant backbone, possibly a polypeptide. Conflicting results[77] obtained in periodate oxidation studies indicate the need for further clarification of the nature of the backbone. The number of oligosaccharide chains attached to this backbone has not been determined precisely, but estimates can be made from available data. When fluoridinitrobenzene reacts with blood group A substance which has been enzymatically inactivated, 110 molecules of dinitrobenzene (DNP) are found to have attached to each mole of blood group substance (300,000 MW). After hydrolysis, about 47 moles of DNP are shown to be associated with galactosamine[61].

Coffee bean α galactosidase inactivates blood group B substance and liberates galactose[60]. If each galactose is liberated from the end of an oligosaccharide chain, then there would be 110 such chains in each molecule.

Structures Involved in Antigenic Specificity

Studies by Carsten and Kabat[85] showed that the amino acid moiety of blood group substances is not responsible for antigenic specificity. Inhibition of activity of isoagglutinins and lectins by the monosaccharide components of blood group substances reveals that blood group A, B and H specificity is dependent on N-acetylgalactosamine[57, 99, 100], galactose[57] and fucose[99-101], respectively. Further information about the antigenic determinants has been obtained by examination of compounds isolated after degradation of blood group substances. Blood group substances have been degraded enzymatically and by alkaline and acid hydrolysis.

The use of enzymes to obtain oligosaccharides with immunologic activity has been largely unsuccessful. Many important observations, however, have resulted from this approach; and these findings have led to a proposed scheme for the biosynthesis of the blood group mucopolysaccharides (see Section IV). The use of alkali to degrade blood group substances was reported by Morgan[94, 95, 97], but these experiments apparently were not pursued. Morgan[77] obtained, by alkaline hydrolysis, an active compound from Le[a] substance which contained fucose, galactose and N-acetylglucosamine. The isolation of an active fucose-containing compound from blood group A substance after alkaline treatment has been reported recently[102].

The use of acid hydrolysis has resulted in the isolation and identification of many oligosaccharides, the most active of which are:

1) α-N-acetylgalactosaminoyl(1–3) βgalactosyl(1–3) N-acetylglucosamine, (A_5II)

2) α-N-acetylgalactosaminoyl(1–3) βgalactosyl(1–4) N-acetylglucosamine

3) αgalactosyl(1–3) βgalactosyl(1–3) N-acetylglucosamine

4) αgalactosyl(1–3) βgalactosyl(1–4) N-acetylglucosamine

Oligosaccharides 1[86, 103, 104] and 2[104] were isolated from blood group A substances, are active in inhibiting precipitation and hemagglutination, and possess Forssman activity. Oligosaccharides 3 and 4 were isolated from blood group B substance[105]. The activities of these four trisaccharides in inhibiting hemagglutination, as compared with those of the most active disaccharides, are presented in Table 2.

The need for a method other than acid hydrolysis was apparent for two reasons. First, the yield of active oligosaccharides from an acid hydrolysate is very small. Less than 50 mg of an active trisaccharide, A_5II, and only 1 mg of an active tetrasaccharide, A_5Id, were isolated from 20 grams of blood group A substance after mild acid hydrolysis[86]. Modifications of the acid hydrolytic procedure have been introduced to increase the yield[106-109], but the yields are still small. Second, the activity of the most active trisaccharides is not much greater than that of the corresponding disaccharides, see Table 2[86, 104, 105] and a tetrasaccharide, A_5Id, is no more active than the trisaccharide A_5II. In analogy to the dextran system,[54, 79] one would have to conclude that the upper

TABLE 2.—*Inhibition of hemagglutination by disaccharides and trisaccharides isolated from blood group substances (data from 104, 105)*

Inhibiting substance	Amount required for inhibition	
	$\mu g/ml$ A-anti-A	$\mu moles/ml$ B-anti-B
α Gal(1–3)β Gal(1–4) N-AcGluc		2.5
α Gal(1–3)β Gal(1–3) N-AcGluc		5
α Gal(1–3)Gal		4
α N-AcGal(1–3) β Gal(1–3) N-AcGluc	600	
α N-AcGal(1–3) β Gal (1–4) N-AcGluc	600	
α N-AcGal(1–3)Gal	600	

limit of the size of the antigenic determinant had been reached. An alternative explanation for these observations is that acid hydrolysis modifies the antigenic determinant by selective cleavage. This possibility could be evaluated only by the use of other methods.

Alkaline degradation in the presence of $NaBH_4$

Two observations led to the use of an alkaline degradative procedure. First, unhydrolyzed blood group substances have a high reducing sugar value (10–15%) which is not depressed by treatment with $NaBH_4$[89]. This finding indicates the existence of bonds labile in the presence of the alkaline conditions of the assay. Second, active oligosaccharides are resistant to degradation by alkali after reduction with $NaBH_4$[86, 110].

Exposure of blood group A substance to 0.1 to 0.2 N NaOH in the presence of 1% $NaBH_4$ causes 75–80% of the treated substance to become dialyzable[87]. The total crude dialysate is a more active inhibitor of A-anti-A precipitation than the most highly purified trisaccharide, A_5II (Figure 1). The crude dialysate could be fractionated by paper chromatography. Fraction A_3 obtained by this method is 10 to 40 times as active as A_5II (Figures 2 & 3).

In similar fashion, dialysis and chromatography of blood group B and H substances after hydrolysis in alkali and reduction with $NaBH_4$ results in the isolation of highly active fractions, B_3 (Figure 4) and H_4. The chemical com-

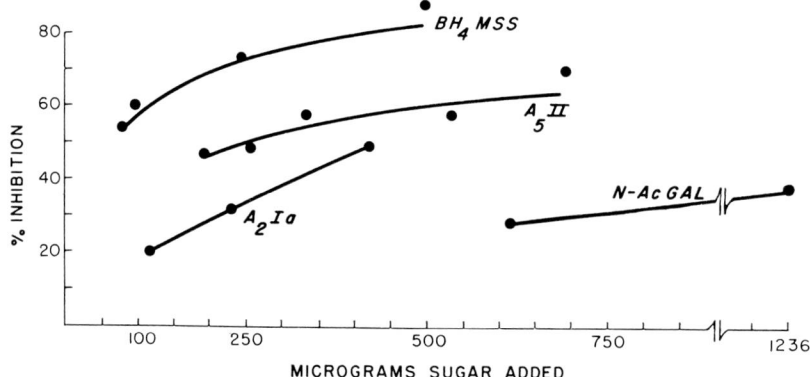

FIG. 1.—Inhibition of A-anti-A precipitation by a dialysate (BH_4 MSS) of alkali-treated human A substance, MSS, as compared with N-acetylgalactosamine, disaccharide A_2I_a, and trisaccharide A5 II. (Reprinted by permission of Schiffman et al. Biochemistry 3: 113, 1964.)

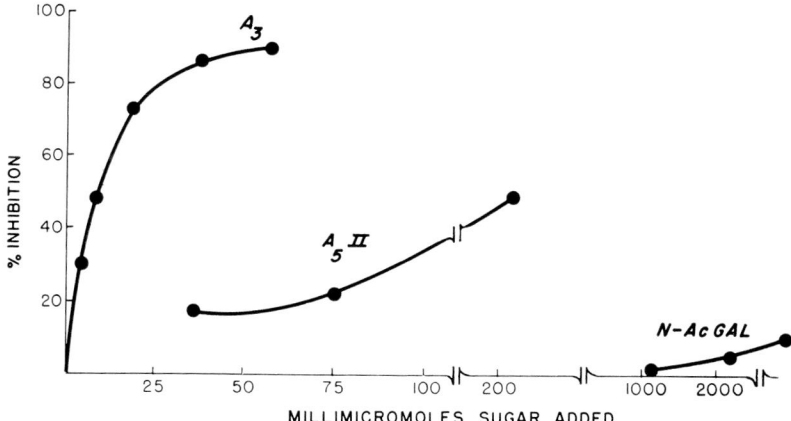

FIG. 2.—Inhibition of A-anti-A precipitation by chromatographic fraction A_3, trisaccharide A_5II and N-acetylgalactosamine. (Reprinted by permission of Schiffman et al. Biochemistry 3: 113, 1964.)

INHIBITION OF HEMOLYSIS OF SHEEP ERYTHROCYTES
0.5 μl Rabbit Anti-Human A Stroma

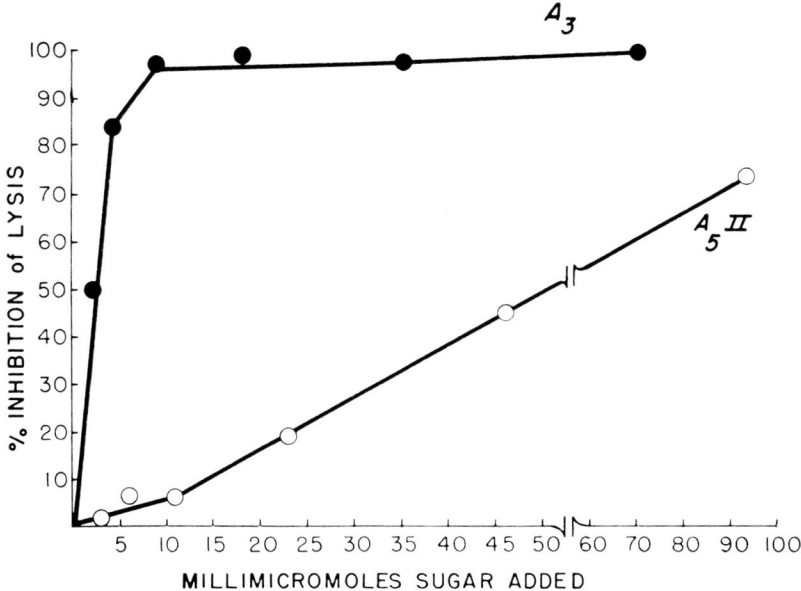

FIG. 3.—Comparison of the activity of A_3 and A_5II in inhibition of lysis of sheep erythrocytes by antibody to human A erythrocyte stromata. (Reprinted by permission of Schiffman et al. Biochemistry 3: 113, 1964.)

position of these partially purified fractions is presented in Table 3. The fractions A_3, B_3 and H_4 are thought to represent the antigenic determinants of blood group A, B and H substances. The immunologic behavior of A_3, B_3 and H_4 are presented in Table 4. Possible structures for A_3, B_3 and H_4 are presented in Figure 5. These structures are based on their chemical composition, their

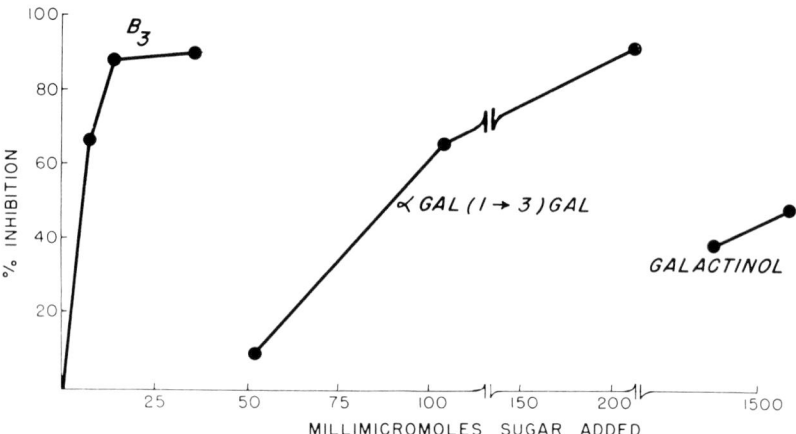

Fɪɢ. 4.—Inhibition of B-anti-B precipitation by B₃, α galactosyl (1–3) galactose and galactinol. (Reprinted by permission of Schiffman et al. Biochemistry 3: 113, 1964.)

SXIV   GAL $\xrightarrow{\beta}$ N–AcGLU.......

Le^a
                                 FUC
                                 αI
              GAL $\xrightarrow{\beta}$ N–AcGLU.......

H
                 FUC   FUC
                 α⋮   α⋮
              GAL $\xrightarrow{\beta}$ N– AcGLU....... (N–AcGLU)

B
                      FUC   FUC
                      α⋮   α⋮
        GAL $\xrightarrow{\alpha}$ GAL $\xrightarrow{\beta}$ N–AcGLU .... (N–AcGLU)

A
                         FUC   FUC
                         α⋮   α⋮
   N–AcGAL $\xrightarrow{\alpha}$ GAL $\xrightarrow{\beta}$ N–AcGLU .... (N–AcGLU)

Fɪɢ. 5.—Structures involved in blood group and blood group-related systems. Compounds active in the type XIV pneumococcal system and in the Leᵃ system have had their structures established unambiguously (77). Structures for the H, B and A antigenic determinants, (H₄, B₃ and A₃) are possible ones based on reasons given in the text and in reference 136.

immunochemical activities and the known structures of active oligosaccharides isolated from blood group substances and other sources[50, 77, 136]. Possible sugar sequences in the carbohydrate chains have been proposed by Rege et al.[137]. The structures of the antigenic determinants of A, B and H substances shown in Figure 5 contain the units proposed by Rege et al but differ in two respects. The structures in figure 5 contain fucose residues whereas those of Rege et al do not; the sequences of sugars in the linear portion of the determinants are extended by Rege et al. to include β galactosyl-N-Acetylgalactosamine in the region in figure 5 now occupied by the dotted line.

III. Blood Group Substances from Erythrocytes

Early attempts to extract ABH substances from intact erythrocytes or from stroma had been reviewed by Kabat[1, p. 118]. In general, the extracts of

TABLE 3.—*Chemical Analysis of Partially Purified Determinants*
(5.0 mg./ml. solutions)

	Galactose	Methyl Pentose	Hexosamine	Acetyl Hexosamine	N
	$\mu moles/ml$	$\mu moles/ml$	$\mu moles/ml$	$\mu moles/ml$	$\mu moles/ml$
A_3	3.2	5.3	8.2	6.0	14
H_4	3.1	4.0	4.6	4.8	8.4
B_3	6.6	6.1	5.1	5.4	6.7

erythrocytes were much less active in hemagglutination inhibition than substances derived from soluble secretions. They differed also in containing glucose, fatty acids and sphingosine, constituents not found in blood group mucopolysaccharides, and in having little or no fucose, glucosamine, or amino acids. The low immunological activity and variable composition of these erythrocyte extracts suggested[1, p. 121] that the observed blood group activity was imparted by traces of material similar to those present in secretions.

The application of new column chromatographic techniques to the resolution of lipid mixtures has provided convincing evidence that the red cell ABH substances are glycolipid in nature[73, 93, 111-115]. They represent, however, only a minute fraction of the glycolipids which are extractable from the erythrocyte membrane. The apparent low activity of the substances from erythrocytes results, at least in part, from the formation of micelles by the glycolipids (see discussion in Section I).

A summary of the composition of several preparations of glycolipid with A or B activity is presented in Table 5. Despite the admitted impurity of this material and the possible heterogeneity arising from the use of pooled units of blood as a starting material, certain general features may be discerned. Among the glycolipids with A activity there is reasonable agreement in the percentages of nitrogen, hexosamine, and reducing sugar. Sialic acid and fucose were found by Koscielak, and by Handa and Yamakawa, but not by Hakomori and Jeanloz. The carbohydrate portion of the glycolipids differs from that of substances from ovarian cysts in containing glucose, sialic acid, a lower content of hexosamine, and very little fucose. All three groups of workers obtained compounds with B activity, and these were similar in composition to the glycolipids with A activity.

The glycolipids isolated by Jeanloz and Hakomori[114] contained a mixture of fatty acids with chain lengths of 16–24 carbon atoms, as did Koscielak's methanol-soluble A glycolipid[116]. The methanol-insoluble glycolipid contained about 90% lignoceric acid and small amounts of C_{22} and C_{23} acids.

There has been little study of the physical properties of these glycolipids. In aqueous solution, Koscielak's methanol-soluble glycolipid had a sedimentation coefficient of 12.4 S at a concentration of 0.15 g per 100 ml; the methanol-insoluble glycolipid had a sedimentation coefficient of 79 S at a concentration of 0.2 g per 100 ml[115]. Sphingolipids of very similar composition—gangliosides—have been purified and characterized more extensively. In aqueous solution they form micellar aggregates with weights of 180,000–450,000, as estimated from sedimentation data, but sedimentation in N,N-dimethylformamide indicated a molecular weight of about 1,500[63-66].

A unit structure for the glycolipids of one molecule each of a fatty acid,

TABLE 4.—*Immunochemical properties of A_3, B_3 and H_4*

Inhibition by of	A_3	$A_31.6$		
Anti-A.	++	+		
Anti-AP1.	−	++		
Forssman Antibody.	++	+		
Anti-SXIV.	−	+		

Inhibition by of	B_3	B_3ET	$B_3 1.6$	$B_3ET 1.6$
Anti-B.	++	−	+	−
Anti-BP1.	−	−	++	−
Anti-SXIV.	−	−	+	++
Ulex (H activity).	−	+	−	−

Inhibition by of	H_4	$H_4 1.6$		
Ulex.	++	−		
Anti-SXIV.	−	+		

++ represents very potent inhibition; + less potent; − not active.

A_3, B_3 and H_4 are the partially purified antigenic determinants of A, B and H activity respectively.

$A_31.6$, B 1.6 and $H_41.6$ are A_3, B_3 and H_4 hydrolyzed at pH 1.6 at 95° for 90 minutes.

B_3ET is B_3 treated with coffee bean α galactosidase.

Ulex is an aqueous extract of *Ulex europeus* seeds which agglutinates O erythrocytes.

Anti-AP1 is human antibody produced in response to immunization with the non-dialyzable portion which remained after mild acid hydrolysis of blood group A substance.

Anti-SXIV is horse antibody to type XIV pneumococcal polysaccharide.

Anti-BP1 is human antibody produced in response to immunization with the non-dialyzable portion which remained after mild acid hydrolysis of blood group B substance.

sphingosine, N-acetylhexosamine, and four hexoses was proposed by Hakomori and Jeanloz[114], and a similar structure with only three hexoses was suggested by Koscielak and Zakrzewski in an early paper[93]. These preliminary formulations, however, do not account for either the fucose or sialic acid. The glycolipids recently isolated by Koscielak had molar ratios of glucose and of sialic acid to sphingosine of 0.57–0.58. He suggested that each molecule may contain two sphingosine residues[116] but it is possible that his preparations were heterogeneous.

Koscielak's methanol-insoluble A-glycolipid and the A-glycolipids of Handa and Yamakawa were of the same order of activity as substances from ovarian

TABLE 5.—*The Composition of Glycolipids with Blood Group Activity*

A activity	Nitrogen	Total reducing sugar	Hexosamine	Sialic acid	Fucose	
Handa and Yamakawa						
E-M[117]	a	38.2[b]	14.5	4.7	2.8	Contained glucose, galactose, glucosamine, and galactosamine.
C-M[117]	a	23.2[b]	9.2	2.5	2.9	
Hakomori and Jeanloz[114]	1.8	44	8–10	a	a	Contained glucose, galactose, galactosamine and very small amounts of glucosamine.
Koscielak[116]						
methanol-insoluble	2.46	43.0	15.8	10.4	1.2	Contained glucose, galactose, glucosamine, and galactosamine.
methanol-soluble	2.48	41.4	12.1	10.9	2.3	
B activity						
Hakomori and Jeanloz[114]	1.89	40	8–10	a	a	Contained glucose, galactose, galactosamine, and very small amounts of glucosamine.
Handa and Yamakawa E-M[117]	a	39.4[b]	12.9	0.8	0.6	Contained glucose, galactose, glucosamine, and galactosamine.

a No value given.

b Reducing sugar value not given; these data represent hexose determinations with a galactose standard.

E-M = Ether-Methanol.

C-M = Chloroform-Methanol.

cysts or hog gastric mucin in precipitin assays or in hemagglutination inhibition[116, 117]. The methanol-soluble and insoluble glycolipids had equal activity in precipitin tests but the latter was 250 times as active in inhibiting hemagglutination. The addition of inactive "carrier" lipid to the methanol-soluble fraction made its activity approximately equal to that of the insoluble material. The latter was not activated by the carrier lipid, and its activity was depressed by mixture with the methanol-soluble fraction[116]. The glycolipids of Hakomori and Jeanloz were relatively less active, but this observation may reflect a failure to achieve optimal assay conditions. Koscielak's A glycolipid possessed Forssman activity, but not H activity, and precipitated with type XIV antipneumococcal serum after treatment with *Trichomonas foetus* enzymes[116]. The A glycolipid of Handa and Yamakawa also had Forssman activity[117].

Watkins, Koscielak, and Morgan have compared the immunological specificity of an A glycolipid with an A substance of ovarian cyst origin[118]. Precipitation of either material by the *Dolichos biflorus* lectin was inhibited by

N-acetylgalactosamine only, and the A-active disaccharide 3-O-α-N-acetyl-galactosaminoyl-D-galactose inhibited the precipitation of either substance by a rabbit anti-A serum. Enzymes present in a partially purified extract of *Trichomonas foetus* destroyed the serological activity of both preparations, and this destruction was inhibited by N-acetylgalactosamine but not by other sugars present in the A substance. Each preparation gave a single precipitin line in agar gel with a rabbit antiserum to human A erythrocytes, and the lines fused completely. The A glycolipid of Handa and Yamakawa gave a single line in agar gel with a rabbit antiserum to human erythrocytes, but the line showed only partial fusion with the band formed by ovarian cyst A substance or by hog gastric mucin[117]. These data, and observations on the parallel enzymatic inactivation of the serological activity of soluble substances and intact erythrocytes[61, 119] indicate that the terminal non-reducing ends of both types of determinant groups are very similar in structure.

IV. Biosynthesis of Blood Group Mucopolysaccharides

Blood group mucopolysaccharides have been treated with specific enzymes to cause the disappearance of one activity and the concomitant appearance of another. Both blood group A and B substances can be altered with loss of A or B activity and appearance of H activity[120-125]. The conversion of A substance into an H-active substance by clostridial enzymes is of especial interest. It has been shown that an initial deacetylation by a purified enzyme, followed by brief exposure to dilute nitrous acid removes the terminal N-acetylgalactosamine and causes the appearance of H activity[61]. Removal of terminal galactose results in the disappearance of B activity concomitant with the appearance of H activity[60, 124].

Similarly, H substance can be inactivated enzymatically with the appearance of Le[a] activity[125, 126]. This conversion is accompanied by the loss of fucose. Le[a] active substance can be converted into a material capable of precipitating with type XIV anti-pneumococcal serum[127]. This latter conversion is also associated with the loss of fucose. These various interconversions are summarized in the following diagram.

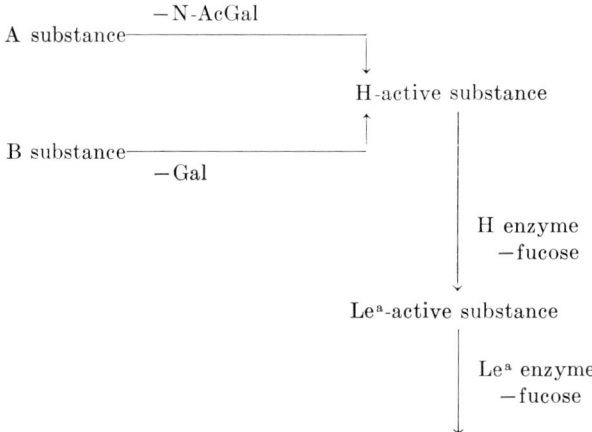

Watkins and Morgan[77, 127-129] and Ceppellini[130] have postulated that in biosynthesis, the reverse sequence of events takes place, and that each step is under genetic control.

The release of galactose from B substance results in the appearance of H activity. Is the H active group the original B determinant minus its terminal α galactosyl residue, or is it an entirely different group which has become accessible? This question can now be answered unambiguously[136]. The dialyzable fraction B_3 does not possess H activity. Treatment with α galactosidase destroys the ability of B_3 to inhibit anti-B and results in the appearance of H activity. After mild acid hydrolysis the α galactosidase-treated B_3 no longer possesses H activity, but will inhibit anti-SXIV (Table 4). Within a small molecule, perhaps no larger than a hexasaccharide, there are at least these three different potential specificities: B, H and cross-reactivity with anti-SXIV. In the light of this observation, one does not have to assume anything more complex than the addition of single sugar residues to mask one activity and to confer a new specificity. These observations answer an objection which had been raised to this biosynthetic scheme. If mild acid hydrolysis removes specifically the antigenic determinants of blood group A and B substances, then the "skeletons" which remain, AP1 and BP1, should not possess different antigenic determinants if they are derived from a common precursor, H substance. The antigenic determinant(s) of BP1 have been thoroughly studied, and found to be different from those of AP1[88]. Both the B and BP1 determinants were shown to possess terminal alpha galactosyl residues, but it was assumed that the BP1 structure was an internal grouping exposed after the removal of the original B determinants. It was demonstrated subsequently, however, that the same galactosyl residue was present in both determinants[136].

All the available data are in accord with the concept that additions of single sugar units confer new specificity on a preexisting molecule. This situation finds parallel in bacterial polysaccharides from streptococci and salmonellas[131-134].

Nature of the cross-reacting antibody in the sera of some O individuals

A fraction of the isohemagglutinins found in certain group O individuals is capable of agglutinating both A and B cells. One such serum has been investigated recently[135]. It was shown that the cross-reacting antibody had a specificity which could best be envisioned as specific for that portion of A_3 and B_3 which is common to both, namely the portion of the molecule not involving carbon 2 of the terminal unit. An examination of the structures postulated for the A and B determinants, A_3 and B_3, (Figure 5) reveals that the major difference between them is the presence of a terminal N-acetylgalactosamine in A and a terminal galactose in B. These two sugars differ only in that the former bears an N-acetyl substituent on carbon 2 in place of an hydroxyl in the latter.

ACKNOWLEDGEMENT

The authors wish to express their gratitude to the many people who have helped in the preparation of this review. In particular, we wish to thank Drs. R. Austrian, D. S. Feingold, R. E. Rosenfield, S. Schlossman, N. M. Abelson, A. J. Rawson, D. K. McCurdy, and G. F. Springer.

REFERENCES

1. Kabat, E. A., *Blood Group Substances*, Academic Press, New York, 1956.
2. Heremans, J. F., Immunochemical studies on protein pathology. The immunoglobulin concept. Clin. Chim. Acta 4: 639, 1959.
3. Heremans, J. F., Les globulines seriques du systeme gamma; leur nature et leur pathologie, Masson et Cie, Paris, 1960.
4. Edelman, G. M., and Benacerraf, B., On structural and functional relations between antibodies and proteins of the gamma-system, Proc. Nat. Acad. Sci. 48: 1035, 1962.
5. Porter, R. R., Gamma-globulin and antibodies, in *The Plasma Proteins*, ed. by Putnam, F., Academic Press, New York, 1960.
6. Kunkel, H. G., Macroglobulins and high molecular weight antibodies, in *The Plasma Proteins*, ed. by Putnam, F., Academic Press, New York, 1960.
7. Franklin, E. C., The structure, function, and significance of the immune globulins, Vox Sang. 7: 1, 1962.
8. Fahey, J. L., Heterogeneity of γ-globulins, Advances in Immunol. 2: 42, 1962.
9. Laurell, A. H. F., Sera from patients with myeloma, macroglobulinemia, and related conditions as studies by ultracentrifugation, Acta Med. Scand. Suppl. 367: 69, 1961.
10. Smith, R. T., Response to active immunization of human infants during the neonatal period, in *Cellular Aspects of Immunity*, Ciba Foundation Symposium, ed. by Wolstenholme, G. E. W., and O'Connor, M., J. and A. Churchill, Ltd., 1960.
11. Bauer, D. C., and Stavitsky, A. B., On the different molecular forms of antibody synthesized by rabbits during the early response to a single injection of protein and cellular antigens, Proc. Nat. Acad. Sci. 47: 1667, 1961.
12. Benedict, A. A., Brown, R. J., and Ayengar, R., Physical properties of antibody to bovine serum albumin as demonstrated by hemagglutination, J. Exp. Med. 115: 195, 1962.
13. Stelos, P., Taliaferro, L. G., and D'Alesandro, P. A., Comparative study of rabbit hemolysins to various antigens, J. Infect. Dis. 108: 113, 1961.
14. LoSpalluto, J., and Miller, W., Jr., The formation of macroglobulin antibodies. I. Studies on adult humans, J. Clin. Inv. 41: 1415, 1962.
15. Fink, C. W., Miller, W. E., Jr., Dorward, B., and LoSpalluto, J., The formation of macroglobulin antibodies. II. Studies on neonatal infants and older children, J. Clin. Inv. 41: 1422, 1962.
16. Uhr, J. W., Dancis, J., Franklin, E. C., Finkelstein, M. S., and Lewis, E. W., The antibody response to bacteriophage ϕX 174 in newborn premature infants, J. Clin. Inv. 41: 1509, 1962.
17. Uhr, J. W., and Finkelstein, M. S., Antibody formation. IV. Formation of rapidly and slowly sedimenting antibodies and immunological memory to bacteriophage ϕX 174, J. Exp. Med. 117: 457, 1963.
18. Bellanti, J. A., Eitzman, D. V., Robbins, J. B., and Smith, R. T., The development of the immune response. Studies on the agglutinin response to Salmonella flagellar antigens in the newborn rabbit, J. Exp. Med. 117: 479, 1963.
19. Bauer, D. C., Mathies, M. J., and Stavitsky, A. B., Sequences of synthesis of γ-1 macroglobulin and γ-2 globulin antibodies during primary and secondary responses to proteins, Salmonella antigens, and phage, J. Exp. Med. 117: 889, 1963.
20. McDuffie, F. C., Kabat, E. A., Allen, P. Z., and Williams, C. A., Jr., An immunochemical study of the relationship of human blood group isoantibodies to γ-1- and γ-2-globulins, J. Immunol. 81: 48, 1958.
21. Abelson, N. M., and Rawson, A. J., Studies of blood group antibodies. I. Fractionation of anti-A and anti-B isohemagglutinins by anion-cation cellulose exchange chromatography, J. Immunol. 82: 435, 1959.
22. Fudenberg, H. H., Kunkel, H. G., and Franklin, E. C., High molecular weight antibodies, Proc. VII Congr. Int. Soc. Blood Transfusion, S. Karger, Basel, p. 522, 1959.
23. Rawson, A. J. and Abelson, N. M., Studies on blood group antibodies. III. Observations on the physicochemical properties of isohemagglutinins and isohemolysins, J. Immunol. 85: 636, 1960.
23a. Rawson, A. J. and Abelson, N. M., Studies on blood group antibodies. VI. The blood group isoantibody activity of γ 1A globulin. In manuscript.
24. Fahey, J. L., and Morrison, E. G., Separation of 6.6S and 18S gamma globulins with isohemagglutinin activity, J. Lab. Clin. Med. 55: 912, 1960.
25. Kochwa, S., Rosenfield, R. E., Tallal, L., and Wasserman, L. R., Isoagglutinins associated with ABO erythroblastosis, J. Clin. Invest. 40: 874, 1961.
26. Yokoyama, M., Finlayson, J. S., Suchinsky, R. T., and Roberts, N. E., Chemical and serological characteristics of blood group antibodies in the ABO and Rh systems, J. Immunol. 87: 56, 1961.
27. Flodin, P., and Killander, J., Fractionation of human-serum proteins by gel filtration, Biochim. Biophys. Acta 63: 403, 1962.
28. Killander, J., and Högman, C. F., Fractionation of human blood group antibodies by gel filtration, Scand. J. Clin. Lab. Invest. 15, Suppl. 69, 1963.
29. Rawson, A. J., and Abelson, N. M., Studies of blood group antibodies, IV. Physiochemical differences between isoanti-A, B and isoanti-A or isoanti-B, J. Immunol. 85: 640, 1960.

30. Polley, M. J., Adinolfi, M., and Mollison, P. L., Serological characteristics of anti-A related to type of antibody protein (7Sγ or 19Sγ), Vox Sang. 8: 385, 1963.
31. Rockey, J. H., and Kunkel, H. G., Unusual sedimentation and sulfhydryl sensitivity of certain isohemagglutinins and skin sensitizing antibody, Proc. Soc. Exp. Biol. & Med. 110: 101, 1962.
32. Kunkel, H. G., and Rockey, J. H., β2A and other immunoglobulins in isolated anti-A antibodies, Proc. Soc. Exp. Biol. & Med. 113: 278, 1963.
33. Speer, R. J., Prager, M. D., Kelley, M. S., and Hill, J. M., Protein fractionation. I. Chromatography of human serum proteins on DEAE-cellulose with special reference to blood group antibodies, J. Lab. Clin. Med. 54: 685, 1959.
34. McDuffie, F. C., and Kabat, E. A., The behavior in the Coombs test of anti-A and anti-B produced by immunization with various blood group A and B substances and by heterospecific pregnancy, J. Immunol. 77: 61, 1956.
35. Muschel, L. H., Osawa, E., and McDermott, D. A., Immune response to blood group A substance, Am. J. Clin. Path. 29: 418, 1958.
36. Owen, R. D., Heterogeneity of antibodies to the human blood groups in normal and immune sera, J. Immunol. 73: 29, 1954.
37. Springer, G. F., Horton, R. E., and Forbes, M., Origin of anti-human blood group B agglutinins in White Leghorn chicks, J. Exp. Med. 110: 221, 1959.
38. Springer, G. F., Inhibition of blood-group agglutinins by substances occurring in plants, J. Immunol. 76: 398, 1956.
39. Pettenkoffer, H. J., Maasen, W., and Bickerich, R., Antigengemeinschaften zwischen menschlichen Blutgruppen und Enterobacteriaceen, Z. Immunitätsforsch. 119: 415, 1960.
40. Springer, G. F., Williamson, P., and Brandes, W. C., Blood group activity of gram-negative bacteria, J. Exp. Med. 113: 1077, 1961.
41. Gonano, F., Modiano, G., and de Andreis, M., Relationships between the somatic antigens of E. coli O$_{86}$B:7 and blood group A and B substances, Vox Sang. 6: 683, 1961.
42. Oliver-Gonzalez, J., Immunological properties of polysaccharides from animal parasites. Ann. Rev. Microbiol. 8: 353, 1954.
43. Muschel, L. H., and Osawa, E., Human blood group substance B and Escherichia coli B 086. Proc. Soc. Exp. Biol. & Med. 101: 614, 1959.
44. Iseki, S., Onuki, E., and Kashiwagi, K., Relationship between somatic antigen and blood group substance, especially B substance of bacterium. Gunma J. Med. Sci. 7: 7, 1958.
45. Young, V. M., Sochard, M. R., Gillem, H., and Ross, S., Infectious agents in infant diarrhea. II. Serological reactions with E. coli 01 through 025, Proc. Soc. Exp. Biol. & Med. 105: 638, 1960.
46. Young, V. M., Gillem, H. C., and Akeroyd, J. H., Sensitization of infant red cells by bacterial polysaccharides of Escherichia coli during enteritis, J. Pediatrics 60: 172, 1962.
47. Makela, O., Studies in hemagglutinins of leguminosae seeds. Academic Dissertation, University of Helsinki, Helsinki, 1957.
48. Makela, O., Structures on the red cell surface reacting with lectins, Proc. 8th Congr. Int. Soc. Blood Transf., S. Karger, Basel, p. 251, 1962.
49. Bhatia, N. M., and Boyd, W. C., Inhibition reactions of fourteen "nonspecific" seed extracts, Transfusion 2: 106, 1962.
50. Watkins, W. M., and Morgan, W. T. J., Further observations on the inhibition of blood-group specific serological reactions by simple sugars of known structure, Vox Sang. 7: 129, 1962.
51. Springer, G. F., and Williamson, P., Limitations of heterologous reagents in the elucidation of blood group H(O) specific structures, Vox Sang. 8: 177, 1963.
52. Lisowska, E., Reaction of erythrocyte mucoproteins with anti-N from phytoagglutinins from Vicia graminea seeds, Nature 198: 865, 1963.
53. Springer, G. F., and Hotta, K., Blood group N specificity and sialic acid, Fed. Proc. 22: 539, 1963.
54. Kabat, E. A., The upper limit for the size of the human antidextran combining site: J. Immunol. 84: 82, 1960.
55. Kabat, E. A., Kabat and Mayer's Experimental Immunochemistry, Charles C Thomas, Inc., Springfield, Illinois, 2nd edition, 1961.
56. Schlossman, S. F., and Kabat, E. A., Specific fractionation of antidextran molecules with combining sites of various sizes. J. Exp. Med. 116: 535, 1962.
57. Kabat, E. A., and Leskowitz, S., Immunochemical studies on blood groups. XVII. Structural units involved in blood group specificity, J. Am. Chem. Soc. 77: 5159, 1955.
58. Marcus, D. M., Kabat, E. A., and Rosenfield, R. E., The action of enzymes from Clostridium tertium on the I antigenic determinant of human erythrocytes, J. Exp. Med. 118: 175, 1963.
59. Morgan, W. T. J., Some immunochemical aspects of the products of the human blood group genes, in Biochemistry of Human Genetics, Ciba Foundation Symposium, ed. by Wolstenholme, G. E. W. and O'Connor, C. M., Little, Brown and Co., 1959.

60. Zarnitz, M. L., and Kabat, E. A., Immunochemical studies on blood groups. XXV. The action of coffee bean α galactosidase on blood group B and BP1 substances, J. Am. Chem. Soc. 82: 3953, 1960.
61. Marcus, D. M., Kabat, E. A., and Schiffman, G., Immunochemical studies on blood groups. XXXI. Destruction of blood group A activity by an enzyme from *Clostridium tertium* which deacetylates N-acetylgalactosamine in intact blood group substances, Biochemistry 3: 437, 1964.
62. Morgan, W. T. J., Some observations on the structure and properties of the blood group specific mucopolysaccharides, in *International Symposium on Biologically Active Mucoids*, Polish Academy of Science, p. 1, Warsaw, 1959.
63. Klenk, E., and Gielen, W., Zur Kenntnis der Ganglioside des Gehirns, Zeit. physiol. Chem. 319: 283, 1960.
64. Egge, H., On the structure of ganglioside 2 from ox-brain/ of some acid oligosaccharides from human milk/ and a new method of methylation, Bull. Soc. Chim. Biol. 42: 1429, 1960.
65. Trams, E. G., and Lauter, C. J., On the isolation and characterization of gangliosides, Biochim. Biophys. Acta 60: 350, 1962.
66. Gammack, D. B., Physicochemical properties of ox-brain gangliosides, Biochem. J. 88: 373, 1963.
67. Hamasoto, Y., The blood group substance in red blood cells. First report. A search for the group (A,B,O)-specific substance in the lipid fragment. Tohoku J. Exp. Med. 52: 17, 1950.
68. Koscielak, J., Reversible inactivation of blood-group A and B substances from red cells, Nature 194: 751, 1962.
69. Rapport, M. M., Lipid-lipid interactions and relation of function to structures of membranes, in *Ultrastructure and Metabolism of the Nervous System*, vol. XL: Research publications, Association for Research in Nervous and Mental Disease, 1962, p. 159.
70. Papirmeister, B., and Mallette, M. F., The isolation and some properties of the Forssman hapten from sheep erythrocytes, Arch. Biochem. & Biophys. 57: 94, 1955.
71. Rapport, M. M., Graf, L., Skipski, V., and Alonzo, N. F., Immunochemical studies of organ and tumor lipids. VI. Isolation and properties of cytolipin H. Cancer 12: 438, 1959.
72. Rapport, M. M., Structure and specificity of lipid haptens of animal cells. J. Lipid Research 2: 25, 1961.
73. Koscielak, J., and Zakrzewski, K., Substance from erythrocytes of blood group A. Nature 187: 516, 1960.
74. Morgan, W. T. J., and Van Heyningen, R., The occurrence of A, B and O blood group substances in pseudo-mucinous ovarian cyst fluids. Brit. J. Exper. Path. 25: 5, 1944.
75. Morgan, W. T. J., Mucopolysaccharides associated with blood group specificity, in Ciba Foundation Symposium "Chemistry and Biology of Mucopolysaccharides". J. and A. Churchill Ltd. London: p. 200–211, 1958.
76. Kabat, E. A., Immunochemical approaches to polysaccharide and mucopolysaccharide structure in Ciba Foundation Symposium "Chemistry and Biology of Mucopolysaccharides". J. and A. Churchill Ltd. London: p. 42–60, 1958.
77. Morgan, W. T. J., A contribution to human biochemical genetics; the chemical basis of blood group specificity. Proc. Royal Soc. London Ser B 151: 308, 1960.
78. Yosizawa, Z., Biochemical studies on blood group mucopolysaccharides, in "Biochemistry and Medicine of Mucopolysaccharides," Muruzen Co. Ltd. Tokyo: p. 117, 1962.
79. Kabat, E. A., Antigenic determinants of dextrans and blood group substances, Fed. Proc. 21: 694, 1962.
80. Morgan, W. T. J., Some observations on the carbohydrate-containing components of human ovarian cyst mucin. N. Y. Acad. Sci. 106: 177, 1963.
81. Stahl, A. J. C., The structure of the specific substance of blood groups. Biol. Med. 52: 283, 1963.
82. Odin, L., Studies on the chemistry of ovarian cyst contents. Acta Soc. Med. Upsaliensis 64: 25, 1959.
83. Dische, Z., Reciprocal relation between fucose and sialic acid in mammalian glycoproteins. Ann. N.Y. Acad. Sci. 106: 259, 1963.
84. Pusztai, A. and Morgan, W. T. J., Studies in immunochemistry 18. The isolation and properties of a sialomucopolysaccharide possessing blood-group Le^a specificity and virus-receptor activity, Biochem. J. 78: 135, 1961.
85. Carsten, M. E. and Kabat, E. A., Immunochemical studies on blood groups. XIX. The amino acids of blood group substances. J. Am. Chem. Soc. 78: 3083, 1956.
86. Schiffman, G., Kabat, E. A. and Leskowitz, S., Immunochemical studies on blood groups XXVI. The isolation of oligosaccharides from human ovarian cyst blood group A substances including two disaccharides and a trisaccharide involved in the specificity of the blood group A antigenic determinant. J. Am. Chem. Soc. 84: 73, 1963.
87. Schiffman, G., Kabat, E. A. and Thompson, W., Immunochemical studies on blood group XXX. Cleavage of A, B and H blood group substances by alkali. Biochem. 3: 113, 1964.
88. Allen, P. Z. and Kabat, E. A., Immunochemical studies on blood groups. XXII. Immuno-

chemical studies on the nondialyzable residue from partially hydrolyzed blood group A, B and O(H) substances (P1 fractions). J. Immunol. 82: 340, 1959.

89. Schiffman, G., Kabat, E. A. and Thompson, W., Immunochemical studies on blood groups XXVII. Periodate oxidation of blood group A, B and O(H) substances. J. Am. Chem. Soc. 84: 463, 1962.

90. Hashimoto, Y., Tsuiki, S., Nisizawa, K. and Pigman, W., Action of proteolytic enzymes on purified bovine submaxillary mucin. Ann. N.Y. Acad. Sci. 106: 233, 1963.

91. Kathan, R. H. and Winzler, R. J., Structure studies on the myxovirus hemagglutination inhibitor of human erythrocytes. J. Biol. Chem. 238: 21, 1963.

92. Howe, C., Avrameas, S., DeVaux St. Cyr, C., Grabar, P. and Lee, L. T., Antigenic components of human erythrocytes. J. Immunol. 91: 683, 1963.

93. Koscielak, J. and Zakrzewski, K.: Blood group ABO substances from red cells, in *International Symposium on Biologically Active Mucoids*, Polish Academy of Science, Warsaw, 1959.

94. Morgan, W. T. J., Nature and occurrence of blood group substances. Brit. Med. Bull. 2: 165, 1944.

95. Morgan, W. T. J., Blood group substances: Biochem. J. 40: xv, 1946.

96. Aminoff, D., Morgan, W. T. J., and Watkins, W. M., Studies in Immunochemistry 11. The action of dilute alkali on the N-acetylhexosamines and the specific blood group mucoids. Biochem. J. 51: 379, 1952.

97. Knox, K. W. and Morgan, W. T. J., The alkaline degradation of the human blood group substances. Biochem. J., 58: v, 1954.

98. Anderson, B., Hoffman, P. and Meyer, K., A serine-linked peptide of chondroitin sulfate. Biochim. Biophys. Acta 74: 309, 1963.

99. Morgan, W. T. J. and Watkins, W. M., The inhibition of the haemagglutinins in plant seeds by human blood group substances and simple sugars. Brit. J. Exp. Path. 34: 94, 1953.

100. Watkins, W. M. and Morgan, W. T. J., Inhibition by simple sugars of enzymes which decompose the blood-group substances. Nature 175: 676, 1955.

101. Watkins, W. M. and Morgan, W. T. J., Neutralization of the anti-H agglutinin in eel serum by simple sugars. Nature 168: 829, 1952.

102. Morgan, W. T. J., Presentation at IX Congress of International Society of Blood Transfusion. Mexico, Sept. 5–12, 1962.

103. Schiffman, G. and Kabat, E. A., Oligosaccharides of blood group A substances, Fed. Proc. 20: 67, 1961.

104. Cheese, I. A. F. L. and Morgan, W. T. J., Two serologically active trisaccharides isolated from human blood group A substance. Nature 191: 149, 1961.

105. Painter, T. J., Watkins, W. M. and Morgan, W. T. J., Isolation of two serologically active trisaccharides from human blood group B substance. Nature 199: 282, 1963.

106. Painter, T. J., Water-soluble polystyrene sulfonic acid as a catalyst in the controlled fragmentation of very labile polysaccharides. Chem. and Ind.: 1214, 1960.

107. Yosizawa, Z. and Sato, T., Hydrazinolysis of simple polysaccharides. Tohoku J. Exper. Med., 76: 100, 1962.

108. Yosizawa, Z., 2-amino sugar-containing oligosaccharides isolated from hydrazinolyzate of blood group A mucopolysaccharide of hog gastric mucus I and II. J. Biochem. (Japan) 51: 1, 145, 1962.

109. Yosizawa, Z. and Sato, T., Hydrazinolysis of blood group A mucopolysaccharide of hog gastric mucus. J. Biochem. (Japan) 51: 233, 1962.

110. Schiffman, G., Kabat, E. A. and Leskowitz, S., Immunochemical studies on blood groups. XXIV. some oligosaccharides isolated from dialysates after mild acid hydrolysis of human blood group B substances from ovarian cyst fluid. J. Am. Chem. Soc. 82: 1122, 1960.

111. Radin, N. S., Discussion, glycolipid chromatography, Fed. Proc. 16: 285, 1957.

112. Yamakawa, T., Irie, R., and Iwanaga, M., The chemistry of lipid of posthemolytic residue or stroma of erythrocytes. IX. Silicic acid chromatography of mammalian stroma glycolipids, J. Biochem. 48: 490, 1960.

113. Yamakawa, T., and Irie, R., On the mucolipid nature of ABO-group substance of erythrocytes, J. Biochem. 48: 919, 1960.

114. Hakomori, S., and Jeanloz, R. W., Isolation and characterization of glycolipids from erythrocytes of human blood A (plus) and B (plus), J. Biol. Chem. 236: 2827, 1961.

115. Koscielak, J., Reversible inactivation of blood-group A and B substances from red cells, Nature 194: 751, 1962.

116. Koscielak, J., Blood group A-specific glycolipids from human erythrocytes, Biochim. Biophys. Acta. 78: 313, 1963.

117. Handa, S., Blood group active glycolipid from human erythrocytes. Japan J. Exper. Med. 33: 347, 1963.

118. Watkins, W. M., Koscielak, J., and Morgan, W. T. J., The relationship between the specificity of the blood-group A and B substances isolated from erythrocytes and from secretions, Proc. IX Cong. Int. Soc. of Blood Transfusion, Mexico City, 1962, (in press).

119. Iseki, S., Changes in group-specific activity in human red cells caused by group sub-

stance-decomposing enzymes, Proc. Eighth Cong. European Soc. Haematol., S. Karger, Basel, 1962, p. 488.

120. Iseki, S. and Masaki, S., Transformation of blood group substance by bacterial enzyme. Proc. Jap. Acad. 29: 460, 1953.

121. Iseki, S. and Ikeda, T., On bacterial enzyme specificity decomposing group B substance. Proc. Jap. Acad. 32: 201, 1956.

122. Iseki, S., Furukawa, K. and Kamamoto, S., B-substance-decomposing enzyme produced by an anaerobic bacterium, Proc. Jap. Acad. 35: 507, 513, 1959.

123. Watkins, W. M., The appearance of H specificity following the enzymic inactivation of blood group substance. Biochem. J. 64: 21P, 1956.

124. Watkins, W. M., Zarnitz, M. L., and Kabat, E. A., Development of H activity by human blood-group B substance treated with coffee bean α galactosides. Nature 195: 1204, 1962.

125. Watkins, W. M., Changes in the specificity of blood-group mucopolysaccharides induced by enzymes from *Trichomonas foetus*. Immunol. 5: 245, 1962.

126. Watkins, W. M., Changes in blood group specificity induced by enzymes. Bull. Soc. Chim. Biol. (Par) 42: 1599, 1960.

127. Watkins, W. M., The serological inactivation of the human blood-group substances by an enzyme preparation obtained from *Trichomonas foetus*. Biochem. J. 54: xxxiii, 1963.

128. Watkins, W. M. and Morgan, W. T. J., Possible genetical pathways for the biosynthesis of blood group mucopolysaccharides Vox Sang. 4: 97, 1959.

129. Watkins, W. M., Some genetical aspects of the biosynthesis of human blood group substances. Ciba Foundation Symposium "Biochemistry of Human Genetics." p. 217 Churchill, London/Little, Brown, Boston, 1959.

130. Ceppellini, R., Physiological genetics of human blood factors, in Ciba Foundation Symposium "Biochemistry of Human Genetics", p. 242, (Churchill, London/Little, Brown, Boston, 1959).

131. McCarty, M., Variation in the group-specific carbohydrate of group A streptococci. J. Exper. Med. 104: 629, 1956.

132. Robbins, P. W. and Uchida, T., Studies on the chemical basis of the phage conversion of O-antigens in the E-group of Salmonellae, Biochem. 1: 323, 1962.

133. Robbins, P. W. and Uchida, T., Determinants of specificity in Salmonella: Changes in antigenic structure mediated by bacteriophage. Fed. Proc. 21: 702, 1962.

134. Uchida, T., Robbins, P. W. and Luria, S. E. Analysis of the serologic determinant groups of the Salmonella E-group O-antigens. Biochemistry 2: 663, 1963.

135. Schiffman, G. and Howe, C., Specificity of AB-cross reacting antibody, presented at American Society of Hematology, Washington, D.C., December 9–10, 1963.

136. Schiffman, G., Kabat, E. A. and Thompson, W., Immunochemical studies on blood groups. XXXII. Immunochemical properties of and possible partial structures for the blood group A, B and H antigenic determinants. Biochem. in press.

137. Rege, V. P., Painter, T. J., Watkins, W. M. and Morgan, W. T. J., Three new trisaccharides obtained from human blood group A, B, H and Le[a] substances: possible sugar sequences in the carbohydrate chains. Nature 200: 532, 1963.

Lead Poisoning: Hematologic Aspects

─────────ROBERT C. GRIGGS─────────

Hematologic alterations have been recognized for many years as prominent manifestations of chronic lead poisoning. These include basophilic stippling of the erythrocytes, anemia, changes in red blood cell fragilities, and abnormal porphyrin excretion. More recently shortened red cell survival, abnormal intracellular iron metabolism, changes in the hemoglobin molecule and specific defects in the biosynthesis of heme have been demonstrated. It is the purpose of this review to present the information available at the present time concerning the structural and metabolic alterations that lead produces in the human red blood cell and to discuss the causes and consequences of such effects.

Historically, clinical lead poisoning has been recognized for centuries. The first description of the disease is attributed to Hippocrates in 370 B.C., who described an attack of colic in a man who extracted metals. The associated anemia was probably first recognized and described by Laennec in 1831. Malassey in 1873 also described the anemia and how the red blood cells were larger and more brittle than normal. The abnormal excretion of porphyrins was observed by Garrod in 1892, and in 1899 Behrend first reported erythrocytic stippling[2, 3]. Readers interested in a more extensive review of the history of lead poisoning are referred to the classic paper of Aub, Fairhill, Minot and Reznikoff[2] published in 1925 and for a more recent review of the toxicology and metabolism of lead, to the review by Kehoe[44, 45, 46].

Despite the extensive knowledge of the cause and prevention of lead poisoning many cases are still seen. These occur in adults from industrial exposure or accidents, and in children because of the ingestion of non-food items from their environments which contain lead usually derived from lead paint. In any large city with old, poorly maintained housing a significant number of children are seen each year with lead poisoning and many more children can be found with subclinical manifestations of increased lead ingestion[31]. It is unusual today to encounter cases caused by lead-contaminated drinking water and wine or due to burning old battery casings for household heating. However, in some areas lead poisoning due to the consumption of lead-contaminated illicit whiskey[12, 16] is still seen. This is not a new problem since Benjamin Franklin[69] noted in 1768 that the "dry belly-ache" was common among punch drinkers and was caused by the use of leaden worms for the distilling of rum. The clinical manifestations of plumbism usually consist of abdominal pain and possibly peripheral nerve involvement in adults and central nervous system involvement in children as manifested by varying degrees of lead encephalopathy.

From the Department of Medicine of Western Reserve University School of Medicine, at Cleveland Metropolitan General Hospital, Cleveland, Ohio.

Supported in part by Public Health Service Research Grant OH 00064, from the Division of Occupational Health.

TABLE I.—*Hematological Values in Chronic Lead Poisoning*
20 Male Adults

	RBC million/cmm	Hgb Gm. %	Hct %	MCV μ^3	MCHC Gm/100 ml	Retics %	Stippled Cells %	Icterus Index
Average	4.21	10.7	35	79	31	4.4	1.8	6.5
Range	3.45–5.36	8.1–12.8	28.8–43	70–92	27–36	1.5–11.6	0.1–7.5	4–10

ROUTINE BLOOD VALUES

The routine hematological values in 20 male adults with chronic lead poisoning from industrial exposure are presented in Table I. They illustrate the mild to moderate microcytic hypochromic anemia, the abnormal number of stippled cells and increased reticulocytes which tend to develop in the adult with lead poisoning[12, 23]. In children the disease is often associated with a more pronounced microcytic, hypochromic anemia and with abnormally low serum iron values[76]. Since nutritional iron deficiency of children has its highest incidence at the same age as lead poisoning, it is usually assumed that the diseases are coincidental, although it has been postulated that the nutritional anemia may predispose to pica or in some manner augment the effect of lead. However, microcytic hypochromic anemia is also seen in children with lead poisoning with normal or elevated serum iron values[51]. In adults serum iron values are usually within the normal range[12]. In general, there is no consistent correlation between degree of anemia, number of stippled cells, or reticulocytosis.

ERYTHROCYTE STIPPLING

The enumeration of stippled erythrocytes in the peripheral blood has been used for many years as a simple and inexpensive method of evaluating the exposure of an individual to lead. Stippling is generally considered an unreliable criterion of lead intoxication since the number of stippled cells does not correlate well with the intensity of exposure. Lead poisoning is seen in patients without stippled red cells, and stippled cells can be found in increased numbers in a variety of hematologic disorders, e.g. various hemolytic anemias, leukemia and after exposure to benzene, aniline, carbon monoxide, arsenic, copper and bismuth[33]. At best stippling should be used as an indication to look more closely for other signs of lead intoxication.

Key[48], McFadzean and Davis[57] and Pirrie[59] have demonstrated in animal experiments that stippled red cells in the peripheral blood were readily and rapidly produced by the administration of lead to rabbits and guinea pigs, but interestingly could not be produced in chickens and cats. They found that the developing erythrocytes were initially affected in the bone marrow since stippling could be seen in the normoblasts during all stages of hemoglobinization. The number of stippled cells was invariably higher in the bone marrow than in the peripheral blood of intact animals; however, after removal of the spleen the number of stippled cells increased in the peripheral blood although there was no change in the bone marrow stippling. The anemia which developed in these lead-poisoned animals was relieved by splenectomy. A variable portion of the basophilic granules gave a positive reaction when stained for iron; granules stained positive for iron with increased frequency after the spleen had been removed. Beritic[8] has recently re-emphasized that in human lead poisoning there are two distinct types of basophilic granulations, since only some give a positive reaction on staining for iron. Bessis and Breton-Gorius[9, 11], using the electron microscope, have demonstrated that in lead poisoning the erythroblasts and erythrocytes present numerous dispersed ferritin molecules or masses of ferritin molecules and characteristic alteration of the erythroblast mitochondria. The mitochondria were all enormous and their cristae were empty. No iron was seen within the mitochondria. Some confusion has arisen over the interpretation of the electron microscopic studies of Bessis in lead poisoning. One report by Bessis and Breton-Gorius[10] has been interpreted to indicate that there is accumulation of ferritin granules in erythroblast mitochondria[12]. However, more recent information[11*] makes it clear that in lead poisoning no iron is found within the mitochondria.

Stippled red cells have an active oxidative energy-producing metabolism. Baikie and Valtis[4] found the oxygen consumption of the stippled cells in lead-poisoned guinea pigs to be as high as that of the reticulocytes produced by bleeding or hemolytic anemia, indicating that the stippled cell is a young cell, since oxygen consumption is negligible in mature red cells.

The information available at present suggests, therefore, that the granulations seen in the erythrocytes of lead-poisoned patients and animals are of two types; one, ferritin deposits or accumulations of excessive iron unusable for hemoglobin formation which give a positive staining reaction for iron, and two, granules which are enlarged and presumedly damaged mitochondria that do not contain iron and, therefore, do not give a positive staining reaction for iron. The fate of these stippled red cells is unknown. The animal experiments cited above indicate that the spleen plays a role in regulating the number of stippled cells in the peripheral blood. Bessis[11] has suggested that the spleen removes these cells from the circulation and matures the cells by some unknown mechanism or removes the granules by a mechanism analogous to that demonstrated by Crosby[15] for red cells with siderocytic granules.

ERYTHROCYTE FRAGILITY

Changes in osmotic and mechanical fragility of the red cells are common in patients with lead poisoning and comparable changes can be produced in vitro by the incubation of normal red blood cells with lead: an increased resistance of the leaded cells to osmotic lysis, and an increased susceptibility of the cells to standard mechanical trauma. The range of these changes are graphically depicted in Figure 1 using the data from ten adult patients in whom red blood cell fragility was measured in our laboratory. The osmotic fragility of unincubated whole blood is only slightly altered from the normal, but in all instances the change was toward increased resistance to the hypotonic sodium chloride solutions. After 24 hours of sterile incubation at 37°C normal erythrocytes are more susceptible to osmotic lysis, the cell population showing a uniform increase in osmotic fragility. All ten cases of lead poisoning showed either

* Personal communication, 1963.

a) increased resistance to lysis after incubation, b) a decrease in resistance which was less than expected for the normal, or c) a combination of these in which some cells apparently became more resistant and some less resistant to osmotic stress. In no case was the osmotic fragility after incubation normal.

Mechanical fragility studies were performed on the same ten patients (Figure 1). The average unincubated mechanical fragility did not differ significantly

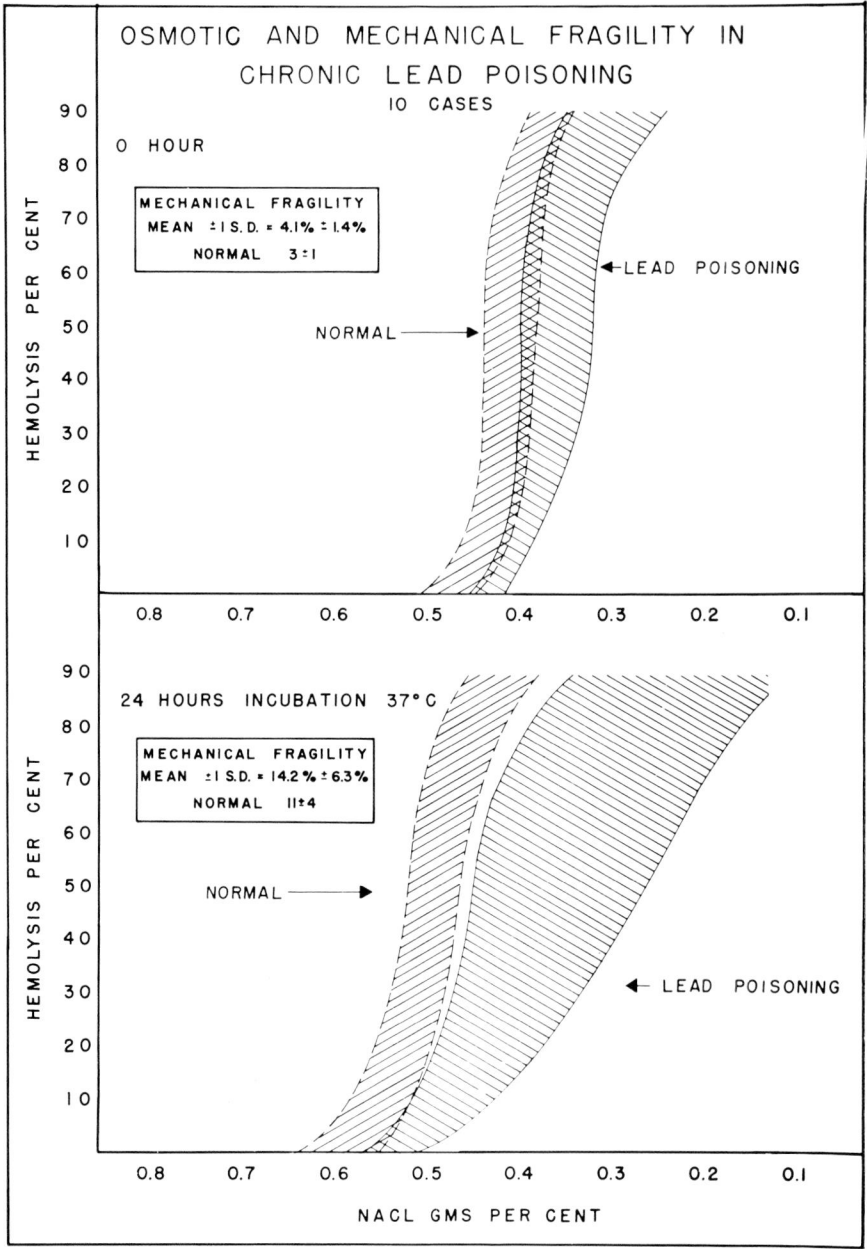

FIG. 1.—Osmotic and mechanical fragility studies in 10 men with lead poisoning from industrial exposure. The ranges are the mean plus or minus one standard deviation.

from the normal range. After 24 hours of incubation the red blood cells from six patients showed an increase in fragility that was within the normal range; four patients showed more than normal increases in fragility, 16.5%, 22.2%, 18.7% and 26% (normal 10.5% ± 3.5%).

In six patients repeat osmotic and mechanical fragility studies were performed during and after therapy with the chelating agent, ethylene diaminetetraacetate (EDTA). Usually during the course of therapy the patients' red blood cells became even more resistant to osmotic lysis and more susceptible to mechanical lysis. After therapy and with time the fragility tests gradually returned to normal. No consistent correlation was found between degree of anemia, stippled cells, reticulocytosis and alterations in mechanical and osmotic fragility.

Aub and associates[2] demonstrated the effect of lead on normal human red blood cells in vitro and showed that lead poisoning in rabbits produced similar increases in resistance of the red cells to lysis by hypotonic saline. Furthermore, the addition of lead chloride to normal human red blood cells suspended in autologous serum or isotonic saline is followed by an increase in the mechanical fragility of the cells and a decrease in susceptibility to osmotic lysis[35]. Four such studies of human erythrocytes suspended in serum and exposed to a concentration of 2.8 mg per cent lead are shown in Figure 2. The results are similar to the changes noted in patients with lead poisoning. Serum seems to protect somewhat against this effect of lead, since concentrations of lead which have no effect upon red cells suspended in serum will produce changes in the fragilities of red cells suspended in saline. The addition of EDTA to the lead chloride solution prior to the addition of the latter to the red blood cell suspensions protects the cells. The molar concentration of EDTA must be three times that of the lead to afford complete protection to the cells. Despite the effect of lead upon the red blood cell fragilities, the addition of lead salts to suspensions of erythrocytes in vitro does not cause the appearance of stippling. Shrinking of red blood cells does occur, however, as indicated by a fall in mean corpuscular volume and increase in mean corpuscular hemoglobin concentration. Objections can be raised to the applicability of these in vitro studies to clinical problems, because the minimum concentration of lead ion that causes changes in the fragilities after incubation in vitro is 1.5 mg per cent when the cells are suspended in serum. This concentration is much above the concentrations present in the blood of patients with lead poisoning. However, recent data have revealed that the concentration of lead in the bone marrow is considerably higher than in the peripheral blood[77]. In one group of patients the blood lead levels ranged from 0.07 to 0.13 mg per cent and the bone marrow lead levels from 4.2 to 9.2 mg per cent. The latter figures are comparable to the concentration necessary to produce changes in the red blood cells in vitro.

Osmotic and mechanical fragility measurements demonstrate alterations in the morphology and permeability of the erythrocyte membrane, but the exact mechanisms of lysis and the effects of incubation are not completely understood. The increased resistance to osmotic lysis seen in both the in vivo and in vitro experiments indicates that more water could enter the cell before the critical spherical form was reached and lysis occurred. The decrease in mean

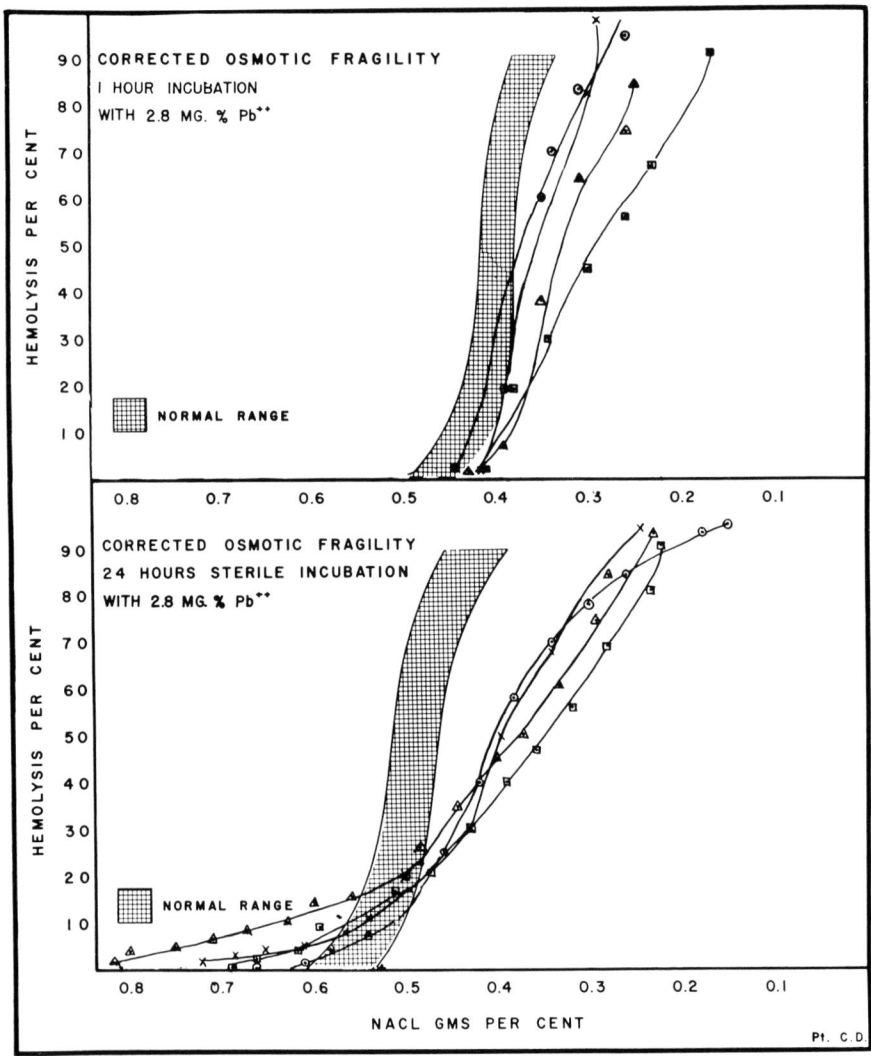

F_IG. 2.—Osmotic fragility changes produced in normal human red blood cells by incubation with lead for one hour and 24 hours.

corpuscular volume, the increase in mean corpuscular hemoglobin concentration, and the increase in specific gravity indicate that the leaded cells are shrunken and therefore have a greater capacity for swelling in hypotonic solutions. It has also been shown that the treatment of human erythrocytes with lead results in a leak of potassium ions from the cell apparently by interfering with the energy-requiring "pump"[41, 73]. In view of the described changes, the characterization by Aub[2] of the red cell in lead poisoning as "contracted, relatively inelastic and brittle", seems quite appropriate.

H_EMOGLOBIN E_LECTROPHORESIS

Electrophoresis has demonstrated an abnormal minor hemoglobin component in some children with lead poisoning, which may represent an increase in hemoglobin A_3[72, 55]*. On filter paper at pH 8.6 it is a faster moving fraction than normal A hemoglobin, but does not separate well from A and probably represents less than 15 per cent of the total hemoglobin. On agar gel, at pH 6.0, this fraction does not separate from hemoglobin A. It apparently is seen in approximately 50 per cent of children with lead poisoning, does not correlate well with the blood lead level, and disappears as the child recovers. Animal experimentation has failed to produce a similar change in hemoglobin.

Red Blood Cell Survival

The mechanism of the anemia of lead poisoning has been debated for many years. Aub[2] reviewed the earlier work in this field and concluded that the anemia was primarily hemolytic. This conclusion was supported by the observations that the bone marrow was usually hypercellular in cases of lead poisoning, that the reticulocytes of the peripheral blood were increased in number, and that increased amounts of the breakdown products of bilirubin metabolism were found in the stool and urine. The work of McFadzean and Davis[57] and of Pirrie[59] with lead-poisoned animals further supported the concept of a hemolytic process since the anemia in such animals was rapid in onset, associated with increased excretion of urobilinogen, and less marked if the spleen was removed. In the experimental animals the anemia was not improved by the administration of ACTH or cortisone although the reticulocytes did increase in number[5].

Sheets and associates[68] studied, by the Ashby technique, the rate of destruction of red blood cells from a patient with lead poisoning after transfusion into a normal recipient. The cells from the patient with lead poisoning were destroyed at an increased rate and apparently destroyed randomly. Fifty per cent of the cells had disappeared in approximately 25 days, compared to a normal half-time of survival by this technique of 55 to 60 days. In our laboratory red cell autosurvival studies have been performed on four adult males with lead poisoning[30]. These were done using the chromium 51 method which gives a half-life of 27–34 days when uncorrected for elution of the radioactive label. The resulting survival curves are shown in Figure 3. Two of the patients had no anemia and two had a very slight reduction in hemoglobin levels. The half-lives of the labeled cells were 20, 20, 25 and 29 days, demonstrating a slight to moderate shortening of red blood cell life span in three of the four patients. Rubino, Prato and Fiorina[62] have reported the most thorough study of erythrocyte survival in lead poisoning. In eight patients the autosurvival of chromium 51 labeled red cells ranged from 12 to 27 days. The labeled red blood cells of three of these patients were also transfused into compatible normal recipients; a short life span was demonstrated which was similar to that in the donor's circulation. Three carefully studied adult cases of anemia due to chronic lead poisoning reported by Hutchison and Stark[37] are of considerable interest. All three patients had a moderate microcytic, hypochromic anemia, elevated reticulocytes (7.5, 5.5 and 22%), normal or elevated serum iron levels with increased bone marrow iron, and increased excretion of urobilinogen in the urine and stool. Haptoglobin levels were normal and the chromium 51 red

---

* Conley, personal communication.

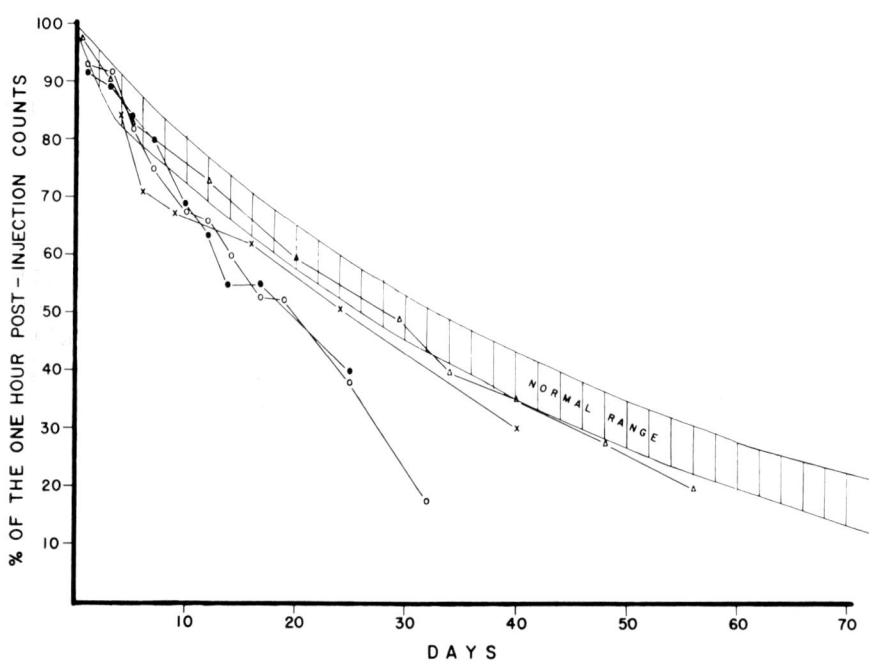

FIG. 3.—Autosurvival of Cr[51] labeled erythrocytes in four men with lead poisoning.

blood cell survival studies were normal in two patients (half-time of survival 26 and 32 days) and shortened to 18 days in the third patient.

Leikin and Eng[51] have recently reported the erythrocyte survival in children with chronic lead poisoning. All children studied had good clinical and laboratory evidence of lead poisoning and did not have concurrent iron deficiency. Red blood cell half-life was shortened in five of seven patients studied using the chromium 51 method; the range was from 13 to 28 days, with a normal range of 25 to 28 days for children by their method. The most pronounced shortening of cell survival was seen in the children with a relatively short history of lead intoxication.

The survival of normal red blood cells exposed to lead in vitro and then returned to the donor's circulation has also been measured[22]. Four survival curves of this type are shown in Figure 4. The cells, labeled with chromium 51, were incubated in vitro for one hour with 2.8 mg% lead. As shown in Figure 2 this amount of lead produced typical changes in the osmotic fragility of these cells. In two cases the survival of these "leaded" cells was moderately shortened. In three similar experiments by Rubino, Prato and Fiorina[62], normal red blood cells, incubated in vitro with lead and reinfused into the normal donor, were found to have a shortened survival.

The above discussion has been confined to patients with chronic lead poisoning. However, the acute administration of large amounts of lead to an individual accidentally, with suicidal intent[42], or therapeutically as was done

AUTOSURVIVAL IN NORMAL SUBJECTS OF Cr⁵¹ LABELED

ERYTHROCYTES TREATED WITH 2.8mg% Pb⁺⁺

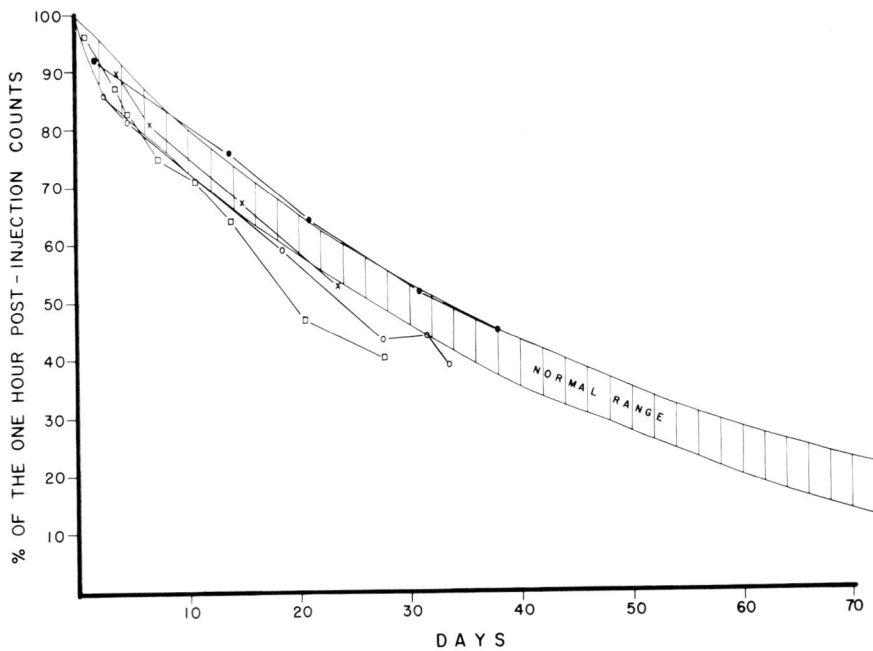

FIG. 4.—Autosurvival in normal adults of Cr⁵¹ labeled erythrocytes incubated in vitro with lead.

at one time in the therapy of cancer[27] can result in the sudden development of anemia. The rapidity of fall in the hemoglobin level, with elevated bilirubin levels and increase in reticulocytes indicates that the anemia is, at least initially, of hemolytic origin. No information on the mechanism of this acute hemolytic process is available but the situation may be analogous to the in vitro exposure of human red cells to a relatively large amount of lead; some permanent damage is apparently produced in the cells leading to an increased rate of destruction when they are retransfused into the circulation.

Coombs' Test

Sutherland and Eisentraut[70] have shown that a positive direct Coombs' test can be found in patients with lead poisoning, if the red cells are separated properly. They studied acute lead intoxication in dogs and noted that, when samples of blood were allowed to sediment, the top fraction of red blood cells containing reticulocytes and stippled cells could be agglutinated with Coombs' serum. Similar results were noted in a group of asymptomatic men with industrial exposure to lead. Crutcher[16] found a positive Coombs' test in three of eight adults with lead poisoning. Jandl and Simmons[38] have found that many multivalent metallic cations, lead included, will produce agglutination of human red blood cells, and that several of these cations possessed the ability to attach proteins to the erythrocyte surface rendering them agglutinable with

Coombs' serum. Lead was not included in this latter group, however. In a later study Jandl[40] reported that the immature red blood cells of man, rabbits and rats are agglutinated by Coombs' serum, which would indicate that the surfaces of these cells contained protein not present on the mature erythrocytes. The increased number and concentration of these sensitized red blood cells, reticulocytes and stippled cells, in the top layer of sedimented blood specimens probably provides an explanation for the positive direct Coombs' test in lead poisoning.

Iron Metabolism

There is no evidence at present that lead interferes with iron absorption, transport of iron by the iron binding protein of the plasma, iron storage, or transfer of the iron from protein to developing red blood cells. Evidence, however, is available which suggests that lead interferes with the intracellular metabolism of iron and the incorporation of iron into protoporphyrin during the synthesis of heme. Jandl, Inman, Simmons, and Allen[39] studied the transfer of iron from human iron binding protein to immature mammalian erythrocytes. They noted, that at high concentrations of lead, cellular uptake of iron was blocked, but at lower concentrations iron uptake was not blocked although the incorporation of iron into heme was. Although a large amount of information is available concerning the mechanisms whereby iron is incorporated into protoporphyrin to form heme, the intermediate steps in the intracellular handling of iron are poorly understood and several alternative pathways have been postulated. The studies of Bessis[11] which show that the mitochondria of developing red blood cells contain increased amounts of iron in certain hematologic conditions associated with abnormal erythrocyte production and the recent studies of Cooper, Webster, and Harris[14] would indicate that mitochondria function as an intermediate in intracellular iron metabolism. Since Bessis has shown that the mitochondria in red blood cells from lead-poisoned animals are distorted and contain no iron, lead may block the metabolism of iron prior to the mitochondria or block incorporation into the mitochondria. In a further study of intracellular iron metabolism, Allen and Jandl[1] found that iron, in being selectively taken up by reticulocytes was first associated with particulate fractions (stroma, mitochondria, and microsomes) and then gradually released to the soluble cytoplasm where it was incorporated into a transient nonhemoglobin protein phase and into hemoglobin. They found that lead in suitable concentrations allowed iron to accumulate in the particulate fraction, presumedly the stroma, but blocked its entry into the nonhemoglobin protein iron phase and into hemoglobin. Lothe and Falbe-Hansen[53] have studied this problem in lead-poisoned rabbit cells and concluded that lead blocks the transfer of iron from a ferritin phase, which was not associated with the stroma, to an electrophoretically fast-moving fraction which they believe is derived from mitochondria.

Recently Cooper* has prepared mitochondria from the reticulocytes of anemic rabbits and has found that lead inhibits mitochondrial uptake of iron. Greenough, Peters and Thomas[29] have studied the effect of lead on the intra-

---

* Personal communication.

cellular metabolism of iron in vitro in a system derived from human and dog bone marrow. They isolated a minor fraction which appeared to be a precursor to hemoglobin. Lead did not block iron incorporation into this fraction but did block incorporation into hemoglobin. Using the technique of short-term marrow culture, Korst, Frenkel and Wilhelm[50] found that serum from anemic animals increased the uptake of iron by the cells; this effect was inhibited by lead.

Boyett and Butterworth[12] have reported studies of iron metabolism in adult males with lead poisoning. In 15 subjects plasma iron clearance was essentially normal, although three patients had a slightly more rapid than normal clearance. The utilization or uptake of iron by the red blood cell mass was normal. In children with lead poisoning, Leikin and Eng[51] found that three of seven children had prolonged plasma iron clearance, decreased iron incorporation and decreased erythrocyte iron turnover. These three children had the longest histories of exposure to lead in contrast to the other four children with short histories and normal or increased iron turnover studies. These in vivo studies are therefore in accord with the in vitro studies and confirm that extracellular iron metabolism is probably normal in lead poisoning. However, with prolonged exposure erythroid hypoplasia may result in decreased turnover of iron.

It is obvious from the above discussion that lead in some manner interferes with the intracellular metabolism of iron although the exact pathways are not clearly defined at present and the precise site of action of lead is unknown. From the information available, it appears that, in lead-poisoned red blood cells, iron is taken up by the stroma in a normal manner, probably transferred to the cytoplasm, but then not incorporated properly into the mitochondria.

PORPHYRIN METABOLISM

The adverse effects of lead on the biosynthesis of heme have been demonstrated in a number of ways, both in clinical and experimental situations and by in vivo and in vitro methods. Industrial workers exposed to lead and children with lead poisoning secondary to the accidental ingestion of lead have typical alterations in the excretory pattern of porphyrins and increased amounts of heme precursors in the bone marrow and red blood cells. Similar changes can be produced in animals and man given lead experimentally. In vivo the deleterious effect of lead on heme synthesis has been demonstrated in a number of biological systems and our knowledge of the mechanism of action of lead on this important pathway is gradually becoming more complete, although we still cannot offer a satisfactory explanation on a biochemical basis for some of the changes that are seen. In the following paragraphs the effects of lead on the biosynthetic steps in heme synthesis will be reviewed followed by a discussion of the effects of lead on porphyrin metabolism in man.

Heme synthesis in vitro

The major steps in the pathway of heme synthesis have been elucidated in recent years. At the present time the origins of all the carbon atoms of the heme molecule have been identified as to their source and the steps of synthesis

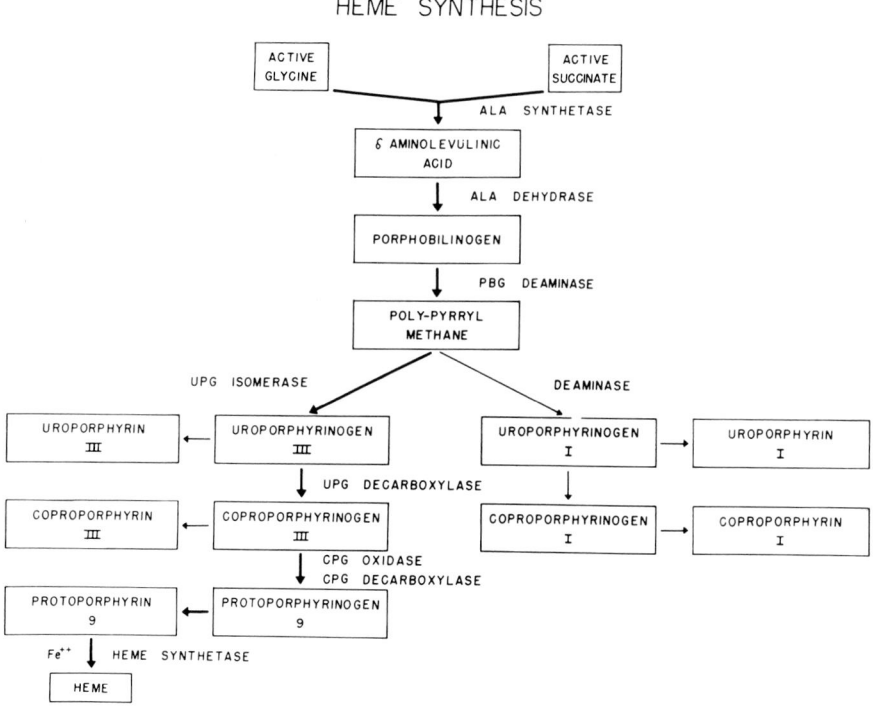

FIG. 5.—Schematic outline of heme synthesis. Heavy arrows indicate major pathway in normal man.

from activated glycine and succinate are fairly well established. Not all the enzymes necessary for this synthesis are present in mature erythrocytes and synthesis of heme, therefore, takes place in the immature nucleated or reticulated cells. Although most of the experimental work has been performed using material derived from the nucleated red blood cells of chickens and ducks, enough work has been performed with human reticulocytes to show that the steps are the same. An outline of this biosynthetic pathway is presented in Figure 5[28, 65]. The basic structural components are glycine and succinate which are joined to form a five carbon chain compound, delta-aminolevulinic acid (ALA). In the next step, two molecules of ALA condense to form a single ring-shaped compound, the monopyrrole, porphobilinogen (PBG). The mechanism of the combination of four PBG monopyrrole rings, to form the tetrapyrrole compound, uroporphyrinogen (UPG), is not clearly understood. It is postulated that a polypyrryl methane is formed which is acted upon by a deaminase to form the type I UPG and by an isomerase to form the type III UPG. Although four isomers are theoretically possible only types I and III have been identified in nature and the type III isomer is the principle compound formed in normal man. A series of decarboxylation reactions then occur resulting in coproporphyrinogen III and protoporphyrinogen 9. The latter is oxidized to protoporphyrin 9 which combines on a mole for mole basis with ferrous iron to form heme. The porphyrinogen compounds, uroporphyrinogen III and coproporphyrinogen III are colorless, nonfluorescing and apparently direct precursors in heme synthesis whereas the oxidative products of these intermediates, uroporphyrin III and coproporphyrin III are pink-colored, fluorescent compounds which are not direct intermediates in heme synthesis.

Many investigators have studied the effect of lead on this synthetic pathway in a variety of in vitro systems, but primarily those derived from avian erythrocytes. Eriksen[21], using an intact duck red blood cell system, showed that lead inhibited the formation of protoporphyrin but did not appear to inhibit the conversion of protoporphyrin to heme. Dresel and Falk[19, 20] studied the effect of lead on both intact and hemolysed chicken erythrocytes and reported that lead inhibited porphyrin synthesis primarily prior to the formation of protoporphyrin at low concentrations, but at higher concentrations heme synthesis from protoporphyrin was also inhibited. They also noted that the most pronounced effect of lead in their system appeared to be on the synthesis of porphyrin from ALA with considerably less inhibition of porphyrin synthesis from PBG. Goldberg and associates[26] concluded that lead inhibited the biosynthesis of heme in at least two locations: prior to the formation of ALA and at the stage of conversion of protoporphyrin to heme. While studying the incorporation of protoporphyrin into heme in chicken red blood cell hemolysates, Grinstein, Bannerman and Moore[32] also noted that there was a partial inhibition of this step by lead. Klein[49], using a system of intact duck red blood cells, found that the principle effect of lead was prior to the formation of protoporphyrin and noted that mercury, cobalt and manganese in similar concentrations had no such effect. Recently Lichtman and Feldman[52] have studied the enzyme, ALA dehydrase, which is necessary for the formation of PBG from ALA and is present in normal mature red blood cells. The activity of this enzyme was found to be reduced in erythrocytes from patients with lead poisoning. Since this reduction in activity could be reversed by preactivation with glutathione, lead was probably effecting the enzyme by inactivating sulfhydryl groups. They too noted that the rate of synthesis of uroporphyrin and coproporphyrin from PBG was decreased and interpreted the results to indicate that lead inhibited porphyrin synthesis at two or more steps between ALA and coproporphyrin. Lead may also exert some deleterious effect on the formation of the globin portion of the hemoglobin molecule. In a duck erythrocyte system Kassenaar, Morrell and London[43] found that lead inhibited the incorporation of glycine into globin.

Porphyrin metabolism in man

The increased excretion of coproporphyrin III in the urine is one of the classical signs of lead toxicity and is used frequently in industrial plants, where there is risk of exposure to lead, for the monitoring and control of such exposure. Another precursor of heme, ALA, has also been shown to be excreted in excessive amounts in individuals with lead poisoning.

The amount of coproporphyrin III in the urine can be measured quantitatively[67] and qualitatively[18]; both methods are used for the detection of lead poisoning. The qualitative test is most useful in clinical applications and should be readily available in all hospital laboratories. Bensen and Chisolm[7] have shown that its reliability can be improved by more careful control of the pH at which the test is performed. It is preferable that the test be done on fresh urine, because coproporphyrin deteriorates rather rapidly in urine left at room temperature and exposed to light. Adjustment of the urine pH to 6.5 to 8.5 by the addition of sodium carbonate[67] and storing the samples in the cold preserves the coproporphyrin for longer periods[33].

Coproporphyrin excretion in the urine is usually elevated in lead poisoning[13, 18, 36, 54, 58, 81] and there is relatively good correlation of increased levels of blood lead and urine lead with increased excretion of coproporphyrin[7, 33]. However, exceptions are not too infrequent and we have seen, for example, one child with severe fatal lead encephalopathy with excretion of normal amounts of coproporphyrin in the urine.

The increased excretion of ALA in the urine of individuals with lead poisoning has been noted only within the past few years, when methods for ALA detection and quantitation became available. Mauzerall and Granick[56] introduced a method for the column chromatographic separation of ALA and porphobilinogen (PBG) and the removal of the interfering urea in 1956, and in 1957 Haeger[34] reported that the ALA excretion was increased in lead workers. This finding has been confirmed by others[30, 71, 79] and more extensive studies by Haeger-Aronsen[33] have indicated its usefulness in the clinical and laboratory study of lead poisoning. ALA has been shown to be relatively stable in urine at a pH of 4 to 7 for several weeks; its concentration is an early and reliable indication of increased tissue concentrations of lead. ALA can also be measured in serum and has been found to be elevated in patients with lead poisoning. There appears to be a fairly good correlation between urine ALA, urine coproporphyrin, and urine lead in the same individual[33]. However, DeKretser and Waldron[17] in a study of 100 workers exposed to lead found no correlation between urinary excretion of ALA and coproporphyrin or between ALA and lead.

The excretion of ALA is also elevated in acute intermittent porphyria and in a few cases of chronic hepatic disease. Figure 6 shows the results of the quantitative determination of ALA in the urine of patients with a variety of conditions possibly associated with changes in heme synthesis. In patients with lead toxicity the ALA has ranged from normal levels to as high as 500 μmoles/ml. Patients with acute intermittent porphyria have varying levels of urinary ALA and may or may not have a concurrent increased excretion of PBG. The increased excretion of ALA is probably a more reliable index of lead toxicity in adults than in children. In our experience the excretion of ALA has been abnormally high in approximately 60% of children with overt lead encephalopathy. In a survey of an area of Cleveland with old housing known to be a source of many cases of childhood lead poisoning, abnormal urinary excretion of coproporphyrin was found in 15% and abnormal ALA excretion in 7% of all children tested, compared to figures of one per cent and 0 per cent respectively for children of similar ages living in good housing[31].

The administration of a chelating agent to a patient for therapy of lead poisoning results in a reduction in the excretion of ALA[33]. Such a study in an adult male is shown in Figure 7. As expected with the administration of versenate there was a marked increase in urine lead. The reduction in the ex-

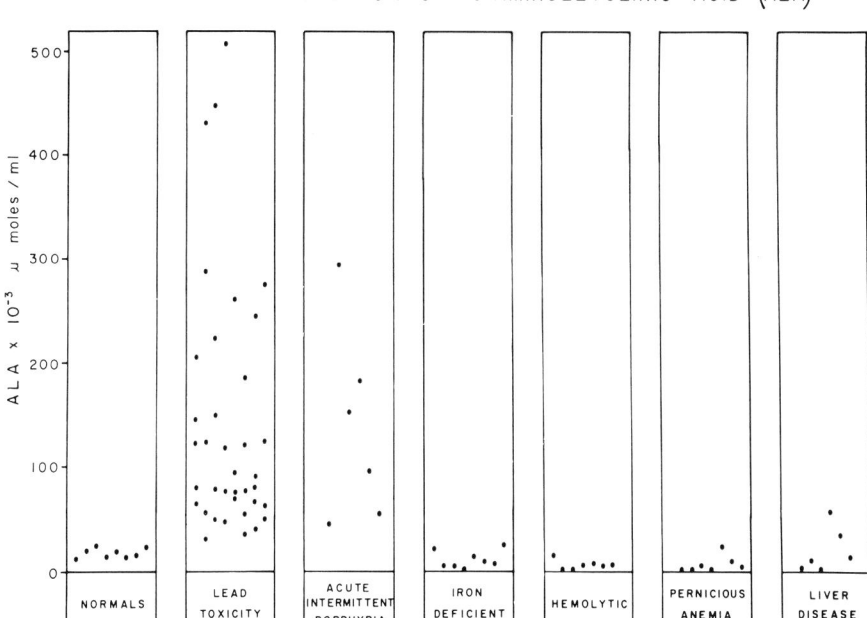

URINARY EXCRETION OF δ-AMINOLEVULINIC ACID (ALA)

FIG. 6.—Urinary excretion of δ-aminolevulinic acid in a variety of conditions. Elevated levels are seen in patients with lead poisoning, acute intermittent porphyria and occasionally in liver disease.

cretion of ALA was maintained for only a few days; within two weeks excretion had returned to pretreatment levels. Saita[64] has reported that elevated serum ALA levels persisted for one to three years after an acute episode of lead intoxication.

In order to determine the time relationships between the changes in ALA, PBG, coproporphyrin and lead excretion, lead was administered to two healthy normal adult male volunteers[79]. The results of these two studies are shown in Figures 8 and 9. Lead was administered daily by mouth in the form of lead chloride. Neither subject showed changes in hematocrit, reticulocyte count, stippled cell count or osmotic and mechanical fragility. In subject 1, Figure 8, excretion of ALA and coproporphyrin became abnormal on the 12th day of study and the administration of lead was discontinued on the 17th day because of the development of crampy abdominal pain. There was a slight rise in PBG excretion but not significantly above the normal range. In subject 2, Figure 9, ALA excretion was first abnormal on the 10th day and coproporphyrin excretion increased on the 29th day, but in less amount than seen in subject 1. No significant change occurred in PBG excretion and no symptoms of lead intoxication developed.

In addition to the abnormalities in ALA and coproporphyrin excretion which have been discussed, PBG excretion is sometimes increased[6, 75]. However, Boyett and Butterworth[12] have pointed out that the reports of excessive excretion of PBG in lead poisoning are based on the qualitative test using

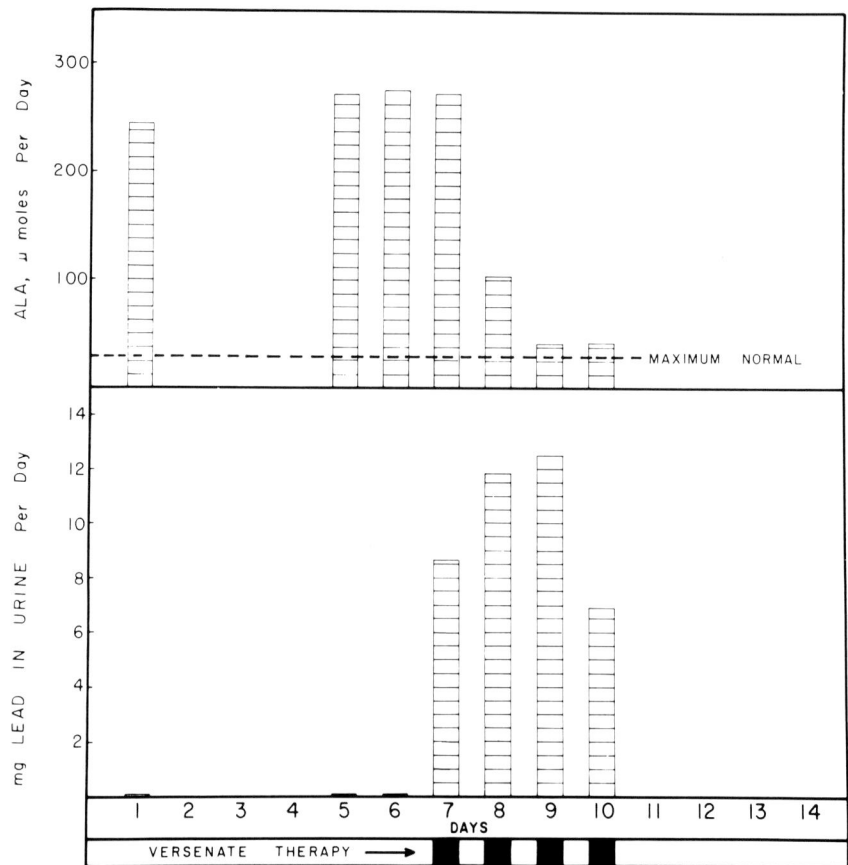

FIG. 7.—Urinary excretion of δ-aminolevulinic acid and lead during the intravenous administration of Versenate.

the Ehrlich aldehyde reaction. More recent studies using the quantitative test have not demonstrated a significant increase in PBG excretion[30, 33] although DeKretser and Waldron[17] did find slight elevations above normal urinary levels in 20 of 100 lead workers. The urinary excretion of coproporphyrin I is also increased in human lead poisoning[47] and the uroporphyrin I concentration of the bone marrow is increased in rabbits poisoned with lead[65].

The concentration of free protoporphyrin is increased in the circulating red blood cells[61, 74, 80]. Rubino[61] found that the erythrocyte protoporphyrin level was high in 21 of 22 patients with lead poisoning and was an early and reliable sign of lead toxicity occurring even prior to a rise in coproporphyrin excretion. Whitaker[78] has shown that the increased amount of protoporphyrin in the blood cells of children with lead poisoning causes 75 to 100% of the red blood cells to fluoresce under the ultraviolet microscope. This simple

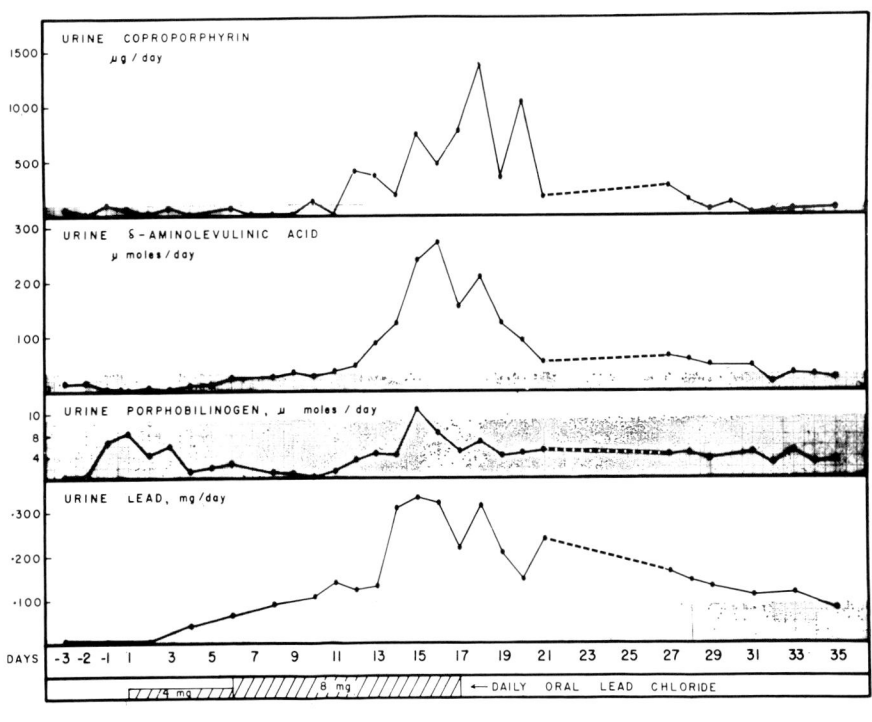

FIG. 8.—Urinary excretion of coproporphyrin III, δ-aminolevulinic acid, porphobilinogen and lead in a normal man given lead by mouth for 17 days, Subject 1.

test can be used as a rapid and reliable aid in the diagnosis of lead poisoning in children.

Richards and Scott[60] have demonstrated that the oral administration of 25 grams of glycine to patients with acute intermittent porphyria will significantly increase the urinary excretion of ALA and PBG. Such a test might be applied to patients with lead poisoning or suspected cases where the porphyrin excretion was normal. Rubino[63] however, found that ALA and PBG excretion was not significantly altered by the administration of glycine in two adults with lead poisoning.

Gajdos[24] has treated patients with porphyria with adenosine-5-monophosphoric acid. He postulates that their partial improvement is due to correction of a deficiency in the phosphorylated derivatives of adenosine secondary to increased porphyrin synthesis. He found that the administration of this drug prevented the occurrence of anemia in lead-poisoned rabbits and decreased the abnormal excretion of ALA, PBG, coproporphyrin and uroporphyrin without change in the high serum ALA or erythrocyte protoporphyrin levels in such animals[25].

The above information would indicate that lead blocks the biosynthesis of heme at several steps with varying degrees of effectiveness. The three principle abnormalities in porphyrin metabolism noted in patients with lead poisoning are: one, the increased excretion of coproporphyrin; two, the increase in

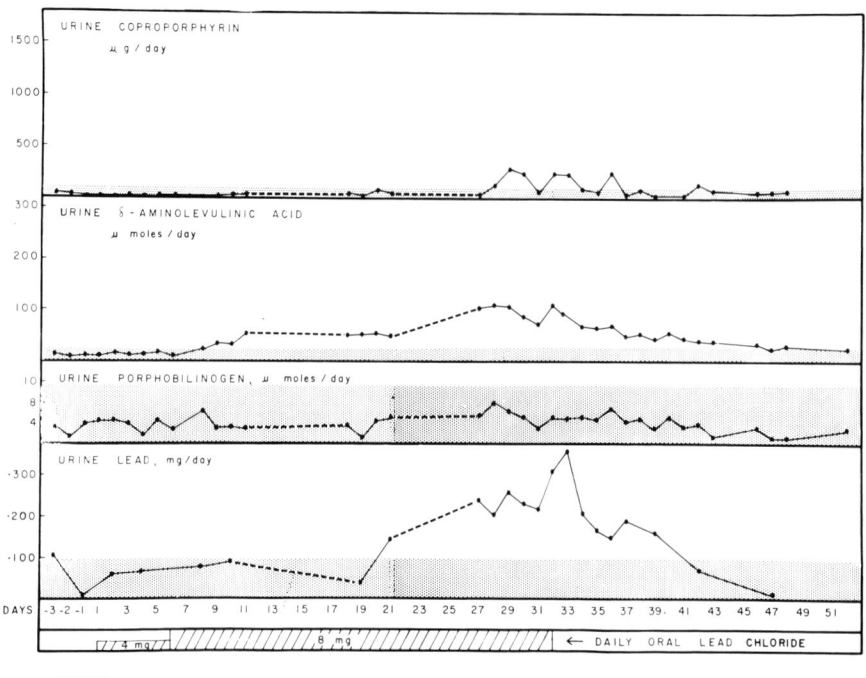

Fɪɢ. 9.—Urinary excretion of coproporphyrin III, δ-aminolevulinic acid, porphobilinogen and lead in a normal man given lead by mouth for 32 days, Subject 2.

free erythrocyte protoporphyrin and; three, the increased serum concentration and urinary excretion of ALA. With the information available at the present time, a reasonable explanation for the increase in ALA can be offered on the basis of a metabolic block at the point of conversion of ALA to PBG and therefore an excessive accumulation and excretion of ALA. The effect of lead on the conversion of protoporphyrin to heme, also, offers a reasonable explanation for the increased protoporphyrin of the red cells. However, no adequate explanation can be put forward at the present time to explain the marked increase in the excretion of coproporphyrin in lead-poisoning. Coproporphyrin is increased in the bone marrow cells[6] but not in the peripheral blood cells[65]; therefore the excessive amount of coproporphyrin may be derived from ineffective erythropoiesis and destruction of red blood cells in the bone marrow. However, there must be some abnormality in heme synthesis which results in increased accumulation of coproporphyrinogen and by auto-oxidation coproporphyrin. This defect has not been pinpointed at the biochemical level.

REFERENCES

1. Allen, D. W., and Jandl, J. H.: Kinetics of intracellular iron in rabbit reticulocytes, Blood 15: 71, 1960.
2. Aub, J. C., Fairhall, L. T., Minot, A. S. and Reznikoff, P.: Lead poisoning, Medicine 4: 1, 1925.
3. Aub, J. C., Reznikoff, P. and Smith, D. E.: Lead Studies. III. The effects of lead on red blood cells. Part 1. Changes in hemolysis, J. Exp. Med. 40: 151, 1924.
4. Baikie, A. G. and Valtis, D. J.: The oxygen consumption of the blood in experimental lead poisoning, Brit. J. Exp. Path. 35: 434, 1954.

5. Baikie, A. G. and Pirrie, R.: The effects of ACTH and cortisone in experimental haemolytic anaemias in guinea-pigs; studies on anaemias due to heterologous anti-red-cell-serum and on the anaemia of chronic lead poisoning, Scot. Med. J. 3: 264, 1958.
6. Bashour, F. A.: Urinary uroporphyrin, porphobilinogen and coproporphyrin excretion in lead-exposed workers, J. Lab. Clin. Med. 44: 764, 1954.
7. Benson, P. F. and Chisolm, J. J., Jr.: A reliable qualitative urine coproporphyrin test for lead intoxication in young children, J. Pediat. 56: 759, 1960.
8. Beritic, T.: Siderotic granules and the granules of punctate basophilia, Brit. J. Haemat. 9: 185, 1963.
9. Bessis, M. and Breton-Gorius, J.: Granules ferrugineaux dans les cellules macrophages et les erythrocytes au cours du saturnisme experimental; examen du microscope electronique, C.R. Soc. Biol. (Paris) 151: 275, 1957.
10. Bessis, M. C. and Breton-Gorius, J.: Ferritin and ferruginous micelles in normal erythroblasts and hypochromic hypersideremic anemias, Blood 14: 423, 1959.
11. Bessis, M. C. and Breton-Gorius, J.: Iron metabolism in the bone marrow as seen by electron microscopy: A critical review, Blood 19: 635, 1962.
12. Boyett, J. D. and Butterworth, C. E., Jr.: Lead poisoning and hemoglobin synthesis, Report of a study of fifteen patients with chronic lead poisoning, Am. J. Med. 32: 884, 1962.
13. Brooks, A. L.: An appraisal of a urinary porphyrin test in detection of lead absorption, Industr. Med. 20: 390, 1951.
14. Cooper, R. G., Webster, L. T., Jr. and Harris, J. W.: A role of mitochondria in iron metabolism of developing erythrocytes, J. Clin. Invest. 42: 926, 1963.
15. Crosby, W. H.: Siderocytes and the spleen, Blood 12: 165, 1957.
16. Crutcher, J. C.: Clinical manifestations and therapy of acute lead intoxication due to the ingestion of illicitly distilled alcohol, Ann. Intern. Med. 59: 707, 1963.
17. DeKretser, A. J. and Waldron, H. A.: Urinary delta aminolevulinic acid and porphobilinogen in lead-exposed workers, Brit. J. Industr. Med. 20: 35, 1963.
18. deLangen, C. D. and ten Berg, J. A. G.: Porphyrin in the urine as a first symptom of lead poisoning, Acta Med. Scand. 130: 37, 1948.
19. Dresel, E. I. B. and Falk, J. E.: Studies on the biosynthesis of blood pigments. 2. Haem and porphyrin formation in intact chicken erythrocytes, Biochem. J. 63: 72, 1956.
20. Dresel, E. I. B. and Falk, J. E.: Studies on the biosynthesis of blood pigments. 3. Haem and porphyrin formation from δ-aminolevulinic acid and from porphobilinogen in haemolysed chicken erythrocytes, Biochem. J. 63: 80, 1956.
21. Eriksen, L.: Lead intoxication: I. The effect of lead on the *in vitro* biosynthesis of heme and free erythrocyte porphyrins, Scand. J. Clin. Lab. Invest. 7: 80, 1955.
22. Fratianne, R. B., Griggs, R. C. and Harris, J. W.: Autosurvival of erythrocytes treated *in vitro* with lead chloride, (Abstract) Clin. Res. 7: 384, 1959.
23. Fullerton, J. M.: Value of haematology in diagnosis of chronic plumbism, Brit. Med. J. 2: 117, 1952.
24. Gajdos, A. and Gajdos-Torok, M.: The therapeutic effect of adenosine-5-monophosphoric acid in porphyria, Lancet 2: 175, 1961.
25. Gajdos, A., Gajdos-Torok, M. and Danieli, G.: Treatment by adenosine-5-monophosphoric acid of experimental saturnism in rabbits, Nature 193: 183, 1962.
26. Goldberg, A., Ashenbrucker, H., Cartwright, G. E. and Wintrobe, M. M.: Studies on the biosynthesis of heme in vitro by avian erythrocytes, Blood 11: 821, 1956.
27. Gould, S. E., Kullman, H. J. and Shecket, H. A.: Effect of lead therapy on blood cells of cancer patients, Am. J. Med. Sci. 194: 1937.
28. Granick, S. and Mauzerall, D.: The metabolism of heme and chlorophyll. In: D. M. Greenberg: Metabolic Pathways 2. New York: Academic Press, 1960, pp. 525 ff.
29. Greenough, W. B., III, Peters, T., Jr. and Thomas, E. D.: An intracellular protein intermediate for hemoglobin formation, J. Clin. Invest. 41: 1116, 1962.
30. Griggs, R. C. and Harris, J. W.: Erythrocyte survival and heme synthesis in lead poisoning, Clin. Res. Proc. 6: 188, 1958.
31. Griggs, R. C., Sunshine, I., Newill, V. A., Newton, B. W., Buchanan, S. and Rusch, C. A.: Environmental factors in childhood lead poisoning, J.A.M.A., in press.
32. Grinstein, M., Bannerman, R. M. and Moore, C. V.: The utilization of protoporphyrin 9 in heme synthesis, Blood 14: 476, 1959.
33. Haeger-Aronsen, B.: Studies on urinary excretion of δ-aminolevulinic acid and other haem precursors in lead workers and lead-intoxicated rabbits, Scand. J. Clin. Lab. Invest. 12: (Supple. 47) 1, 1960
34. Haeger, B.: Increased content of a δ-aminolevulinic acid-like substance in urine from workers in lead industry, Scand. J. Clin. Lab. Invest. 9: 211, 1957.
35. Harris, J. W. and Greenberg, M. S.: Erythrocyte fragilities in plumbism (Abstract), Clin. Res. Proc. 2: 55, 1954.
36. Holecek, V.: Excretion of urinary coproporphyrin in lead poisoning, I & II, Brit. J. Industr. Med. 14: 198, 1957.
37. Hutchison, H. E. and Stark, J. M.: The anemia of lead poisoning, J. Clin. Path. 14: 548, 1961.
38. Jandl, J. H. and Simmons, R. L.: The agglutination and sensitization of red cells by

metallic cations: Interactions between multivalent metals and the red-cell membrane, Brit. J. Haemat, 3: 19, 1957.

39. Jandl, J. H., Inman, J. K., Simmons, R. L. and Allen, D. W.: Transfer of iron from serum iron-binding protein to human reticulocytes, J. Clin. Invest. 38: 161, 1959.

40. Jandl, J. H.: The agglutination and sequestration of immature red cells, J. Lab. Clin. Med. 55: 663, 1960.

41. Joyce, C. R. B., Moore, H. and Weatherall, M.: Effects of lead, mercury, and gold on the potassium turnover of rabbit blood cells, Brit. J. Pharmacol. 9: 463, 1954.

42. Karpatkin, S.: Lead poisoning after taking Pb acetate with suicidal intent. Report of a case with a discussion of the mechanism of anemia, Arch. Environ. Health 2: 679, 1961.

43. Kassenaar, A., Morell, H. and London, I. M.: The incorporation of glycine into globin and the synthesis of heme in vitro in duck erythrocytes, J. Biol. Chem. 229: 423, 1957.

44. Kehoe, R. A.: The metabolism of lead in man in health and disease. I. The normal metabolism of lead. J. Roy. Inst. Public Health, 24: 81, 1961.

45. Kehoe, R. A.: The metabolism of lead in man in health and disease. 2. The metabolism of lead under abnormal conditions. J. Roy. Inst. Public Health 24: 129, 1961.

46. Kehoe, R. A.: The Harben Lectures, 1960: The metabolism of lead in man in health and disease. 3. Present hygienic problems relating to the absorption of lead. J. Roy. Inst. Public Health 24: 177, 1961.

47. Kench, J. E., Lane, R. E. and Varley, H.: Urinary coproporphyrins in lead poisoning, Brit. J. Industr. Med. 9: 133, 1952.

48. Key, J. A.: Lead studies. IV. Blood changes in lead poisoning in rabbits with especial reference to the stippled cells, Am. J. Physiol. 70: 86, 1924.

49. Klein, J. R.: Depression of heme formation and production of free porphyrin in duck erythrocytes, Am. J. Physiol. 203: 971, 1962.

50. Korst, D. R., Frenkel, E. P. and Wilhelm, J. E.: Studies using short-term bone marrow culture. I. Ferrokinetics and erythropoietin. In: Jacobsen, L. D. and Doyle, M: Erythropoiesis. New York: Grune & Stratton, 1962.

51. Leikin, S. and Eng, G.: Erythrokinetic studies of the anemia of lead poisoning, Pediatrics 31: 996, 1963.

52. Lichtman, H. C. and Feldman, F.: *In vitro* pyrrole and porphyrin synthesis in lead poisoning and iron deficiency, J. Clin. Invest. 42: 830, 1963.

53. Lothe, K., Falbe-Hansen, I.: Incorporation of 59-Fe into erythrocyte nonhaem iron and haemoglobin in anaemic and lead-poisoned rabbits, Clin. Sci. 24: 47, 1963.

54. Maloof, C. C.: Role of porphyrins in occupational diseases. I. Significance of coproporphyrinuria in lead workers, Arch. Industr. Hyg. 1: 296, 1950.

55. Marder, V. J. and Conley, C. L.: Electrophoresis of hemoglobin on agar gels. Frequency of hemoglobin D in a Negro population. Bull. Johns Hopkins Hosp. 105: 77, 1959.

56. Mauzerall, D. and Granick, S.: The occurrence and determination of δ-aminolevulinic acid and porphobilinogen in urine, J. Biol. Chem. 219: 435, 1956.

57. McFadzean, A. J. S. and Davis, L. J.: On the nature and significance of stippling in lead poisoning, with reference to the effect of splenectomy, Quart. J. Med. 18: 57, 1949.

58. Pinto, S. S., Einert, C., Roberts, W. J., Winn, G. S. and Nelson, K. W.: Coproporphyrinuria; study of its usefulness in evaluating lead exposure, A.M.A. Arch. Industr. Hyg. 6: 496, 1952.

59. Pirrie, R.: The effect of splenectomy and reticuloendothelial blockade upon the anaemia of lead poisoning in guinea-pigs, J. Path. Bact. 64: 211, 1952.

60. Richards, F. F. and Scott, J. J.: Glycine metabolism in acute porphyria, Clin. Sci. 20: 387, 1961.

61. Rubino, G. F., Pagliardi, E., Prato, V. and Giangrandi, E.: Erythrocyte copper and porphyrins in lead poisoning, Brit. J. Haemat. 4: 103, 1958.

62. Rubino, F. G., Prato, V. and Fiorina, L.: L'anemia da plombo: sua natura e patogenesi, Folia Med. (Napoli) 42: 1, 1959.

63. Rubino, G. F., Rossetti, L. and Giarrusso, P.: Effect of glycine administration on δ-aminolevulinic acid and porphobilinogen excretion in lead poisoning, Panminerva Med. 4: 388, 1962.

64. Saita, G. and Moreo, L.: The concentration of serum δ-aminolevulinic acid in lead poisoning, Med. Lavoro 54: 183, 1963.

65. Schmid, R., Hanson, B. and Schwartz, S.: Experimental porphyria. I. Isolation of uroporphyrin I from bone marrow of lead-poisoned rabbits, Proc. Soc. Exp. Biol. Med. 79: 459, 1952.

66. Schmid, R.: The Porphyrias. In: Stanbury, J. B., Wyngaarden, J. B. and Frederickson, D. S.: The Metabolic Basis of Inherited Disease. New York, McGraw-Hill, 1960. pp. 939 *ff*.

67. Schwartz, S., Zieve, L. and Watson, C. J.: An improved method for the determination of urinary coproporphyrin and an evaluation of factors influencing the analysis, J. Lab. Clin. Med. 37: 843, 1951.

68. Sheets, R. F., Janney, C. D., Hamilton, H. E. and DeGowin, E. I.: Studies with in-

agglutinable erythrocyte counts. III. Kinetics of erythrocyte destruction in human beings, J. Clin. Invest. 30: 1272, 1951.

69. Smyth, A. H.: The writings of Benjamin Franklin, Vol. 5, New York: The MacMillan Company, 1906. pp. 101 ff.

70. Sutherland, D. A. and Eisentraut, A. M.: The direct Coombs' test in lead poisoning, Blood 11: 1024, 1956.

71. Tishkoff, G. W., Granville, N. B., Rosen, R. and Dameshek, W.: Excretion of δ-aminolevulinic acid in lead intoxication, Acta Haemat. 19: 321, 1958.

72. Tuttle, A. H. and Fitch, C.: Alteration in the electrophoretic characteristics of hemoglobin in "paint eaters", Am. J. Dis. Child. 96: 503, 1958.

73. Vincent, P. C. and Blackburn, C. R. B.: Effects of heavy metal ions on the human erythrocyte. I. Comparisons of the action of several heavy metals, Aust. J. Exp. Biol. Med. Sci. 36: 471, 1958.

74. Watson, C. J.: The erythrocyte coproporphyrin: Variation in respect to erythrocyte protoporphyrin and reticulocytes in certain of the anemias, Arch. Int. Med. 86: 797, 1950.

75. Watson, C. J., Hawkinson, V. and Bossenmaier, I.: Some studies of the nature and clinical significance of porphobilinogen, Trans. Ass. Am. Physicians 66: 144, 1953.

76. Watson, R. J., Decker, E. and Lichtman, H.: Hematologic studies of children with lead poisoning, Pediatrics 21: 40, 1958.

77. Westerman, M. P., Pfitzer, E. A. and Jensen, W. N.: Bone marrow lead stores and a comparison of the chelating efficacies of EDTA and D-penicillamine in plumbism (Abstract), Clin. Res. 11: 201, 1963.

78. Whitaker, J. A. and Vietti, T. J.: Fluorescence of the erythrocytes in lead poisoning in children: an aid to rapid diagnosis, Pediatrics 24: 734, 1958.

79. Widmann, D. E., Newton, B. W., Sunshine, I., Griggs, R. C. and Harris, J. W.: Effect of lead ingestion in the daily urinary excretion of δ-aminolevulinic acid, porphobilinogen, coproporphyrin III and lead, Clin. Res. 6: 393, 1958.

80. Wranne, L.: Free erythrocyte copro—and protoporphyrin: A methodological and clinical study, Acta. Paediat. 49 (Suppl. 124) 1, 1960.

81. Wyllie, J.: Urinary porphyrins in lead absorption. A.M.A. Arch. Industr. Health 12: 396, 1955.

Chloramphenicol Toxicity: Clinical Features and Pathogenesis

——ADEL A. YUNIS* and GORDON R. BLOOMBERG——

Sɪɴᴄᴇ the introduction of chloramphenicol as an antimicrobial agent in 1948 reports of bone marrow aplasia in association with its use have continued to appear. Chloramphenicol is now the leading single cause of drug-induced aplastic anemia in man. Although the mechanism by which this antibiotic injures the bone marrow is not well understood, many important studies dealing with the problem have recently appeared in the literature. It is the purpose of the present review to summarize these studies with particular emphasis on pathogenetic mechanisms and on some of the effects of chloramphenicol in certain biological systems. A large number of the reported cases will be surveyed. This review, however, is not intended to be an exhaustive clinical analysis but rather a framework for discussion of pathogenesis. Several reviews on the subject of aplastic anemia and drug-induced blood dyscrasias have recently appeared[1-3]. The problem of detecting and preventing drug-induced blood dyscrasias has been succinctly summarized by Erslev and Wintrobe[4].

Bɪᴏᴄʜᴇᴍɪsᴛʀʏ ᴀɴᴅ Pʜᴀʀᴍᴀᴄᴏʟᴏɢʏ ᴏғ Cʜʟᴏʀᴀᴍᴘʜᴇɴɪᴄᴏʟ

Chloramphenicol (D-(−)-threo-1-p-nitrophenyl-2-dichloro acetamido 1–3-propanediol)[5] (Fig. 1) is an antibiotic originally obtained from the species of Actinomycetes called Streptomyces Venezuela, an organism first isolated by Burholder in 1947. The drug was subsequently chemically synthesized. It is the only antibiotic known with a nitrobenzene moiety. It is stable to boiling and its activity is unaffected over a pH of 2 to 9[6]. Only the D-stereo isomer is biologically active, and among the structural derivatives available chloramphenicol possesses the greatest antimicrobial activity[7]. The structure of the propanediol moiety is critical for activity. Any one of the following structural modifications results in almost complete loss of activity: Replacing either hydroxyl groups by hydrogen atoms, esterification of either hydroxyl group[8], substitution of a methyl group for the hydrogen atom on carbon 2[9], complete removal of the dichloroacetamide side chain[5], or replacing the free hydrogen on the nitrogen atom with a methyl group[9]. There is no absolute requirement for the chlorine atoms and the aryl nitro group is not essential for activity, although substitution of this group may result in partial loss of activity[7].

Chloramphenicol has both a bacteriostatic and bacteriocidal effect; in the usual therapeutic concentrations it is bacteriostatic[10]. Among the organisms inhibited by relatively low concentrations of the drug are the gram negative

From the Department of Medicine and Pediatrics, Washington University, St. Louis, Missouri.

* The investigations by one of the authors (A.A.Y.) were supported by U. S. Public Health Service Grant No. CA 06213-04.

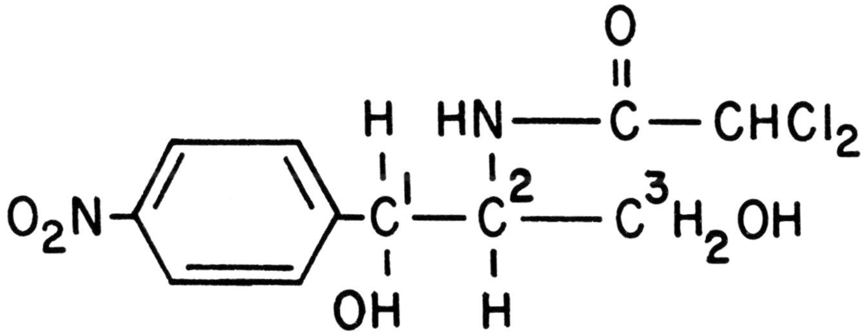

$$O_2N - \text{phenyl} - \overset{H}{\underset{OH}{\overset{|}{C^1}}} - \overset{HN - C - CHCl_2}{\underset{H}{\overset{|}{C^2}}} - \overset{O}{\underset{}{C^3H_2OH}}$$

Fig. 1.—Structure of chloramphenicol.

bacteria, A. aerogenes, E. coli, K. pneumonia, H. pertussis, S. typhosa, Proteus, Neisseria, Salmonella, Shigella, Brucella, and V. cholera[6]. Chloramphenicol is also effective against rickettsial organisms and the Psittacosis-lymphogranuloma venereum group of viruses. Sensitive organisms are completely inhibited by concentrations of 1–10 $\mu g/ml$[8].

Bacterial resistance to chloramphenicol has been described, but the biochemical basis for this resistance is not clear. Many bacterial species have the capacity to reduce the nitro group of chloramphenicol to an arylamine or to hydrolyze the amide linkage, thus reducing markedly the activity of the drug[10]. For instance, Smith and Worrel[11] have reported that reduction of the nitro group on the chloramphenicol molecule to an amino group is a major degradative pathway used by E. coli. Merkel, et al.[12] showed a direct correlation between resistance to chloramphenicol and "chloramphenicol reductase" activity in E. coli at certain stages of resistance. However, the increase in enzymatic activity did not account for all the resistance which can be developed. The possibility of decreased cell permeability to the drug as one mechanism for resistance remains to be investigated.

METABOLISM OF CHLORAMPHENICOL

Chloramphenicol appears to be completely absorbed from the gastrointestinal tract. Maximum serum concentrations range from 20–40 $\mu g/ml$ after a 2 gm. dose and 40–60 $\mu g/ml$ after a 4 gm. dose[6]. In the body chloramphenicol is concentrated in the kidneys, liver and lungs[13] as determined by microbiologic assays. This pattern of distribution was recently confirmed in rats using C^{14}-labeled chloramphenicol; the concentration in the bone marrow follows that in the plasma[14]. The major site of degradation of chloramphenicol is the liver where the drug is conjugated with glucuronic acid. Reduction of the nitro group of chloramphenicol by human liver homogenates has also been demonstrated[15]. Over 85 per cent of a given dose is excreted in the urine in 24 hours. About 10 per cent of this material is biologically active; the remainder is in the form of glucuronic acid conjugate and hydrolysis products. In contrast to man, the major pathway of excretion in the rat is the biliary system[16]. Kunin, et al.[17] have demonstrated that the half-life of the metabolic products of chloramphenicol is prolonged in severe renal disease, while in liver disease there is prolongation of the half-life of active chloramphenicol due to a slower rate of glucuronide conjugation.

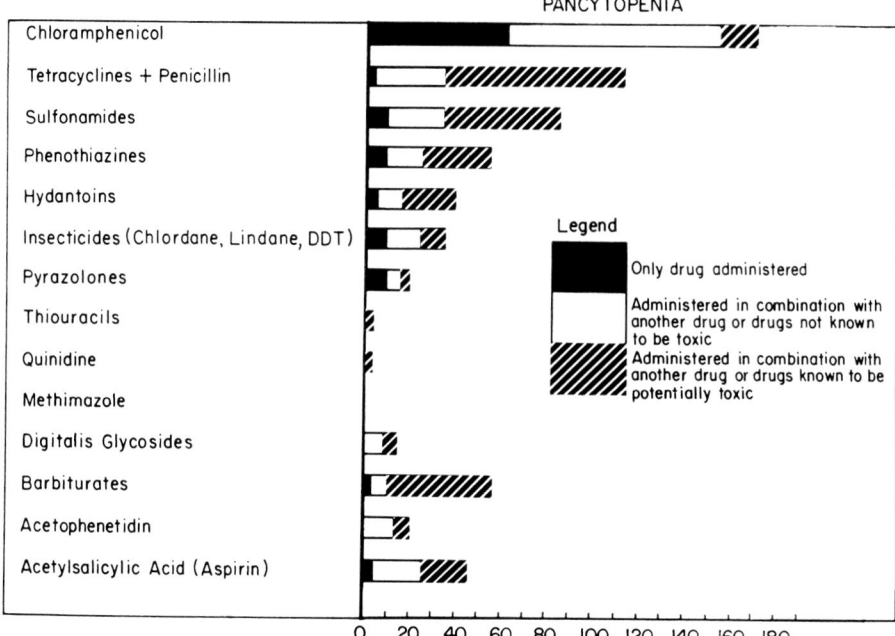

FIG. 2.—Drugs commonly associated with development of pancytopenia (Courtesy of Erslev and Wintrobe[4]).

CHLORAMPHENICOL TOXICITY

In spite of the obvious difficulty in establishing a cause-effect relationship in any single case, the association of bone marrow toxicity with chloramphenicol therapy has been frequent enough that the cumulative evidence leaves no doubt about the direct causation of aplastic anemia by this drug. In a series of 607 cases of aplastic anemia and pancytopenia reported by Welch[18] a history of exposure to drugs was obtained in 279 people, 92 of whom had taken chloramphenicol alone or with other drugs. Among the 1195 cases of blood dyscrasias reported to the Council on Drugs in this country between 1955 and 1962 chloramphenicol was the most frequent of 14 drugs commonly associated with pancytopenia[4]. (Fig. 2).

Analysis of Reported Cases

Several hundred cases of blood dyscrasia associated with chloramphenicol therapy have been reported. They fall into three general catagories: 1) Patients in whom a blood dyscrasia was an incidental finding during or after chloramphenicol therapy. 2) Those who received chloramphenicol for a particular indication, but also were studied closely for drug toxicity. 3) Patients in whom chloramphenicol toxicity was experimentally induced.

To exclude bias on the part of the reporter only the first group is included in this analysis, although reference to the other two groups of patients will be made under the heading, "Pathogenesis". Furthermore, among patients in the first category only those who were described in enough detail to allow analysis

TABLE I.—*Drug Intake and Bone Marrow Cellularity in 94 Cases of*
Chloramphenicol-Induced Blood Dyscrasias

	All Cases	Bone Marrow Cellularity[‡]	
		Aplasia/ Hypoplasia	Normocellular/ Specific Depression
Chloramphenicol only*.............	67	42	20
Chloramphenicol			
With Other Drugs†...............	27	19	7
Sulfonamides...................	18	12	5
Antihistamines..................	3	3	
Chloroquine....................	1	1	
Methimazole...................	1	1	
Meprobamate...................	2		2
"Naphtha"....................	1	1	
Not Stated....................	1	1	

* Includes other drugs that are not considered potentially myelotoxic e.g. Penicillin, Tetracycline.

† Excludes drugs taken more than one year prior to onset of dyscrasia.

‡ 6 cases not evaluated.

were included. For instance, from among the large series of blood dyscrasias associated with chloramphenicol reported by Welch[18] only those few cases that were singled out and described in detail were analyzed. All the relevant data were extracted and recorded on data cards; the cards were then coded and the pertinent information assembled. It was felt that assembling all such cases reported over a 15-year period would introduce a certain degree of randomness from which a clearer picture of chloramphenicol toxicity would emerge.

With these criteria in mind, 94 cases[1, 19-54] of blood dyscrasias* associated with chloramphenicol therapy were available for study (Table I). In 67 cases chloramphenicol was the only drug that could be incriminated; in the remaining 27 cases other drugs known to be potentially toxic to the bone marrow had also been given, most significant among which were the sulfonamides. However, none of these drugs was believed to have contributed to the development of the blood dyscrasia in these cases, although this possibility could not be entirely excluded.

Incidence

The incidence of blood dyscrasias from chloramphenicol cannot be determined with reasonable accuracy since neither the population at risk is known nor are all cases of drug-induced dyscrasias reported. From the total sale of chloramphenicol during 1958 and 1959 and the reported cases of associated aplastic anemia, Welch estimated an incidence of 1/156,000 and 1/227,000 for the two years respectively[51]. While these figures may not be accurate, they emphasize the fact that aplastic anemia is a rare complication of chloramphenicol therapy.

Aplastic anemia from chloramphenicol is more common in females. In Welch's series of 198 cases of blood dyscrasia associated with chloramphenicol the ratio of females to males was 1.6:1[51]. In the present series there was

* Blood dyscrasia is defined as a transient or persistent depression of bone marrow or peripheral blood elements.

TABLE II.—*Sex Distribution in 94 Cases of Chloramphenicol-Induced Blood Dyscrasias*

Sex		Marrow		
		Aplastic/Hypoplastic	Normocellular/Specific Depression	Marrow Not Evaluated
Male	41	23	16	2
Female	49	36	11	2
Sex Not Stated	4	2		2
Total	94	61	27	6

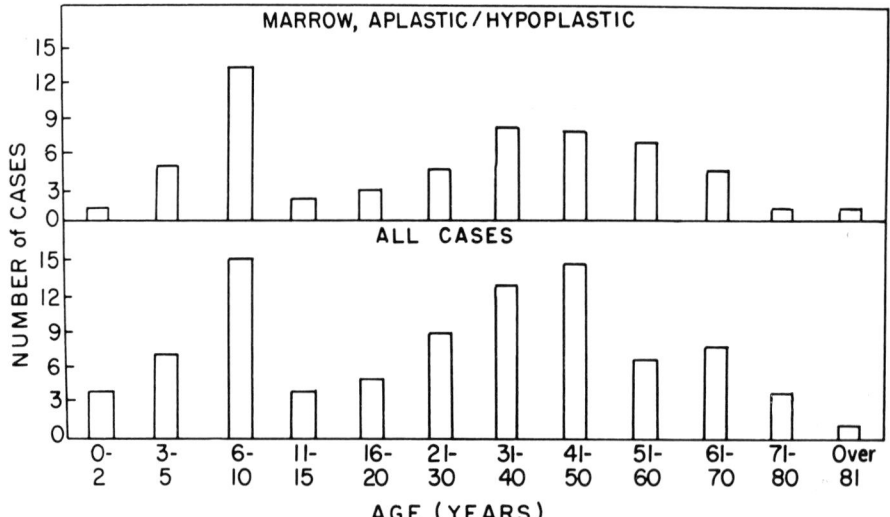

FIG. 3.—Age distribution in 95 cases of blood dyscrasias associated with chloramphenicol administration.

slight predominance of females, the difference being more appreciable when only the cases with aplastic marrow are considered (Table II).

Over 60 per cent of Welch's cases were children under 10 years of age. The age distribution of the present series is shown in Fig. 3. About 30 per cent of the cases were 10 years of age or under. The appearance of peak incidence in the first and 4th decade of life is probably more apparent than real.

Bone Marrow Cellularity

In 88 cases the bone marrow could be evaluated. In 61 subjects the marrow was hypoplastic or aplastic; the remaining cases had normocellular marrows with or without a specific depression in one of the cellular elements (Table I). This distribution is not necessarily characteristic of chloramphenicol-induced dyscrasia; indeed, chloramphenicol toxicity with a normally cellular bone marrow is a much more frequent occurrence than bone marrow aplasia from the drug.

Major Cytologic Changes in the Peripheral Blood

The relation of the peripheral blood findings to bone marrow cellularity is shown in Table III. Among the 61 patients with aplastic/hypoplastic marrow

TABLE III.—*Relation of Peripheral Blood Abnormalities to Bone Marrow Cellularity*

	All Cases	Marrow Cellularity		
		Aplastic	Normo-cellular	Not Done
Presenting Peripheral Blood Pattern	94	61	27	6
Pancytopenia	62	57	5	
Anemia without Pancytopenia	25	2	22	1
Alone	14	2	11	1
With Leukopenia/Neutropenia	10		10	
With Thrombocytopenia	1		1	
Leukopenia/Neutropenia	6	2		4
Thrombocytopenia	1			1

57 (93%) had pancytopenia, while only 5 (18%) of the 27 subjects with normocellular marrow presented with pancytopenia; almost all the remaining cases showed anemia with or without leukopenia. Leukopenia alone was present in 6 of the 94 patients, two of whom had a hypoplastic bone marrow; in the remaining four cases bone marrow was not evaluated. In the single case of thrombocytopenia[42] marrow examination was not done; this child was given one gram of chloramphenicol on each of two consecutive days for pertussis. The relation of the thrombocytopenia to chloramphenicol administration remains very doubtful. Leukopenia and/or thrombocytopenia occurring without anemia seem to be infrequent even though most early reports on chloramphenicol toxicity emphasized leukopenia and neutropenia[19, 21, 55, 56].

Relation to Dose and Duration of Therapy

The relation of blood dyscrasia to the total dose and duration of chloramphenicol therapy is shown in Fig. 4. A difference in the dose distribution is noted between those patients with bone marrow aplasia and those with normocellular marrow. The total dose tended to be directly proportional to the duration of therapy for the first group, i.e., larger doses were given over longer periods of time; in those with normocellular marrows relatively large doses were given within shorter periods, indicating a dose-effect relationship.

Time Relation of Onset of Symptoms to Therapy

In all cases with normocellular marrow the dyscrasia appeared during therapy (Table IV). In sharp contrast, in 73% of the cases with bone marrow aplasia the clinical onset of the blood dyscrasia occurred two weeks to five months after the last dose.

Course and Outcome

Since toxicity occurring concurrently with chloramphenicol therapy is usually associated with a normocellular marrow, this group of patients might be expected to have a more favorable prognosis. This relationship is clearly illustrated in Table V where all cases are divided between concurrent and late toxicity. Among the 49 cases in the first group 38 had complete recovery. Of the 11 patients who died 8 had aplastic bone marrows; the remaining 3 subjects had normocellular marrows and died of unrelated causes. In all 43 patients in

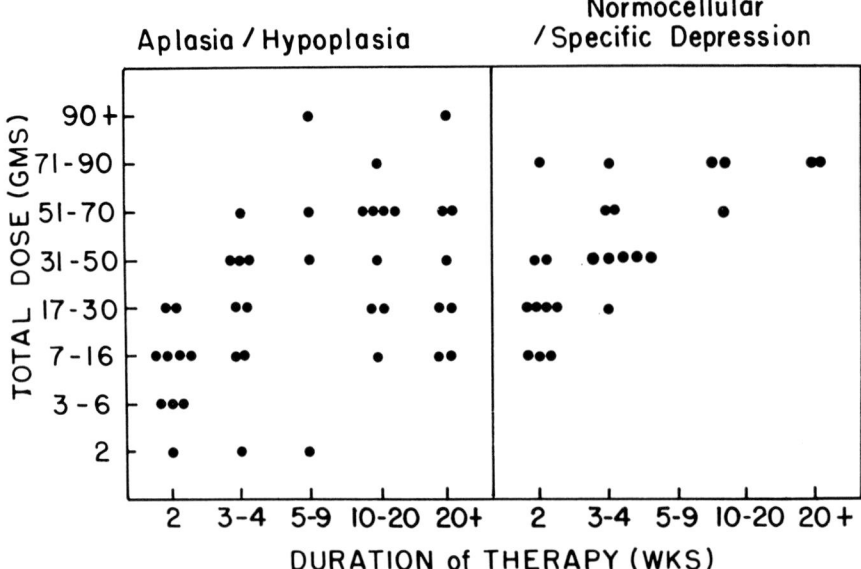

FIG. 4.—Relation of chloramphenicol toxicity to total dose and duration of therapy.

TABLE IV.—*Relation of Bone Marrow Cellularity to the time of Clinical Onset of Chloramphenicol Toxicity*

Time Relation of Toxicity to Chloramphenicol Therapy	Marrow Cellularity	
	Aplasia/Hypoplasia	Normal
4–5 months*	6	
2–3 months*	22	
2–7 weeks*	14	
< 2 weeks*	1	
Concurrent Relationship	16	27

* After suspension of treatment.

whom the onset of toxicity was delayed, the bone marrow was aplastic; of these patients 38 (90%) died and only two subjects had complete recovery.

A division of these cases into two groups according to outcome, i.e., fatal versus recovered, allows comparison of certain features not previously appreciated (Table VI). In general, the two groups fall into patterns determined by bone marrow cellularity. The bone marrow was aplastic in 46 of the 49 fatal cases. No particular relation of toxicity to total dose or duration of therapy is noted. Drug administration was intermittent in 37 cases. In only 8 patients did the dyscrasia appear during therapy; all eight subjects, however, had received chloramphenicol on one or more occasions within the five months preceding symptoms. The most common presenting symptom was purpura and/or hemorrhage. The most common cause of death was cerebral or gastrointestinal hemorrhage. The duration of life after onset of symptoms was usually short; 45% were dead in 7 weeks, 63% died in 7 months and all were dead within 18 months.

TABLE V.—*Relation of Time of Onset of Toxicity and Bone Marrow Cellularity to the Outcome of Disease*

Outcome	Time Relation of Toxicity to Therapy			
	Concurrent		2 wks – 5 mos. after last dose	
	Number of Cases			
	49†		43	
	Marrow Cellularity			
	Cellular 27	Aplastic 16	Cellular 0	Aplastic 43
Fatal..............................	3*	8		38
Partial Recovery..................		2		2
Complete Recovery................	24	3		2
No Change........................		3		1

* Death due to unrelated causes.

† Bone marrow was not evaluated in 6 cases who had complete recovery.

Thirty-five patients had complete recovery; 8 had pancytopenia, 5 of whom had an aplastic bone marrow. In 24 cases the bone marrow was normocellular. In general the total chloramphenicol doses were large and given within relatively short periods of time. In 32 of the 35 cases toxicity appeared during drug therapy. The most common presenting symptom was anemia. Recovery usually took place within two weeks after discontinuation of chloramphenicol. In three cases the onset of recovery occurred one year after the appearance of symptoms.

Comments

It is clear from the above analysis that chloramphenicol produces two types of bone marrow toxicity, the characteristics of which are summarized in Table VII. One type of toxicity occurs during chloramphenicol treatment, is usually dose related, and is characterized by a normocellular bone marrow and anemia with or without leukopenia or thrombocytopenia all of which are usually reversible when administration of the drug is discontinued. The second type of toxicity has a later onset (2 weeks to 5 months), is not necessarily dose related, and is characterized by an aplastic bone marrow, pancytopenia, and a fatal outcome.

PATHOGENESIS

In discussing pathogenesis, separate consideration for each of the two types of toxicity described above is warrented. Several recent contributions throw light on the mechanism by which chloramphenicol induces reversible hematopoietic depression. However, the mechanism by which this antibiotic causes irreversible bone marrow aplasia is still completely unknown.

In his classification of agents that are associated with the occurence of pancytopenia, Wintrobe[57] lists two categories: 1) Agents which regularly produce marrow hypoplasia and aplasia if a sufficient dose is given, e.g., ionizing

TABLE VI.—*Clinical Features in Cases of Fatal and Non-fatal Chloramphenicol Toxicity*

	Fatal	Complete Recovery
No. of patients	46	35
Peripheral Blood Findings	Pancytopenia..............44 Anemia only.............. 0 Leukopenia................ 1 Unknown.................. 1	Pancytopenia............... 8 Anemia only...............11 Anemia & Leukopenia.......10 Anemia & Thrombocytopenia 1 Leukopenia & Neutropenia... 4 Thrombocytopenia.......... 1
Age	Over 15 years.............26 Under 15 years............20	Over 15 years.............23 Under 15 years............12

	Fatal			Complete Recovery		
		Child	*Adult*		*Child*	*Adult*
Sex	Male..........17	6	11	Male..........19	6	13
	Female.........27	14	13	Female.........14	4	10
	Not Stated..... 2			Not Stated..... 2		

	Fatal	Complete Recovery
Relation of Onset to Last Dose	Concurrent................ 8 2–7 weeks.................13 2–3 months...............21 4–5 months............... 4	Concurrent................32 2–7 weeks................. 2 4 months.................. 1
Continuity of Therapy	Constant.................. 9 Intermittent...............37	Constant..................27 Intermittent............... 8
Initial Symptoms	Anemia/Pallor............. 7 Leukopenia/Neutropenia.... 3 Purpura/Hemorrhage.......36	Anemia/Pallor.............23 Leukopenia/Neutropenia..... 7 Purpura/Hemorrhage........ 5
Marrow Cellularity	Aplasia/Hypoplasia.........46 Normocellular............. 0	Aplasia/Hypoplasia.......... 5 Normocellular and/or Specific Depression................24 Not Done.................. 6
Major Cause of Death	Intracranial Hemorrhage....20 Massive G.I. hemorrhage...18 Infection.................. 8	

radiation, antimetabolites, etc.; and 2) Agents which are only occasionally associated with bone marrow aplasia such as chloramphenicol and other drugs. Most agents under the first category have a certain more or less predictable effect, and a direct toxic action on bone marrow cells can be demonstrated. The second group of agents depress hematopoiesis in a small fraction of the population and their toxic effect is totally unpredictable. Likewise, the mechanism by which they exert their toxic effect is poorly understood. Two theories have been advanced.

1. *Autoimmune Process*—It has been postulated that a drug may act as a hapten combining with some specific protein in the cell resulting in the formation of a new antigen to which antibodies are subsequently formed. An antigen-antibody reaction thus will result in cell injury[58]. Such a mechanism has been demonstrated in thrombocytopenia caused by sedormid (allyl-isopropyl-

TABLE VII.—*Clinical Features of Two Types of Chloramphenicol Toxicity*

Bone Marrow Cellularity	I Normocellular	II Hypoplastic or Aplastic
Peripheral Blood	Anemia with or without Leukopenia or Thrombocytopenia	Pancytopenia
Drug Dosage	Usually large and given within a short period	No particular relation to dose. Frequently intermittent therapy
Time Relation of Toxicity to last dose	Concurrent	2 wks.—5 months later
Most Common Presenting Symptoms	Anemia, Pallor	Purpura and/or Hemorrhage
Outcome	Recovery is the rule	Fatal in most cases

acetyl carbamide)[59] and quinidine[60] and in amidopyrine agranulocytosis[61]. Leukoagglutinins have been demonstrated in few instances of pancytopenia[62-64] where evidence of peripheral cellular destruction was also present. The role of these agglutinins in acquired bone marrow aplasia is questionable. Furthermore, in most instances of acquired aplastic anemia no significant peripheral cellular destruction can be detected[1]. The occurrence of aplastic anemia following intermittent chloramphenicol therapy and the history of allergic manifestations in some of the patients reported[31] tend to favor an underlying immunological mechanism. There is, however, no substantial evidence to support this possibility.

2. *Direct Toxicity*—Increasing evidence for a direct toxic action of chloramphenicol on bone marrow elements has recently appeared, and is derived from both *in vitro* studies and clinical observations. Lengthy attempts to find suitable experimental models to further our understanding of chloramphenicol toxicity have been unsuccessful. Mild erythroid hypoplasia and reticulocytopenia have been described in ducks given the antibiotic[65]. Anemia without leukopenia has also been described in dogs receiving the drug intramuscularly[66].

Studies in Human Subjects

As early as 1949 Volini[19] described chloramphenicol-induced bone marrow depression in man which remitted upon withdrawal of the drug. In 1955 Krakoff[67] induced reticulocytopenia in 4 patients with advanced cancer by the administration of 12 gms. of the antibiotic daily for 20–22 days. The pancytopenia was reversible in all patients upon discontinuing medication. Attempts to reproduce these hematologic changes in one patient by the readministration of 2 gms. of the drug were unsuccessful. Subsequent studies on patients receiving chloramphenicol have clearly indicated that erythropoietic depression from this drug is more frequent than has been previously recognized. Rubin, et al. demonstrated early changes in iron metabolism indicative of depressed erythropoiesis during chloramphenicol therapy[68-69]. These changes consisted of elevation in plasma iron levels with an abnormally high saturation of the plasma iron binding globulin (Fig. 5), a delay in the disappearance of radioactive iron from the plasma (Fig. 6) and failure of the radioactive iron to appear in the

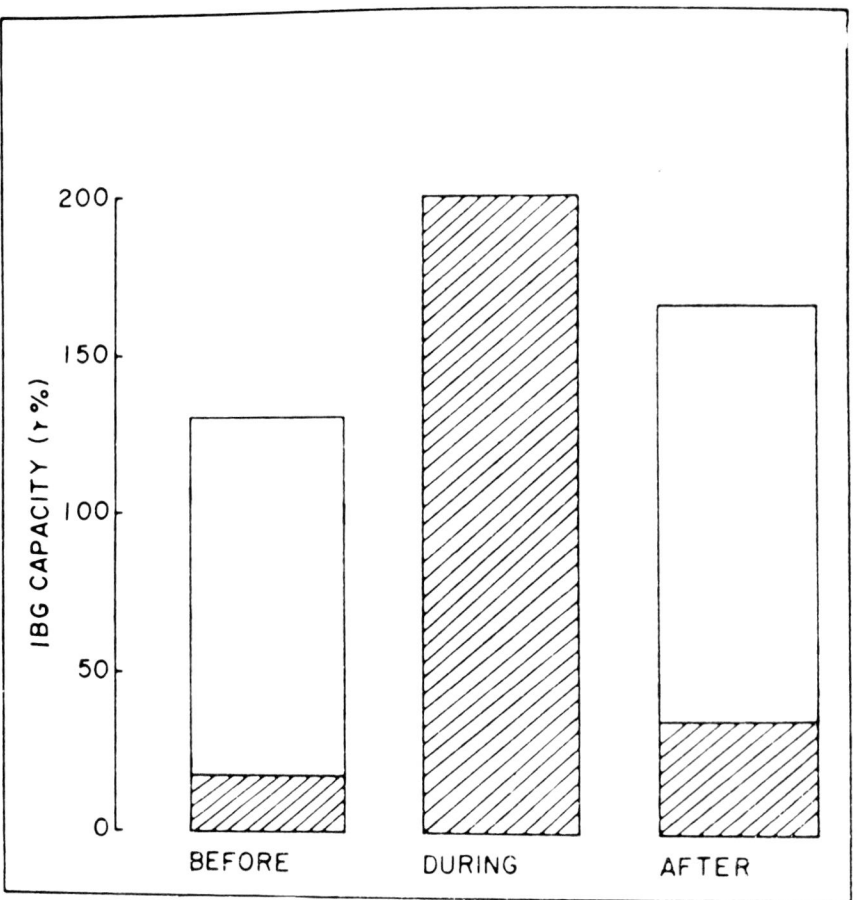

Fig. 5.—Saturation of iron binding globulin during chloramphenicol therapy (Courtesy of Rubin et al.[68])

circulating red cells for a period of 8 or more days. These authors were able to demonstrate definite erythropoietic depression in 2 per cent and borderline toxicity in 6 per cent of 50 healthy volunteers receiving the drug[69].

More recently striking morphologic changes in the bone marrow along with erythroid hypoplasia have been described in patients receiving chloramphenicol. In 10 of 22 patients given the drug at the rate of 40–85 mgm/kg/day for 4–27 days for various infections, Saidi, et al. described large vacuoles (Fig. 7) in the primitive erythroblasts associated with anemia and reticulocytopenia[70]. Twelve patients received the drug in a dose of 11–45 mgm/kg/day for 4–59 days without developing hematologic changes, thus indicating a dose-effect relationship. These authors also observed a delay or interruption in the reticulocyte response in 4 patients with pernicious anemia on vitamin B_{12} therapy and in 2 patients with iron deficiency anemia on iron therapy when chloramphenicol was added to the therapeutic regimen.

Vacuolization of proerythroblasts accompanied by depressed erythropoiesis and reticulocytopenia (henceforth referred to as the erythropoietic lesion)

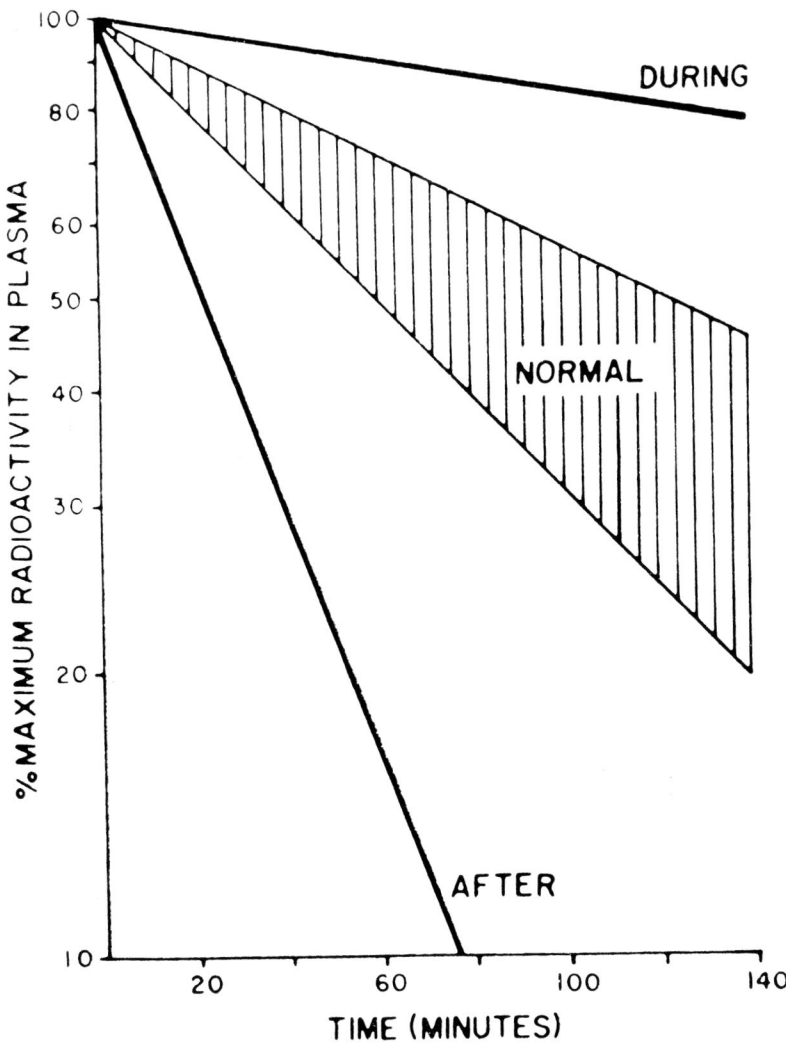

FIG. 6.—Plasma clearance of intravenously administered Fe[59] during Chloramphenicol therapy (Courtesy of Rubin et al[68]).

occurring with chloramphenicol therapy have subsequently been observed repeatedly[47, 48, 53, 71]. McCurdy[72] was able to correlate these changes with the levels of free chloramphenicol in the blood. More recently Jiji, et al.[71], demonstrated elevation of serum iron, reticulocytopenia, and vacuolization of proerythroblasts in 10 volunteers who received chloramphenicol in a dose of 49–68 mgm/kg/day for 13–42 days. These authors offered evidence that the development of these toxic changes was dose and time dependent. In agreement with these observations and those of McCurdy are those of Suhrland and Weisberger who found increased frequency of toxicity in patients with liver disease along with higher levels of free chloramphenicol in the blood[73]. It is of interest that neither B$_{12}$ nor folinic acid corrected these changes when given concomitantly with chloramphenicol. Both Saidi, et al. and Jiji, et al. observed that chloram-

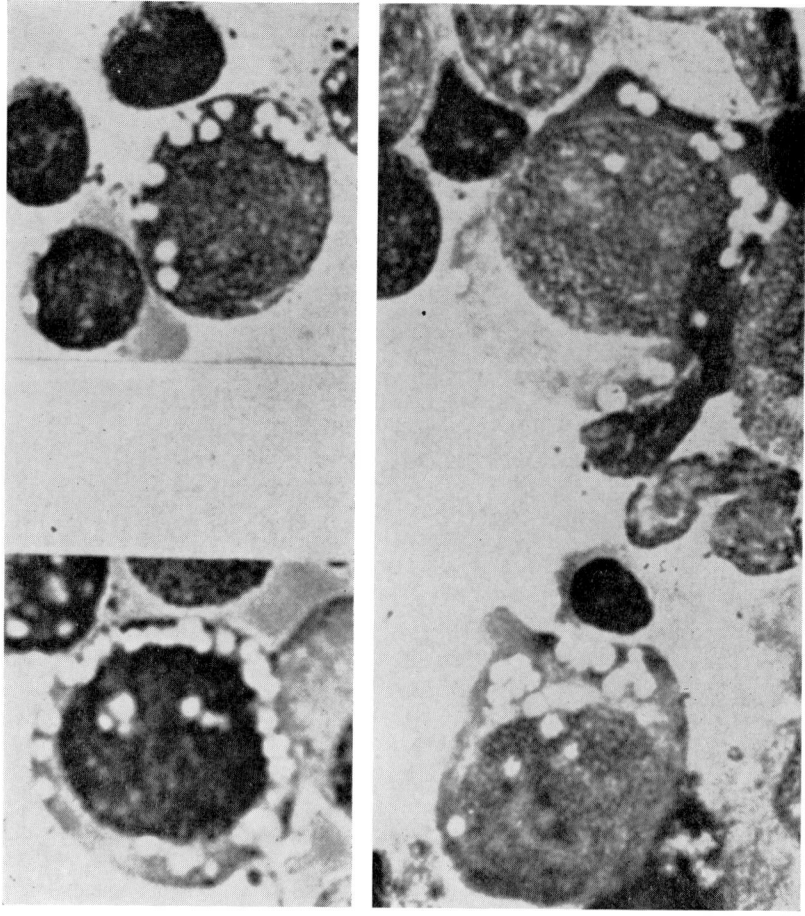

FIG. 7.—Vacuolization of erythroblasts during chloremphenicol administration (Courtesy of Saidi et al.[70])

phenicol given with B_{12} to patients with pernicious anemia did not inhibit the transformation of megaloblasts into normoblasts even though it blocked the reticulocyte response. This suggested to them that the site of action of the drug is not on nucleic acid synthesis which is presumably involved in this transformation.

To evaluate the relation of structure to this type of toxicity from chloramphenicol several p-substituted analogues of the drug were studied. It was found that replacing the nitro group in the para position by sulfamoyl

$$\left(NH_2 - \overset{\overset{\displaystyle O}{\|}}{\underset{\underset{\displaystyle O}{\|}}{S}} - \right),$$

methylsulfonyl

$$\left(CH_3 - \overset{\overset{\displaystyle O}{\|}}{\underset{\underset{\displaystyle O}{\|}}{S}} \right),$$

or methyl mercapto (CH$_3$—S—) radicals increased the toxicity of the drug indicating that the para nitro group is not the determining factor in reversible toxicity from chloramphenicol[71, 74].

The most important question with regard to the erythropoietic lesion induced by chloramphenicol is whether it is related in any way to the development of bone marrow aplasia from the drug. In all cases in which this lesion has been described it has been completely reversible. These depressive effects of chloramphenicol clearly fall under the type of toxicity that occurs concurrently with drug therapy, is dose related, is associated with a normally cellular bone marrow and is reversible upon withdrawal of medication. There is also good evidence that these toxic effects can be induced in all cases given enough of the drug[71]. Wallerstein has emphasized that "reversible depression of erythropoiesis following the use of chloramphenicol cannot be considered a side reaction; it must be recognized as a pharmacological effect".[75]. Furthermore, at least part of the erythropoietic lesion may be nonspecific since similar vacuolization of proerythroblasts has been described in 8 of 13 patients with acute alcoholism[76]. Aplastic anemia from chloramphenicol, on the other hand, is rare, has its onset typically 5 weeks or longer from the last dose, without any constant relationship to dose or duration of therapy and is irreversible in most instances. Of all the cases in the literature in which the erythropoietic lesion has been described none developed bone marrow aplasia[71]. It seems reasonable to conclude that no relation can be discerned between these two types of chloramphenicol toxicity; the occurrence of the erythropoietic lesion with chloramphenicol therapy should not at present be construed as a warning of impending aplastic anemia.

In Vitro Studies

It is difficult to envision bone marrow aplasia from chloramphenicol without implicating some fundamental disturbance in cell metabolism. Yet, extensive in vitro studies with the drug have failed to provide a biochemical explanation for observed end results. Thus, there is very little experimental evidence for a direct effect of chloramphenicol on the metabolism of bone marrow cells. A striking difference exists between the sensitivity of microorganisms and of mammalian cells to the biochemical effects of this antibiotic. The metabolic effects of chloramphenicol in microorganisms have been reviewed recently by Brock[8].

Effects of Chloramphenicol on Bacterial Cell Metabolism

In sensitive bacteria chloramphenicol in concentrations of 10 μg/ml or higher causes complete inhibition of protein synthesis while synthesis of nucleic acids continues[77, 78]. Thus, numerous enzymes fail to be synthesized in the presence of the drug[8]. It is not known which intermediate step in protein synthesis is inhibited. Neither amino acid activation[79] nor the transfer of activated amino acids to soluble RNA[80] is affected. The drug does not interfere with the release of newly formed protein from the ribosomes into the supernatant fluid[81]. Hence, it is believed that chloramphenicol inhibits the transfer of amino acids from soluble RNA to protein, but the exact site of action has not yet been determined.

Both DNA and RNA continue to be synthesized in the presence of chloramphenicol. However, the synthesis of nucleic acids may be inhibited by the drug under certain conditions. In synchronized cultures DNA synthesis can be inhibited if the antibiotic is added just before cell division; RNA synthesis can be blocked if the antibiotic is added just after cell division. This is presumably brought on by inhibition of the synthesis of enzymes involved in nucleic acid synthesis at certain stages of cell division[82], thus indirectly blocking nucleic acid production.

DNA synthesized in the presence of chloramphenicol appears to be biologically active[83, 84]. RNA formed in the presence of the antibiotic is unstable and is degraded rapidly by the cell[85] and more recently has been shown to resemble in some respects messenger RNA[86]. Rendi and Ochoa[81] suggested that chloramphenicol might inhibit protein synthesis by interfering with the attachment of messenger RNA to the ribosomes. These authors believe that chloramphenicol may selectively affect bacterial ribosomes; the inactivity of the antibiotic in animal systems would be based on a genetically controlled difference in structure of the ribosomes.

Carbohydrate assimilation and bacterial energy metabolism are unaffected by chloramphenicol[87].

Effects on Mammalian Cell Metabolism

In contrast to microorganisms, the mammalian cell is much less sensitive to chloramphenicol. Attempts to demonstrate inhibition of protein synthesis in mammalian cells using comparable pharmacologic concentrations of the drug generally have failed[88,89]. Inhibition of amino acid incorporation by mammalian reticulocytes *in vitro* occurs only when drug concentrations greatly exceed therapeutic levels[90]. A similar situation is observed when one examines other metabolic effects of chloramphenicol on mammalian cells including human bone marrow cells. In thymic nuclei considerably higher drug concentrations are required to inhibit nucleic acid synthesis[91]. In testing the effect of chloramphenicol on leukocyte respiration, Follette, et al.[92] observed moderate inhibition of oxygen uptake only at a drug concentration of 10^{-3}M (323 μg/ml); inhibition was progressively greater at higher concentrations and complete at a concentration of 6.1×10^{-3}M. Chloramphenicol levels well above 100 μg/ml are needed to inhibit DNA and RNA synthesis by normal human bone marrow[46] and to suppress the uptake and intracellular utilization of Fe^{59} by human bone marrow cells and reticulocytes[93].

Using a cell free system of ribosomes prepared from mammalian reticulocytes, Weisberger[94] could demonstrate no significant inhibition of incorporation of leucine-C^{14} into ribosomal protein by chloramphenicol concentrations as high as 2 μmoles/ml. The addition of polyuridylic acid to this system stimulated the incorporation of C^{14} L-phenylalanine into the ribosomes. This stimulation could be inhibited by very small concentrations of chloramphenicol depending on the amount of polyuridylic acid added; the incorporation of phenylalanine induced by 1 μg of polyuridylic acid was significantly inhibited by 0.005 μmoles of the drug per ml (1.6 μg/ml). Weisberger suggested that chloramphenicol may either prevent the binding of polyuridylic acid to the ribosomes or combine and inactivate polyuridylic acid. However, it is not known if this action of chloramphenicol also applies to natural messenger RNA from mammalian sources or is specific for polyuridylic acid. If it does apply to natural mammalian messenger RNA, it would be important to know if this action is specific for chloramphenicol since other antibiotics such as erythromycin[99] have been shown to exert a similar effect on bacterial protein synthesis and are not known to be particularly myelotoxic.

No clear biochemical explanation for the observed toxic effect of chloramphenicol has been discovered. However, all the biochemical studies described represent short term experiments; the length of exposure of the hemopoietic tissue to the drug could be a more important factor. The findings of Weisberger, et al., if shown to be specific for chloramphenicol, may offer a good biochemical explanation for the reversible pharmacologic effects observed from the drug.

The most puzzling problem of how chloramphenicol produces irreversible bone marrow aplasia in only an occasional individual who receives the drug remains completely unanswered. Almost certainly one has to implicate an individual susceptibility, the nature of which could be on a biochemical level. Patients who develop bone marrow aplasia from chloramphenicol may: 1) be unable to excrete the drug normally thereby attaining higher blood levels; 2) selectively concentrate the drug in their bone marrow; 3) metabolize the drug in an abnormal way thus giving rise to toxic metabolites; or 4) have an inborn error of metabolism such as an enzymatic deficiency which makes them susceptible to the toxic action of chloramphenicol. Unfortunately, studies directed to these possibilities have to be performed on patients who have aplastic anemia from chloramphenicol or who have recovered from this disease. For obvious reasons, most of these problems are not at present amenable to investigation and are at best limited to *in vitro* testing. Other than a statement by Erslev (referring to a personal communication with Glasko[4] that in few patients with chloramphenicol-induced pancytopenia the drug was found to be detoxified and excreted normally, no metabolic data are available on patients with bone marrow aplasia from the drug. Although chloramphenicol is not concentrated in rat bone marrow[14], it is not known if the same observation applies to subjects who develop aplastic anemia from the antibiotic.

Since bone marrow aplasia does not appear to be dose related a more likely possible mechanism of toxicity would be a biochemical susceptibility involving some essential metabolic pathway. This could be on the basis of an enzymatic defect analogous to G6PD deficiency. An inhibitory effect of chloramphenicol on the metabolic activity of normal bone marrow cells can be demonstrated *in vitro* only if the drug is used in concentrations 3–10 times the pharmacologic levels. To examine the possibility of a biochemical predisposition to chloramphenicol-induced bone marrow aplasia, Yunis and Arimura[95] studied the uptake of C^{14}-formate into DNA and RNA of bone marrow obtained from 5 patients who had recovered partially or completely from bone marrow aplasia believed to be due to chloramphenicol. In all 5 patients a 20–30% inhibition of formate uptake into both DNA and RNA could be demonstrated at drug concentrations of 25–50 $\mu g/ml$. (Fig. 8). Control studies on three

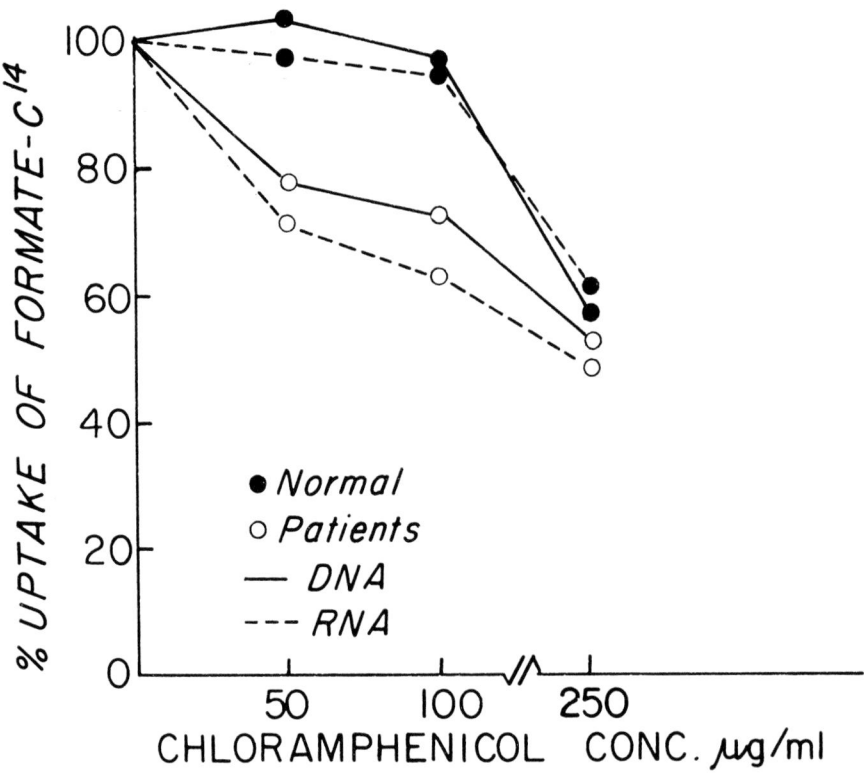

FIG. 8.—The effect of chloramphenicol on the in vitro uptake of Formate—C14 into DNA and RNA of bone marrow obtained from 5 subjects who have recovered from chloramphenicol-induced bone marrow aplasia.

patients with aplastic anemia not known to be related to chloramphenicol showed a pattern of inhibition similar to normal marrow[46], i.e., no inhibition until drug concentrations well above 100 μg/ml were used. Thus, it appeared that patients who develop aplasia from chloramphenicol demonstrate inhibition of nucleic acid synthesis at pharmacologic concentrations of the drug. The biphasic character of this inhibitory effect as seen in Fig. 8 may reflect a different level of sensitivity among the different cell populations; i.e., the inhibition at 50 μg/ml may represent a selective effect on the erythroid cells, other cells being unaffected until higher concentrations are attained. This possibility is now under investigation using tritiated nucleic acid precursors and autoradiography. The difference from normal in the pattern of inhibition observed here strongly suggests a biochemical predisposition to chloramphenicol-induced bone marrow aplasia involving the pathway of nucleic acid synthesis. However, further studies are needed to clarify the nature of this inhibition to be able to establish its importance in the pathogenesis of bone marrow aplasia from chloramphenicol. The above findings do not answer the question of why and how aplasia begins long after the drug has been discontinued. Several possibilities may be mentioned. Small amounts of the drug may remain within susceptible cells and exert their effect slowly. In the susceptible individual chloramphenicol may combine with the genetic makeup of the cell or DNA and thereby produce a lethal cellular effect. Chloramphenicol is incapable of penetrating the mature red cell to a significant degree[96]. It is not known if the same situation exists with relation to immature red cells. In the susceptible individual, the primary defect could be in the cell membrane which becomes abnormally permeable to chloramphenicol. These and other possibilities are under investigation.

Concluding Remarks

The problem of chloramphenicol toxicity as presented in this review can best be summed up in three important questions: 1) What are the characteristics and nature of myelotoxicity from this drug? 2) What is the mechanism by which chloramphenicol exerts its toxic effects? 3) In the light of present knowledge concerning the nature and mechanism of this toxicity, are there any preventive or precautionary measures that could be used effectively in patients receiving chloramphenicol?

It is clear from the present data that a distinction should be made between the reversible hematopoietic depression which frequently accompanies chloramphenicol therapy and the aplastic anemia from the drug. The existence of these two types of lesions from chloramphenicol raises several questions that are of both clinical and pathogenetic importance. Evidence has been presented that reversible toxicity from chloramphenicol is a pharmacological action of the drug which can be induced in most if not all subjects receiving large doses of the antibiotic. The biochemical mechanism for this effect is not well understood. In short-term *in vitro* experiments, chloramphenicol has no demonstrable effect on nucleic acid and protein synthesis unless used in concentrations many times the therapeutic level. However, this does not preclude a direct metabolic effect of the antibiotic *in vivo* since the length of exposure to the drug could be a more important determining factor. The evidence, provided by Weisberger, for an interaction of chloramphenicol with messenger RNA and inhibition of protein synthesis on that basis may offer a good biochemical explanation for the observed pharmacologic effects; however, further studies are needed in order to evaluate the importance of these findings.

Much less understood is the mechanism by which chloramphenicol causes irreversible bone marrow aplasia. There is no indication that this disastrous complication of chloramphenicol therapy is related clinically or pathogenetically to the reversible erythropoietic lesion from the drug. Since bone marrow aplasia is rare and has no constant relationship to drug dosage, an individual susceptibility is the most likely basic mechanism involved. A biochemical defect involving some essential metabolic pathway could be the determining factor. The significant inhibition of nucleic acid synthesis by pharmacologic concentrations of chloramphenicol observed in bone marrows from patients who have recovered from chloramphenicol-induced bone marrow aplasia tends to support this hypothesis.

The final and perhaps the most important question is whether there are any practical measures that could be instituted to prevent the onset of bone marrow aplasia in the patient receiving chloramphenicol therapy. It has been suggested that chloramphenicol administration should be monitored with blood tests and that the appearance of early toxic changes necessitates discontinuation of antibiotic[97]. Since no relation can be established between the reversible erythropoietic lesion and the development of aplastic anemia, the value of such an approach remains doubtful. Furthermore, no evidence exists that continued administration of the drug would lead to bone marrow aplasia nor is there evidence that early discontinuation of therapy would prevent the subsequent development of aplastic anemia. Even if it is assumed that the basic mechanism of toxicity is the same in both lesions, and that one is only an exaggerated form of the other occurring in occasional susceptible individuals, it is not possible by present means to foretell such individuals. The present authors believe that if chloramphenicol is given only when the drug is clearly indicated, it should not be discontinued because of the appearance of early toxic changes. The most important step in preventing bone marrow aplasia from chloramphenicol is not the monitoring of its administration, but the initial judgement of the physician as to whether the drug should or should not be given.

Most physicians recognize that chloramphenicol is an important addition to the list of antimicrobial agents and an excellent broad spectrum antibiotic. However, in view of the clearcut risk involved in its use, the antibiotic should be given only for life-threatening infections in which no other antibiotic is effective. An example of such a situation is typhoid fever. Unfortunately, in spite of repeated warnings by clinical investigators, the AMA Council on Drugs, and the manufacturers, reports[98] indicate that the drug is given for minor infections and even for conditions as trivial as malaise and iron deficiency anemia! In a great number of cases of fatal aplastic anemia from chloramphenicol, the drug need never have been given.

REFERENCES

1. Scott, J. L., Cartwright, G. E. and Wintrobe, M. M.: Acquired aplastic anemia. An analysis of 39 cases and review of the pertinent literature. Medicine 38: 119, 1959.
2. Mohler, D. N. and Leavell, B. S.: Aplastic Anemia: An analysis of 50 cases. Ann. Int. Med. 49: 326, 1958.
3. Huguley, C. M.: Drug-induced blood dyscrasias. Disease-a-Month. Oct., 1963.
4. Erslev, A. J. and Wintrobe, M. M.: Detection and prevention of drug-induced blood dyscrasias. J.A.M.A. 181: 114, 1962.
5. Rebstock, M. C., Crooks, H. M., Controulis, J. and Bartz, Q. R.: Chloramphenicol. IV. Chemical Studies. J. Am. Chem. Soc. 71: 2458, 1949.
6. Goodman, L. S. and Gilman, A.: The Pharmacological Basis of Therapeutics. Second Ed. The McMillan Company, 1960, p. 1394.
7. Hahn, F. E., Hayes, J. E., Wissman, C. L., Jr., Hopps, H. E., and Smadel, J. E.: Mode of Action of chloramphenicol. VI. Relation between structure and activity in the chloramphenicol series. Antibiotics and Chemotherapy 6: 531, 1956.
8. Brock, T. D.: Chloramphenicol. Bacteriological Reviews. 25: 32, 1961.
9. Collins, R. J., Ellis, B., Hansen, S. B., Mackenzie, H. S., Moualim, R. J., Petrow, V., Stephenson, O. and Sturgeon B.: Structural requirements for antibiotic activity in the chloramphenicol series II. J. Pharm. and Pharmacol. 4: 693, 1952.
10. Jackson, G. G.: Current concepts in therapy: Antibiotics IX Chloramphenicol. New Eng. J. Med. 259: 1172, 1958.
11. Smith, G. N. and Worrel, C. S.: The decomposition of chloromycetin by microorganisms. Arch. Biochem. 28: 232, 1950.
12. Merkel, J. R. and Steers, E.: Relationship between chloramphenicol reductase activity and chloramphenicol resistance to E. coli. J. Bacteriol. 66: 389, 1958.
13. Glazko, A. J., Wolf, L. M., Dill, W. A. and Bratton, A. C.: Biochemical studies on chloramphenicol. II. Tissue distribution and excretion studies. J. Pharmacol. Exp. Therap. 96: 445, 1949.
14. Yunis, A. A.: Unpublished observations.
15. Collins, Z. H.; and Beutler, E.: Personal communication.

16. Glazko, A. J., Dill, W. A. and Wolf, L. M.: Observations on the metabolic disposition of chloramphenicol in the rat. J. Pharmacol. Exp. Therap. 104: 452, 1952.
17. Kunin, C. M., Glazko, A. J., and Finland, M.: Persistence of antibiotics in blood in patients with acute renal failure. II. Chloramphenicol and its metabolic products in the blood of patients with severe renal disease or hepatic cirrhosis. J. Clin. Invest. 38: 1498, 1959.
18. Welch, H., Lewis, C. N. and Kerlan, I.: Blood dyscrasias, a nationwide survey: Antibiotics and Chemotherapy 4: 607, 1954.
19. Volini, I. F., Greenspan, I., Ehrlich, I., Gonner, J. A., Felsenfeld, O., and Schwartz, S. O.: Hematopoietic changes during administration of chloramphenicol. J.A.M.A. 142: 1333, 1950.
20. Rich, M. L., Ritterhof, R. J., and Hoffman, R. J.: A fatal case of aplastic anemia following chloramphenicol therapy. Ann. Int. Med. 33: 1459, 1950.
21. Gill, P. F.: Agranulocytosis following chloromycetin: Report of two cases. Med. J. Aust. 1: 768, 1950.
22. Rheingold, J. J. and Spurling, C. L.: Chloramphenicol and aplastic anemia. J.A.M.A. 149: 1301, 1952.
23. Smiley, R. K., Cartwright, G. E., Wintrobe, M. M.: Fatal aplastic anemia following chloramphenicol administration. J.A.M.A. 14: 914, 1952.
24. Sturgeon, P.: Fatal aplastic anemia in children following chloramphenicol therapy. J.A.M.A. 149: 918, 1952.
25. Wilson, L. E., Harris, M. S., Henstell, M. H., Witherbee, O. O. and Kahn, J.: Aplastic anemia following prolonged administration of chloramphenicol. A report of 2 cases, one a fatality. J.A.M.A. 149: 231, 1952.
26. Wolman, B.: Fatal aplastic anemia after chloramphenicol. Brit. Med. J. 2: 426, 1952.
27. Claudon, D. B. and Holbrook, H. A.: Fatal aplastic anemia associated with chloramphenicol therapy—Report of two cases. J.A.M.A. 149: 912, 1952.
28. Cone, T. E. and Abelson, S. M.: Aplastic anemia following two days of chloramphenicol therapy. J. Ped. 41: 340, 1952.
29. Recant, L. and Hartroft, S.: Clinical Pathology Conference: Aplastic anemia in a patient receiving chloramphenicol. Am. J. Med. 13: 782, 1952.
30. Dameshek, W., Campbell, E. W.: Hypoplastic anemia following continued administration of chloramphenicol—Report of a case. Bull. N. Eng. Med. Center 14: 181, 1952.
31. Hargraves, M., Mills, S. D. and Heck, F. J.: Aplastic anemia associated with administration of chloramphenicol. J.A.M.A. 149: 1293, 1952.
32. Hawkins, L. A. and Lederer, H.: Fatal aplastic anemia after chloramphenicol treatment. Brit. Med. J. 2: 423, 1952.
33. Loyd, E. L.: Aplastic anemia due to chloramphenicol—Antibiotics and Chemotherapy 2: 1, 1952.
34. Thompson, H. E., and Rowe, H. J.: A case of hypoplastic anemia with secondary thrombocytopenic purpura following the use of chloramphenicol. Ann. Int. Med. 39: 1124, 1952.
35. Erslev, A.: Hematopoietic depression induced by chlormycetin. Blood 8: 170, 1953.
36. Rankin, N. E.: Disseminated aspergillosis and moniliasis associated with agranulocytosis and antibiotic therapy. Brit. Med. J. 1: 918, 1953.
37. Ley, A. B.: Bone marrow depression from chloramphenicol. A.M.A. Arch Int. Med. 91: 43, 1953.
38. Todd, R. M.: The treatment of hypoplastic anemia after chloramphenicol. Arch. Dis. Child. 29: 575, 1954.
39. Hodgkinson, R.: Blood dyscrasias associated with chloramphenicol. An investigation into cases in the British Isles. Lancet 1: 285, 1954.
40. Pickard, K. and Rosenblatt, P.: Aplastic anemia due to chloromycetin toxicity. N.Y. State J. Med. 54: 1784, 1954.
41. Peyman, M. A.: Medical Memoranda. A fatal case of pernicious anemia associated with chloramphenicol treatment. Brit. M. J. 1: 1135, 1955.
42. Poulton, E. M.: Medical Memoranda. Thrombocytopenic purpura during chloramphenicol therapy. Brit. M. J. 2: 106, 1955.
43. Shaw, R. G., McLean, J. H.: Chloramphenicol and aplastic anemia. M. J. of Austral. 44: 352, 1957.
44. Johnston, A. W.: Aplastic anemia following treatment with chloramphenicol—Transfusion of polycythemic blood using sequestrene. Lancet 2: 319, 1959.
45. Ozer, F., Truax, W. E. and Levin, W. C.: Erythroid hypoplasia associated with chloramphenicol therapy. Blood 16: 997, 1960.
46. Yunis, A. A. and Harrington, W. J.: Patterns of inhibition by chloramphenicol of nucleic acid synthesis in human bone marrow and leukemic cells. J. Lab. Clin. Med. 56: 831, 1960.
47. Rosenbach, L., Caviles, A. and Mitus, W. J.: Chloramphenicol toxicity reversible vacuolization of erythroid cells. N. Eng. J. Med. 263: 724, 1960.
48. McCurdy, P. R.: Chloramphenicol bone marrow toxicity. J.A.M.A. 176: 588, 1961.

49. Nuguid, T. and Bacon, H. E.: Aplastic anemia following chloramphenicol therapy in chronic ulcerative colitis. A report of a case. Diseases of the Colon and Rectum 4: 269, 1961.
50. Jacobziner, H. and Raybin, H. W.: Poison control; chloromycetin poisoning. Arch. Ped. 78: 159, 1961.
51. Leiken, S. L., Welch, H. and Guin, G.: Aplastic anemia due to chloramphenicol. Clin. Proc. Children's Hosp. Wash. D.C., 17: 171, 1961.
52. Ghitis, J.: Acute benign erythroblastopenia possibly chloramphenicol-induced. J. Ped. 60: 566, 1962.
53. Gussoff, B. D., Lee, S. L. and Lichtman, H. C.: Erythropoietic changes during therapy with chloramphenicol. Arch. Int. Med. 109: 176, 1962.
54. Bjorkman, S. E.: Case of aplastic anemia caused by chloramphenicol with recovery after twenty-two months. Acta Hematologica. 27: 124, 1962.
55. Recinos, A., Ross, S. and Olshaker, T. E.: Chloromycetin in the treatment of pneumonia in infants and children (A preliminary report in 33 cases) N. Eng. J. Med. 241: 733, 1949.
56. Låpresti, J. M., Kaufman, P. and Olshaker, B., Ross, S. and Stevens, S.: Use of chloramphenicol in the treatment of urinary tract infections in childhood. Clin. Proc. Child. Hosp. Wash. D.C. 6: 177, 1950.
57. Wintrobe, M. M.: Clinical Hematology, Philadelphia, Lea and Febiger, 1956.
58. Osgood, E. E.: Drug-induced hypoplastic anemias and related syndromes. Ann. Int. Med. 39: 1173, 1953.
59. Ackroyd, J. F.: Allergic purpura including purpura due to foods, drugs and infections. Am. J. Med. 14: 605, 1953.
60. Bolton, F. G.: Thrombocytopenic purpura due to quinidine. II. Serologic mechanisms. Blood 11: 547, 1956.
61. Moeschlin, S., Meyer, H., Israels, L. G. and Tarr-Gloor, E.: Experimental agranulocytosis. Its production through leukocyte agglutination by antileukocytic serum. Acta Haemat. 11: 73, 1954.
62. Dausset, J., Nenna, A. and Brecy, H.: Leukoagglutinins in chronic idiopathic or symptomatic pancytopenia and in paroxysmal nocturnal hemoglobinuria. Blood. 9: 696, 1954.
63. Moeschlin, S., Siegenthaler, W., Gasser, C. and Hassig, A.: Immunopancytopenia associated with incomplete cold hemagglutinins in a case of primary atypical pneumonia. Blood 9: 214, 1954.
64. Matoh, Y., Elian, E., Nelken, D. and Nevo, A. C.: Specificity of lytic factors for erythrocytes, leukocytes, and platelets in a case of pancytopenia. Blood 11: 735, 1956.
65. Rigdon, R. H., Crass, G., and Mailin, N.: Anemia produced by chloramphenicol in the duck. A.M.A. Arch. Path. 58: 85, 1954.
66. Smith, R. M.: Chloromycetin. Biological studies. J. Bacteriol. 55: 425, 1948.
67. Krakoff, I. H., Karnofsky, D. A. and Burchenal, J. H.: Effects of large doses of chloramphenicol on human subjects. New Eng. J. Med. 253: 7, 1955.
68. Rubin, D., Weisberger, A. S., Botti, R. E. and Storaasli, J. P.: Changes in iron metabolism in early chloramphenicol toxicity. J. Clin. Invest. 37: 1286, 1958.
69. Rubin, D., Weisberger, A. S. and Clark, D. R.: Early detection of drug induced erythropoietic depression. J. Lab. & Clin. Med. 56: 453, 1960.
70. Saidi, P., Wallerstein, R. O. and Aggeler, P. M.: Effect of chloramphenicol on erythropoiesis. J. Lab. & Clin. Med. 57: 247, 1961.
71. Jiji, R. M., Gangarosa, E. J. and DelaMacorra, F.: Chloramphenicol and its sulfamoyl analogues. Report of reversible erythropoietic toxicity in healthy volunteers. Arch. Int. Med. 111: 70, 1963.
72. McCurdy, P. R.: Plasma concentrations of chloramphenicol and bone marrow suppression. Blood 21: 363, 1963.
73. Suhrland, L. G., and Weisberger, A. S.: Chloramphenicol toxicity in liver and renal disease. Arch. Int. Med. 112: 747, 1963.
74. Suhrland, L. G. and Weisberger, A. S.: Hematologic toxicity of a chloramphenicol analogue. Amer. J. Med. Sci. 244: 54, 1962.
75. Wallerstein, R. O.: Chloramphenicol. Calif. Med. 97: 180, 1962.
76. McCurdy, P. R., Pierce, K. E. and Rath, C. E.: Abnormal bone marrow morphology in acute alcoholism. New Eng. J. Med. 266: 505, 1962.
77. Gale, E. F., and Folkes, J. B.: The assimilation of amino acids by bacteria 15. Actions of antibiotics on nucleic acid and protein synthesis in staphylococcus aureus. Biochem. J. 53: 493, 1953.
78. Wissman, C. L., Jr., Smadel, J. E., Hahn, F. E. and Hopps, H. E.: Mode of action of chloramphenicol. I. Action of chloramphenicol on assimilation of ammonia and on synthesis of proteins and nucleic acids in Escherichia coli. J. Bacteriol. 67: 662, 1954.
79. Demoss, J. A. and Novelli, D.: An amino acid dependent exchange between P^{32} labelled inorganic pyrophosphate and ATP in microbial extracts. Biochim. et Biophys. Acta. 22: 49, 1956.
80. Lacks, S. and Gros, F.: A metabolic study of the RNA-amino acid complexes in Escherichia coli. J. Molecular Biol. 1: 301, 1960.

81. Rendi, R., and Ochoa, S.: Effect of chloramphenicol on protein synthesis in cell free preparations of Escherichia coli. J. Biol. Chem. 237: 3711, 1962.
82. Doudney, C. O.: Inhibition of nucleic acid synthesis by chloramphenicol in synchronized cultures of Escherichia coli. J. Bacteriol. 76: 122, 1960.
83. Thomas, R.: Effects of chloramphenicol on genetic replication in bacteriophage. Virology 9: 275, 1959.
84. Goodgal, S. H. and Melechen, N. E.: Synthesis of transforming DNA in the presence of chloramphenicol. Biochem. Biophys. Res. Commun. 3: 114, 1960.
85. Horowitz, J., Lombard, A. and Chargaff, E.: Aspects of the stability of a bacterial ribonucleic acid. J. Biol. Chem. 233: 1517, 1958.
86. Dagley, S., White, A. E., Wild, D. G. and Sykes, J.: Synthesis of Protein and Ribosomes in Bacteria. Nature. 194: 25, 1962.
87. Hahn, F. E., Wissman, C. L., Jr., and Hopps, H. E.: Mode of action of chloramphenicol. III. Action of chloramphenicol on bacterial energy metabolism. J. Bacteriol. 69: 215, 1955.
88. Rendi, R.: The effect of chloramphenicol on the incorporation of labelled amino acid into proteins by isolated subcellular fractions from rat liver. Exp. Cell Res. 18: 187, 1959.
89. Von Ehrenstein, G., Lipmann, F.: Experiments on hemoglobin biosynthesis. Proc. Nat. Acad. Sci. 47: 941, 1961.
90. Borsook, H., Fischer, E. H. and Keighley, G.: Factors affecting protein synthesis in vitro in rabbit reticulocytes. J. Biol. Chem. 229: 1059, 1957.
91. Breitman, T. R. and Webster, G. C.: Effect of chloramphenicol on protein and nucleic acid synthesis in isolated thymus nuclei. Biochim. et Biophys Acta. 27: 408, 1958.
92. Folette, J. H., Shugarman, P. M., Reynolds, J., Valentine, W. N. and Lawrence, J. S.: The effect of chloramphenicol and other antibiotics on leukocyte respiration. Blood 11: 234, 1956.
93. Erslev, A. J. and Iossifides, I. A.: In vitro action of chloramphenicol and chloramphenicol analogues on the metabolism of human immature red blood cells. Acta Hemat. 28: 1, 1962
94. Weisberger, A. S., Armentrout, S. and Wolfe, S.: Protein synthesis by reticulocyte ribosomes. I. Inhibition of polyuridylic acid-induced ribosomal protein synthesis by chloramphenicol. Proc. Nat. Acad. Sci. 50: 86, 1963.
95. Yunis, A. A. and Arimura, G. K.: Biochemical predisposition to chloramphenicol-induced bone marrow aplasia. Clin. Res., April, 1963.
96. Watson, K. C.: Penetration of human red cells by penicillin, chloramphenicol and tetracycline. J. Lab. & Clin. Med. 51: 778, 1958.
97. Hartmann, R. C.: Chloramphenicol and the code of Hammurabi. American Practitioner 13: 497, 1962.
98. A.M.A. Council on Drugs Report. J.A.M.A. 172: 2044, 1960.
99. Wolfe, A. D. and Hahn, F. E.: Erythromycin mode of action. Science 143: 1445, 1964.

Myeloma Proteins and Macroglobulins: Hallmarks of Disease and Models of Antibodies

——GEORGE M. BERNIER and FRANK W. PUTNAM——

1. *Introduction*

ONE hundred and seventeen years before this review was written, a chemical pathologist named Henry Bence Jones began the literature of the myeloma proteins by describing the urinary protein that bears his name.[64] More recently, investigators have accorded this time-hallowed protein a special place in their quest of antibody structure. Through these many years, Bence-Jones proteins and myeloma globulins have had a dual scientific importance. They have been of diagnostic value for clinicians and, because of their relative purity and accessibility, they have been of great interest to protein chemists. In the last few years this interest has heightened because study of the myeloma globulins and Bence-Jones proteins has enabled the antigenic classification of the human immunoglobulins and has facilitated the understanding of their chemical structure. The purpose of this review is to summarize recent advances in biochemical understanding of the myeloma proteins and to discuss the relatively newfound role of these proteins as models of antibodies. For a more clinical viewpoint, the reader is referred to recent reviews by Waldenström[124] and Osserman and Takatsuki[76] which deal with both clinical and chemical aspects of multiple myeloma and macroglobulinemia.

Since the reviews of this topic in 1959 and 1960 by Putnam,[87, 88] the single most significant advance in structural study was Porter's demonstration that the γ-globulin molecule could be cleaved into biologically active fragments by limited enzymatic hydrolysis.[81] This finding opened new avenues of research into the subunit structure of the γ-globulins; these have since been extended to include methods of polypeptide chain separation by reductive cleavage[25] and have led to the postulation of a model of the multichain structure of γ-globulin.[34] Parallel studies of this sort utilizing homogeneous myeloma globulins[24] rather than the heterogeneous γ-globulin population have shed light on the structure not only of myeloma proteins but of γ-globulins in general.

Extensive studies have also been carried out on the series of murine plasmacytomas which are transmissible within an inbred strain of mice.[27, 28, 83, 84] Despite the great importance of this animal system for experimental investigation of the pathogenesis of multiple myeloma and macroglobulinemia, this review will be restricted to the human disease. However, many of the observations on human myeloma proteins have been confirmed by analogy in the mouse system.

A related series of investigations has dealt with genetic markers on human

From the Department of Biochemistry, University of Florida College of Medicine, Gainesville, Florida.

Support is acknowledged from Public Health Service Research Grant CA-02803 from the National Cancer Institute.

γ-globulin molecules.[49, 50, 105, 115] The finding that γ-globulin from some normal individuals, but not from others, can inhibit red cell agglutination by certain rheumatoid sera has led to the elucidation of the Gm and InV factors. At present, the demonstration of the presence or absence of these allotypic factors rests upon indirect biological testing; however, the detection of these factors provides a discriminating tool for locating inherited differences in γ-globulins in world populations[106, 116] and for localizing individual genetic factors to specific portions of the γ-globulin molecule.[19, 40, 51]

Chemical study of the myeloma proteins and of γ-globulin has been greatly facilitated by the application of the peptide mapping techniques earlier applied to normal and abnormal hemoglobins by Ingram.[62] In particular, elucidation of the relationship of Bence-Jones proteins to one another and to myeloma globulins and normal γ-globulins has been possible.[89]

In the following sections, these approaches will be discussed as they apply to the different classes of human myeloma proteins. For ease in identification, the myeloma proteins will be referred to as "pathological proteins." This is not intended to imply that the protein is abnormal in structure or composition (though it may be). The label here reflects more the source of the protein rather than the protein itself. Nomenclature is a problem in this field as it is in so many others, and table I is included to list synonymous terms used by various workers. For example, the letter "A" is used in at least seven designations and in several different senses. As more information is obtained, it should be possible to devise a more uniform nomenclature which reflects chemical structure and biological properties.

2. The Immunoglobulin Family

It has long been known that the term γ-globulin encompassed a diverse group of protein molecules, but it was not appreciated just how diverse this was until

TABLE I.—Synonyms of Terms Used in this Review

Term	Synonym
7S γ-globulin	γ_2 , γ_{SS} , 6.6S γ
β_{2A}-globulin	γ_{1A} , γ_1
β_{2M}-globulin	γ_{1M} , 19S γ
γU	γ_L , gamma-related urinary protein
Antigenic type I	Antigenic type B, type 1
Antigenic type II	Antigenic type A, type 2
F (Fast) fragment	Piece III*, fragment B, acidic fragment
S (Slow) fragment	Pieces I and II*, fragments A and C, basic fragment
Gm	Gm_1
InV	Gm_2
H (Heavy) chain	A chain*
L (Light) chain	B chain*

* Used in descriptions of rabbit antibody.

TABLE II.—*Chemical Composition and Physical Constants of Normal Immunoglobulins*

Class	Pathological counterpart	Range of mobility*	$s_{20,w}$†	Approx. molecular weight	Carbo-hydrate content	Normal serum concentration (range)‡
7S γ-globulin	7S γ myeloma globulin	0.5–1.3	6.6S	150,000	3%	0.8–1.5
β_{2A}-globulin	β_{2A} myeloma globulin	1.2–3.6	7S, 10S, 14S	150,000 and multi-ples	10%	0.056–0.195
β_{2M}-globulin	Waldenström macroglob-ulin	0.5–2.3	19S	1,000,000	10%	0.039–0.117
γU	Bence-Jones proteins		2S	22,000	0§	—

    * Values expressed as 10^{-5} cm² volt^{-1} sec^{-1} at pH 8.6 in Veronal buffer refer to the normal component.

    † Expressed in Svedberg units.

    ‡ Given in gm per 100 ml.

    § Inferred from study of Bence-Jones proteins.

the advent of immunoelectrophoresis.[47, 127] As a consequence, three related yet distinct classes of γ-globulins have been described[55]—the β_2-macroglobulin (β_{2M}), the fast migrating γ-globulin (β_{2A}), and an electrophoretically, extremely heterogeneous population (7S γ). Each class has been shown to possess antibody activity,[31, 59] hence the name immunoglobulins. Each class also has been found to have two kinds of antigenic portions: one which is highly characteristic of the class and one which is common to all three classes. Low molecular weight urinary proteins normally excreted in small amounts (γ_U) are antigenically related to these immunoglobulins and are here considered as a fourth class (table II). Thus, the immunoglobulins include both proteins with antibody activity and proteins having an antigenic specificity in common with them. The reference to a common antigenic specificity permits the inclusion of proteins whose antibody activity has not been demonstrated, such as "normal γ-globulin" and the pathological myeloma globulins, macroglobulins, and Bence-Jones proteins. This brings up the very interesting point of whether any of the immunoglobulins are truly devoid of antibody activity, including both normal γ-globulins and the pathological proteins.

In plasma cell malignancies, one or more of these immunoglobulins may be greatly increased, resulting in the production of a highly homogeneous 7S γ or β_{2A} myeloma globulin, a Waldenström macroglobulin, and/or a Bence-Jones protein. Some of the characteristic electrophoretic patterns obtained in multiple myeloma are illustrated in figure 1. The electrophoretic patterns in macroglobulinemia are similar to those illustrated for multiple myeloma. Starch gel electrophoresis and immunoelectrophoresis, though not quantitative in nature, enable the ready identification of myeloma globulins and macroglobulins and afford much better resolution of other serum components (fig. 2). The myeloma globulins exhibit sharp bands in starch gel electrophoresis, whereas macroglobulins fail to move from the origin or migrate slowly. The most reliable physical

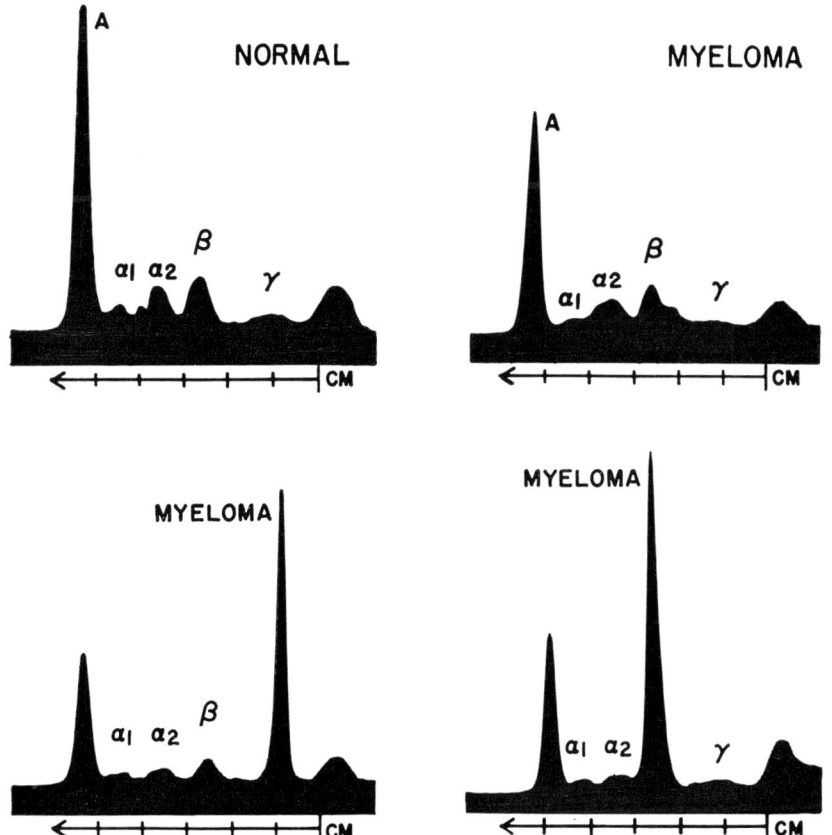

FIG. 1.—Tiselius electrophoretic patterns of normal and myeloma sera. Note that the pathological protein may have differing electrophoretic mobilities in different patients, although the mobility of the pathological protein in any individual myeloma patient is rather constant with time. The serum diagram in the upper right is that of a myeloma patient without hyperglobulinemia but with a Bence-Jones urinary protein.

method for distinguishing the myeloma globulins and macroglobulins is analytical ultracentrifugation, illustrated in figure 3.

Most commonly, patients with plasma cell malignancies have one pathological serum globulin and/or a urinary Bence-Jones protein. (The latter, of course, also traverses the serum.) However, there are reports of myeloma patients with more than one pathological serum globulin[61, 107, 123] and also patients with no demonstrable pathological proteins in the serum or urine.[76]

Immunoelectrophoresis and immunodiffusion permit identification and classification based on the characteristic antigenic determinants of the various immunoglobulins. Korngold and Lipari[66] in this country and Burtin et al.[14] in France found Bence-Jones proteins to be of two distinct antigenic types, now designated I and II. Subsequent antigenic analysis of many myeloma globulins and macroglobulins with antisera prepared against a type I or a type II Bence-Jones protein revealed that any given pathological protein could be typed either as antigenic type I or type II.[69, 74] It was thus found that each pathological serum globulin

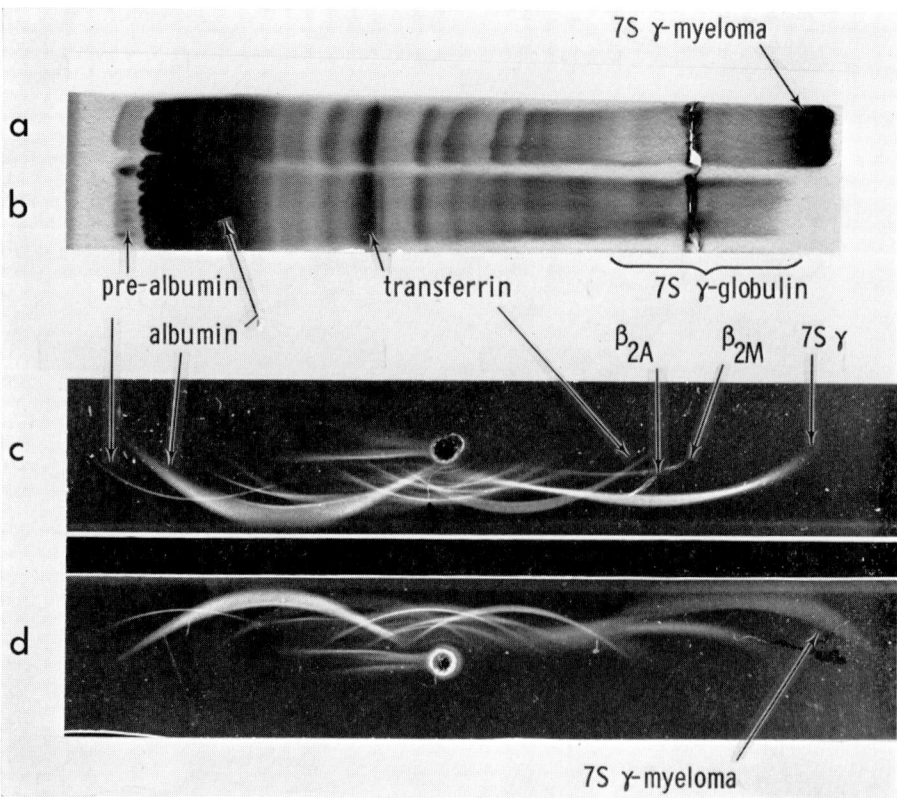

FIG. 2.—Starch gel electrophoretic and immunoelectrophoretic comparison of a normal serum (b, c) and the serum of a patient with 7S γ myeloma (a, d). Some of the normal serum constituents are identified. The 7S γ myeloma protein shown here (pt. Be) is an extremely basic one. It is identifiable as a band in starch gel electrophoresis (a) and as an arc of antigen excess in immunoelectrophoresis against anti-human serum (d).

has two portions, one which is class specific (i.e., 7S γ, β_{2A}, or β_{2M}) and one which is antigenic type I or type II. This means that there are in all eight kinds of pathological proteins. These are illustrated schematically in figure 4. Immunoglobulins from normal persons may also be grouped into these two antigenic types.[30, 39, 71, 119] Present evidence indicates that approximately 60% of the 7S γ-globulin molecules from a normal individual are of antigenic type I and 40% are of antigenic type II.[30, 71] Precise quantitation of the relative amounts of type I and type II normal β_{2A}, β_{2M}, and γ_U has been reported by Fahey,[30] and in each case the connection of type I molecules was approximately twice that of type II. The following three sections deal with the pathological proteins in detail and stress the chemical basis for the antigenic classification.

3. Bence-Jones Proteins

The oldest known and most frequently studied of the myeloma proteins, the Bence-Jones proteins, have emerged as the common antigenic and structural thread throughout the immunoglobulin family. Earlier work has been reviewed.[86]

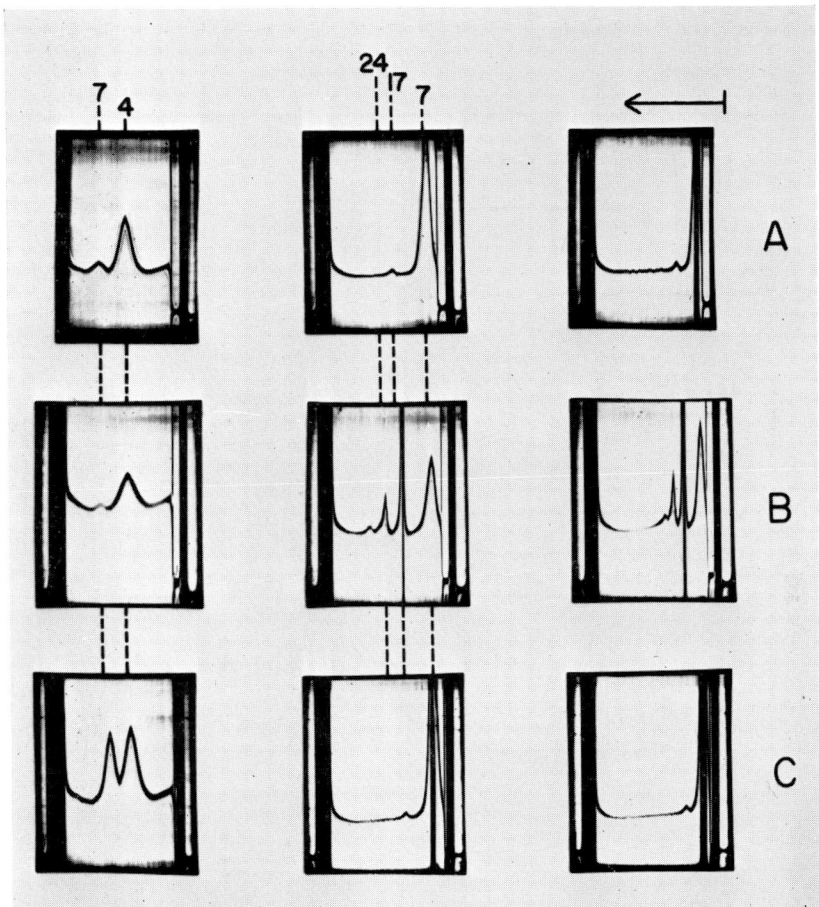

FIG. 3.—Ultracentrifugal diagrams of a normal serum (A), a Waldenström's macro-globulinemic serum (B), and a serum with increased 7S γ-globulin (C). The latter serum, though not from a myeloma patient, shows the sedimentation pattern observed in ultra-centrifugation of 7S γ myeloma sera. The analyses were done at 59,780 r.p.m. in a pH 8.6 Veronal buffer and photographs have been selected to demonstrate the progressive separa-tion of the several components at approximately the same time after acceleration to top speed. The dotted lines are references drawn in to indicate the approximate s_{20} . The s_{20} values 24 and 17 refer to macroglobulins, 7 to the 7S γ-globulin, and 4 to albumin and other minor serum components. Note that in A and C, the high molecular weight component is present but is quantitatively less than in the serum of Waldenström's macroglobulinemia. (Reprinted with permission of author and publisher from Cooper, G. R., Electrophoretic and ultracentrifugal analysis of normal human serum. *In* Putnam, F. W. (Ed.) The Plasma Proteins. Vol. I., Isolation, Characterization, and Function. New York, Academic, press, 1960.)

Recent studies have dealt with the question of homogeneity,[7, 121, 126] with physical properties,[7, 21, 120] antigenic characteristics,[67, 70, 114] chemical composition,[6, 16, 120] and the relationships of Bence-Jones proteins to one another and to the myeloma globulins.[66, 69, 74, 89] Another important advance has been the demonstration of the normal counterpart of Bence-Jones proteins—the γ_U .[37, 117, 125]

a. *Homogeneity.*—Although Bence-Jones proteins may differ rather markedly

PATHOLOGICAL IMMUNOGLOBULINS

Schematic Antigenic Map

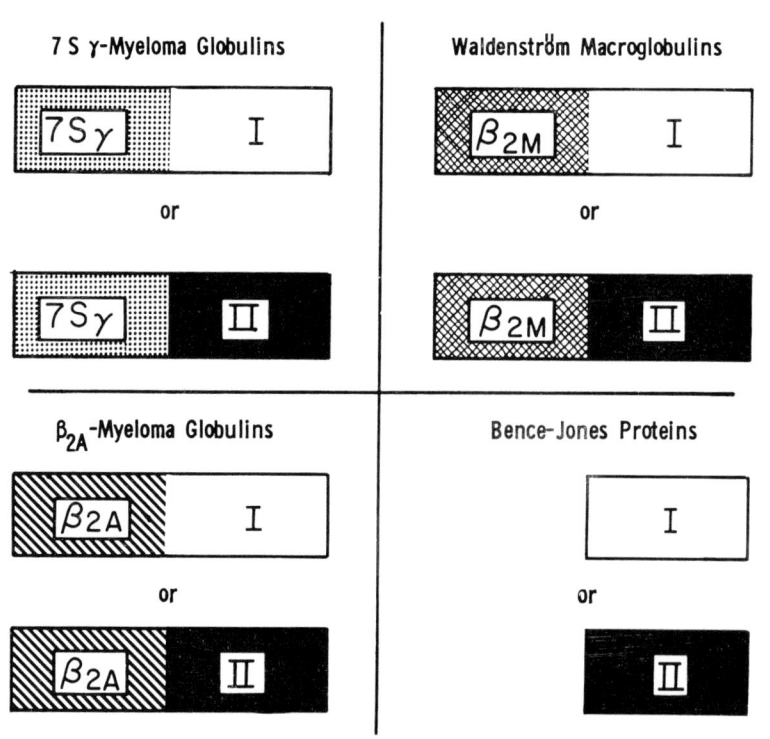

FIG. 4.—Schematic antigenic representation of the pathological immunoglobulins, showing the common type I or type II portions and the class-specific determinants. In the normal individual, molecules of all eight classes are present. The patient with multiple myeloma may produce more than one pathological protein. Thus far, these have always been of a single antigenic type, e.g., type I β_{2A} myeloma globulin and type I Bence-Jones protein.

from one another in terms of electrophoretic charge,[54, 96] the protein excreted by a single myeloma patient is quite constant from day to day. A Bence-Jones protein preparation, isolated from the urine by ammonium sulfate precipitation, may appear quite homogeneous by several criteria (free boundary and paper electrophoresis and ultracentrifugation). However, when electrophoresed in starch gel, most Bence-Jones proteins exhibit a multiple banding phenomenon.[26, 35] By a combination of ion exchange chromatography and gel filtration, several laboratories have been able to prepare Bence-Jones proteins which migrate as single bands in starch gel electrophoresis.[7, 24, 120] By isolation of minor components the multiple banding has been shown to result both from the presence of polymeric and polymorphic forms and from contamination with non-Bence-Jones proteins.[7]

 b. *Physical properties.*—Most Bence-Jones proteins have a sedimentation

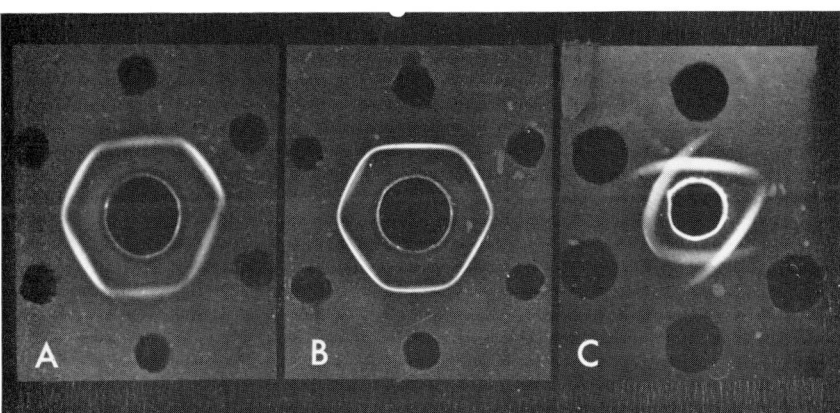

Fig. 5.—Ouchterlony double diffusion experiments with Bence-Jones proteins and anti-7S γ-globulin: A) type I Bence-Jones proteins from different individuals giving a reaction of identity to one another, B) type II Bence-Jones proteins from different individuals also giving a reaction of identity, and C) reactions of non-identity between three type II Bence-Jones proteins and two type I Bence-Jones proteins.

coefficient of 3.6S (molecular weight of approximately 45,000), although $s_{20,w}$ values ranging from 1.8S to 5.5S have been reported for some Bence-Jones proteins.[93] Recent evidence suggests that the monomer unit of these proteins is about 22,000 and that the usual 3.6S unit is a dimer.[6, 7] Bence-Jones proteins with $s_{20,w}$ values of 5.5S would then be tetramers. Moreover, some Bence-Jones proteins exhibit the curvilinear concentration dependence curves of $s_{20,w}$ characteristic of a rapidly interacting monomer-dimer system. When monomer and dimer have been isolated from a single preparation of Bence-Jones protein, they have been found to be virtually identical by amino acid composition, peptide mapping, antigenic analysis, and thermal solubilities. However, the report of Heimer et al.[53] is at variance with this general scheme.

c. *Antigenic characteristics.*—As has been mentioned, Korngold and Lipari[66] found Bence-Jones proteins to belong to either one of two antigenic classes (I and II); this classification has been extended to the myeloma globulins and macroglobulins as well.[69, 74] When several type I Bence-Jones proteins are reacted in Ouchterlony immunodiffusion plates against anti-7S γ-globulin, a reaction of identity results (fig. 5A). The same is true for type II Bence-Jones proteins (fig. 5B), but when a Bence-Jones protein of each type is used, a reaction of nonidentity occurs (fig. 5C). Although all Bence-Jones proteins may be grouped into these two types, each protein also appears to have antigenic determinants specific to itself. Mannik and Kunkel[70] have shown that antisera prepared against a particular Bence-Jones protein, e.g., of type I, will react only with that specific protein after the antiserum has been absorbed with pooled 7S γ-globulin. Thus, a specific "signature" is present upon each Bence-Jones protein, as well as determinants designating it as type I or II. Stein et al.[114] have presented evidence for individual and subgroup antigenic specificity of Bence-Jones proteins.

d. *Chemical composition.*—Neither in the Bence-Jones proteins nor in the myeloma globulins have any unique constituents been found. Amino acid analyses have failed to demonstrate any consistent difference between type I and type II Bence-Jones proteins, except possibly the absence of methionine in the type II proteins. However, peptide mapping (two-dimensional chromatography-electrophoresis) of the tryptic peptides obtained from these proteins has proven of great value in the establishment of similarities and differences between Bence-Jones proteins.

Under their conditions, Putnam and co-workers[94] found that the peptide maps of type I Bence-Jones proteins are totally dissimilar to maps of type II. Moreover, Bence-Jones proteins of a given antigenic type share many peptides in common but have a variable number of peptides apparently specific for the protein. The use of peptide mapping in establishing the relationship between Bence-Jones proteins and the myeloma globulins will be dealt with in a later section.

The reports of variable carbohydrate content of Bence-Jones proteins have been clarified by the findings of Clamp et al.[16] that these proteins are carbohydrate-free and that variable amounts of carbohydrate-rich contaminants may be present in individual preparations.

e. *Normal counterparts.*—For the biologist who sees byproducts of disease as the overproduction of normal metabolites, some recent findings make Bence-Jones protein seem to be a less anomalous substance.

Stevenson,[117] Berggård and Edelman,[4] and Franklin[37] have shown that normal individuals excrete in their urine small amounts of an electrophoretically heterogeneous, low molecular weight protein, antigenically related to γ-globulin. This has been termed γ_U. It is also possible to isolate such proteins from normal serum by ultrafiltration,[4] and it is probable that the γ_U has the same relationship to normal γ-globulins as the Bence-Jones proteins have to myeloma globulins. Takatsuki and Osserman[119] and Fahey[30] have recently shown that the γ_U proteins may be classed as type I and type II; that is, they possess the antigenic determinants of Bence-Jones proteins and lack the 7S γ specific determinants.

Although Bence-Jones proteins were first recognized by their remarkable thermal solubility properties, it is not surprising that many other proteins have been found to have specific temperatures for precipitation and for redissolution. The difference between most of the Bence-Jones class and other proteins is the higher temperature required for the latter to dissolve (greater than 110° in most cases). However, "pseudo Bence-Jones proteins," which are chemically and antigenically like any other Bence-Jones protein, also require temperatures higher than the boiling point of water for dissolution.[7] In this connection attention should be directed to a practical thermal test for the detection of Bence-Jones protein in which the importance of the adjustment of the pH of the urine is recognized.[93] A micro-modification of this test employing a sealed capillary tube has been reported.[7] The most important criterion is the precipitation of the protein below 60°. Paper electrophoresis with the finding of a major urinary protein component other than albumin is a desirable verification test.

4. *Myeloma Globulins*

Each class of normal immunoglobulin (7S γ, β_{2A}, β_{2M}) may be further divided, as has been said, into two antigenic types (I and II). Each subgroup (e.g., 7S γ, type I) is far from homogeneous electrophoretically and in all likelihood consists of many antibody populations which differ from one another by differences in primary sequence. As is the case with Bence-Jones proteins, each antibody population may have its own "signature" in addition to the class and type determinants.

Myeloma globulins and Waldenström macroglobulins, on the other hand, probably represent a highly homogeneous overproduction of one such population or "clone," and the individual molecules closely resemble one another. It had been believed for some time that the resemblance was that of absolute identity, but recent studies by Fahey[29] have demonstrated electrophoretic heterogeneity of myeloma globulins in starch gel when high pH's are used. The basis for this heterogeneity has not as yet been explained.

In this section, studies pertaining to the subunit structure of the myeloma globulins will be reviewed. The structure of 7S γ myeloma proteins will be considered first. The term "myeloma globulins" as used herein will refer to the 7S γ and β_{2A} myeloma globulins and not macroglobulins.

a. *7S γ myeloma globulins.*—It had been suspected for some time that the 7S γ myeloma proteins were multichain structures because of the presence of more than one N-terminal amino acid.[85] However, only in the past few years has the subunit structure of antibodies and myeloma proteins been investigated vigorously. Three procedures have been used to elucidate the subunit structure of the γ-globulins: (1) limited enzymatic cleavage, (2) chemical cleavage, and (3) comparison of the chemical and antigenic properties of Bence-Jones proteins with those of fragments or polypeptide chains obtained by cleavage of the normal and pathological proteins.

(1) Limited enzymatic cleavage—The principal impetus to subunit investigation was Porter's finding[81] that papain in the presence of a reducing agent would cleave specific rabbit antibody into three chromatographically separable fragments (I, II, and III). These fragments (Porter pieces) are of approximately equal size, and two of them (I and II) continue to possess specific activity as univalent antibody. Subsequent investigation[23, 78, 110] has shown that fragments I and II have similar physical, chemical, and biological properties, but they are derived from different electrophoretic populations of molecules. Since fragments I and II have similar antigenic properties, they *do not* correspond to antigenic types I and II in the human immunoglobulin system. The papain products of rabbit 7S γ-globulin are currently referred to as Porter fragment I and Porter fragment III (see table I). Some of the secondary biological activities of γ-globulin have been found to reside in fragment III (complement fixation, skin fixation, and placental transfer), but only fragment I and fragment II combine specifically with antigen. All three fragments possess some antigenic determinants of rabbit 7S γ-globulin.

When papain cleavage was applied to human 7S γ-globulins, and in particular to myeloma globulins, analogous fragments were produced.[38, 92] These have been termed "Fast" (F) and "Slow" (S) because of their relative mobilities in immuno-electrophoresis at pH 8.6. The F fragment was found to resemble fragment III of the rabbit in that it contained the carbohydrate and the factors for skin fixation and complement fixation.[38] It has further been shown to possess the genetically determined Gm factors[19, 40, 51] and to contain the class-specific anti-

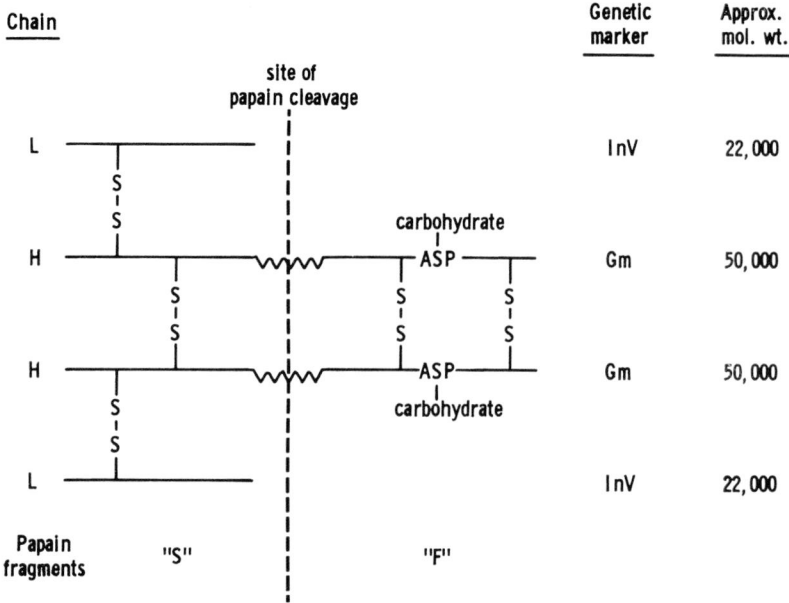

FIG. 6.—Modification of Porter's[82] model of the polypeptide chain structure of 7S γ-globulin. The L chains are similar to Bence-Jones proteins and possess the InV activity and the antigenic type I or type II determinants. A single 7S γ-globulin molecule has either type I L chains or type II L chains but not both. However, the serum of normal individuals contains both kinds of 7S γ-globulin. The H chains possess the secondary biologic characteristics of the molecule, the Gm activity, and the carbohydrate. The jagged line in the middle of each of the H chains represents the site of papain cleavage and indicates the possibility that the H chain may really be two polypeptide chains instead of one.

genic determinants of 7S γ-globulin. The S fragment is similar to piece I in that it retains combining activity when prepared from an antibody[38] but lacks the secondary biological activities. Studies on the myeloma proteins have shown that the S fragment has both the genetically determined InV factor[40, 51] and the determinants responsible for antigenic type (I or II).[69, 74] It is this portion of the 7S γ molecule, therefore, which is antigenically related to the rest of the immunoglobulin family. The structural relationship of the S and F fragments to the multichain structure of 7S γ-globulin is later illustrated schematically in figure 6.

Comparative peptide mapping of F fragments of myeloma globulins shows them to be closely alike regardless of the antigenic type of the original protein.[90] The S fragment of a 7S γ myeloma is quite different from the F by peptide mapping and contains virtually all the tryptic peptides of the Bence-Jones protein from the same individual. The S fragment contains other peptides as well, some of which are common to both antigenic types I and II. These results are in accord with the concept[89] that the Bence-Jones protein represents one of the polypeptide chains of the myeloma globulin, as is described in a later section.

(2) Chemical cleavage—A rather different approach to the subunit structure of antibodies and myeloma globulins has involved chemical cleavage without splitting of peptide bonds. In this approach, disulfide bonds are split by reducing

agents, the free sulfhydryl groups are blocked by alkylation, and the resultant chains are separated by gel filtration or ion exchange chromatography in the presence of dispersing agents such as urea,[25] detergent,[63] or propionic acid.[34]

By reductive cleavage of myeloma globulins Edelman and co-workers[24, 109] obtained two kinds of polypeptide chains. The larger (molecular weight = approximately 50,000) is called "H" for heavy and the other "L" for light (molecular weight = approximately 22,000). The L chains from a reduced-alkylated myeloma globulin were virtually indistinguishable from the Bence-Jones protein of the same patient in terms of electrophoresis in starch-urea gel, amino acid composition, peptide mapping, and antigenic and spectrofluorometric studies. The H chain was wholly dissimilar to both the L chain and the Bence-Jones protein. On the basis of these findings, Edelman and Gally[24] postulated that the usual 3.5S Bence-Jones protein was a dimer of unincorporated L chains. Recent findings on monomer-dimer forms of Bence-Jones proteins further substantiate this possibility (see Section 3). The concept that the Bence-Jones proteins are unincorporated chains accords with earlier metabolic studies by isotopic methods.[95]

Using somewhat different methods of reductive cleavage on horse and rabbit antibody, Porter[82] has proposed a model of the chain structure of γ-globulin. This model has found general acceptance although some aspects of it are unresolved. In figure 6 the postulated polypeptide chain structure of a 7S γ myeloma globulin is depicted in a schematic form based on Porter's model. The diagram takes into account the additional information available from study of the chemical and antigenic relationships of myeloma globulins and Bence-Jones proteins and the distribution of genetic markers among the subunits. The proposed structure consists of two heavy (H) chains of 50,000 molecular weight which are 7S γ specific, contain the carbohydrate, have the Gm sites, and secondary biological characteristics. The light (L) chains are Bence-Jones-like, possess InV factors, and are of antigenic types I or II; hence, they represent the common structural and antigenic portion of the immunoglobulins. There is still disagreement as to which of the two kinds of chains in antibodies possesses the combining activity. At present, there is evidence for the heavy chain,[34] the light chain,[103] or both chains[36, 102] being involved in the antigen-combining site.

(3) Franklin's disease—As details of the substructure of the 7S γ-globulins were unfolding, a new disease entity became recognized. Described originally by Franklin[42] and later and more fully by Osserman and Takatsuki,[76] the disease bears closer clinical resemblance to malignant lymphoma than to myeloma. However, as with the myelomas, a pathological protein is synthesized in large amount and appears in the serum and urine. The Franklin protein is of low molecular weight (approximately 53,000) but is unrelated to Bence-Jones proteins or L chains. The Franklin protein is chemically and antigenically related to the H chain of 7S γ-globulin but more closely resembles the F fragment than the intact H chain. To date, five cases of Franklin's disease have been investigated.[42, 76, 77] It is anticipated that the disease will be found to be more common as it is looked for, and that low molecular weight proteins bearing exclusively β_{2A} or β_{2M} determinants will also be found, both in serum and urine. Using antisera prepared against two of the Franklin proteins, Ballieux et al.[2] have demon-

strated the presence of two populations of normal and myeloma 7S γ-globulins which differ to some extent in the antigenic characteristics of the H chains. Previous studies by Korngold[65] and Peetoom and Kramer[80] have indicated that the scheme illustrated in figure 4 is probably an oversimplification.

b. *β_{2A} myeloma globulins.*—The study of human serum with immunoelectrophoresis by Williams[127] and by others[47, 55, 58] demonstrated the existence of a β-globulin which was antigenically related to 7S γ-globulin. This is at present termed the β_{2A}- or γ_{1A}-globulin. In normal individuals, β_{2A}-globulin is present at concentrations of 56–195 mg/100 ml of serum[55] and constitutes approximately 10% of the immunoglobulins. The antibody role of the β_{2A}-globulin class has been demonstrated.[33, 59, 108] This class is probably identical to an intermediate size antibody frequently increased in allergic states.[101]

First distinguished from 7S γ myeloma globulins by Heremans,[56] the β_{2A} myeloma globulins tend to exhibit polymer type heterogeneity both in the ultracentrifuge (s_{20} = 7S, 10S, 14S) and in starch gel electrophoresis.[29] Because of their relatively high sedimentation coefficients, β_{2A} myeloma globulins were first considered to be "atypical macroglobulins" but were later[60] shown to be distinct from the pathological macroglobulins described by Waldenström.

β_{2A} myeloma globulins are distinguished from 7S γ myeloma globulins by relatively greater amounts of carbohydrate, a faster electrophoretic mobility, and the above-mentioned polymer type heterogeneity, as well as by their antigenic characteristics. Whether or not this heterogeneity is a simple polymerization of a basic unit has not yet been established.

(1) Subunit structure—There is, at present, less chemical information on the subunits of the β_{2A} class of normal and pathological proteins than there is for the 7S γ-globulins. Franklin[39] has demonstrated the occurrence of two antigenic types (I and II) of normal β_{2A}, and antigenic mapping of β_{2A} myeloma globulins has suggested the schematic structure depicted in figure 4. Comparative peptide maps of β_{2A} myeloma globulins and the Bence-Jones proteins from the same individual have shown most of the Bence-Jones peptides to be contained in the autologous globulin.[8] Certain peptides absent in the Bence-Jones protein but present in the autologous β_{2A}-globulin are also found in other β_{2A} myeloma globulins but are lacking in the 7S γ proteins. These peptides may be characteristic of a β_{2A} chain analogous to the H chain of 7S γ.

Attempts to perform limited papain hydrolysis of human β_{2A} myeloma globulins under conditions used for 7S γ-globulins have met with less success.[8, 20] Papain, in this case, apparently cleaves random peptide bonds with the production of free peptides and a 3.5S fragment containing both Bence-Jones-like and β_{2A} specific determinants. Peptide mapping of this fragment also shows β_{2A} and Bence-Jones specific peptides present. Reductive cleavage of β_{2A} myeloma globulins has been undertaken using acetic acid and detergent as dispersing agents.[8, 17, 30] Evidence suggests that there are $H^{\beta_{2A}}$ chains which are class specific and L chains which possess the type I or II determinants and closely resemble the Bence-Jones protein from the same patient. At present, not enough detailed quantitative data are available to permit an estimate of the number of chains present. Consequently, the model for 7S γ-globulins (fig. 6), though instructive as a guide for study of the structure of β_{2A}-globulins, is not necessarily applicable.

5. Macroglobulins

Normal human serum contains two kinds of high molecular weight proteins, which differ completely from each other except in terms of size (molecular weight = approximately 1,000,000). One is a fast migrating α_2-globulin which is frequently elevated in the nephrotic syndrome. The other is an antibody-active, β-globulin member of the immunoglobulin family: β_2-macroglobulin (β_{2M}). In the normal individual, macroglobulin antibody appears to be the first antibody synthesized in response to antigenic stimulation.[111, 118] The macroglobulin antibody binds less tenaciously to antigen than does 7S γ antibody, and its activity can be destroyed by treatment with reducing agents. β_2-macroglobulin is usually present at a concentration range of approximately 35–120 mg/100 ml of normal serum.[41, 55] Fahey[30] has shown the normal β_2-macroglobulin to consist of both type I and type II molecules. The β_{2M}-globulins are distinguished by a high carbohydrate content and an extremely high intrinsic viscosity,[68] as well as by their antigenic characteristics.

In 1944 Waldenström[122] reported ultracentrifugation studies on the sera of patients diagnosed as having multiple myeloma. A number of these sera which by electrophoresis had been shown to have a homogeneous fast γ-globulin peak contained large amounts of rapidly sedimenting 19S protein. In retrospect, the patients were found to have a rather different clinical and cytopathological picture, and Waldenström termed the disorder "macroglobulinemia." The incidence of this disorder is about 10–20% that of 7S γ and β_{2A} myeloma combined.[1] Occasionally, patients with Waldenström's macroglobulinemia excrete a Bence-Jones protein.

The β_2-macroglobulin was the first of the pathological immunoglobulins to be successfully broken into smaller units. Deutsch and Morton[22] showed that treatment with reducing agents broke the 19S protein into 7S subunits which were antigenically identical to one another and to the parent molecule. With removal of the reducing agent, the 19S polymer reformed; however, by alkylating the reduced protein, stable monomers could be obtained. With this in mind reducing agents have been administered intravenously to patients in order to alleviate the untoward effects of the high serum viscosity due to the elevated macroglobulin.[100] Although transient success has been obtained, the procedure is impractical for long term therapy. Although treatment of macroglobulins with papain readily produces 3.5S fragments,[97] the localization of biological functions in the fragments has not yet been demonstrated in a manner analogous to that for 7S γ-globulin. As with β_{2A} myeloma globulins, free peptides and a fragment possessing both β_{2M} and type specific determinants have been produced by papain cleavage.[97]

Successful reduction and alkylation of pathological and normal β_2-macroglobulins into two kinds of chains has been reported by Cohen,[17] Fahey,[30] and Gross and Epstein.[48] Data quantitative enough for construction of a model have not as yet been presented, but the L chains of the macroglobulin have been shown to possess the type I or type II determinants. Gross and Epstein[48] have demonstrated a close similarity between the L chains of a reduced-alkylated Waldenström macroglobulin and the autologous Bence-Jones protein. Hence, in all four classes of immunoglobulins, antigenically related L chains are present;

and, furthermore, in the three classes of pathological immunoglobulins, close similarity between the L chains and the autologous Bence-Jones protein has been demonstrated. Thus, there is cumulative evidence that the Bence-Jones proteins represent one of the types of polypeptide chains in all of the immunoglobulins.

6. *Chemical Structure*

In the preceding sections the antigenic and biosynthetic relationships among the immunoglobulins have been explained in terms of their polypeptide structure in which the L chain is common to the four classes and the H chain is characteristic of the class. This classification rests on chemical structure as well as on similarities in immunological and physical properties. The chemical evidence derives largely from comparison of the tryptic peptide maps of Bence-Jones proteins and of the immunoglobulins and their constituent polypeptide chains and to a lesser extent from amino acid analysis of the isolated peptides.

Because of its heterogeneity and its high molecular weight, normal 7S γ-globulin is not amenable to amino acid sequence analysis similar to that applied to hemoglobin and other proteins. The 7S γ molecule has a molecular weight of about 150,000 and is thought to consist of the two pairs of identical chains depicted in figure 6: H with a molecular weight of about 50,000, L about 22,000, and carbohydrate totalling about 5,000. In all, this corresponds to about 1,300 amino acids of 20 different types plus about 27 carbohydrate residues of five different types. Furthermore, normal 7S γ-globulin consists of a family of closely related but unresolvable molecules, and there are two types of L chains, L^I and L^{II}, and two antigenic types of H chains. The same considerations apply to β_{2A}- and β_{2M}-globulins. It is not surprising then that no amino acid sequence information is yet available on the human immunoglobulins, and only a single pentapeptide sequence is known in rabbit γ-globulin. However, the greater homogeneity of the myeloma globulins and macroglobulins, as well as the availability of free L chains (the Bence-Jones proteins) has greatly facilitated structural study of the normal human immunoglobulins.

a. *Peptide maps of Bence-Jones proteins.*—Despite their similar biosynthetic origin and structural role in the immunoglobulins, Bence-Jones proteins differ individually in amino acid sequence, though they fall into two structural types in accord with the two antigenic types. The first evidence for structural differences among Bence-Jones proteins came from end group assay which revealed the frequent presence of N-terminal aspartic acid in type I proteins and its absence in type II.[93] Column chromatography of the tryptic peptides later indicated extensive structural differences among Bence-Jones proteins.[43] However, it was the procedure of two-dimensional electrophoresis-chromatography (peptide mapping or fingerprinting) which first established that in accord with their lack of common antigenic determinants Bence-Jones proteins of types I and II have no tryptic peptides in common.[94] (This is not to say that they have no structural features in common, for the α and β chains of human hemoglobin have a 45% overlap in sequence though they share no tryptic peptides.)

When tryptic peptide maps are compared for a series of Bence-Jones proteins of type I, some 20 peptide spots are obtained—about the number predicted from the specificity of the enzyme, the arginine and lysine content of the protein, and an assumed monomer molecular weight of 22,000. The peptide maps of different type I proteins resemble each other in possessing many common spots but also differ in multiple positions. This indicates Bence-Jones proteins of the same antigenic type differ in sequence though they contain many common peptides. The type I peptides have been designated B_1, B_2, etc.; however, in figure 7 they are indicated by vertical lines. Of these, some ten to twelve seem present in all Bence-Jones proteins of type I and appear to represent a fixed portion of the sequence. The remaining peptides are variable and seem characteristic of the specimen studied, as if they reflected a mutable part of the L chain. The same findings obtain with type II Bence-Jones proteins although this group appears to be more variable in structure than type I. These generalizations hold whether the Bence-Jones protein is obtained from a patient having a 7S γ or β_{2A} myeloma globulin, or from a patient without hyperglobulinemia.

b. *Peptide maps of normal and myeloma 7S γ-globulins.*—The structural relationships of normal and myeloma 7S γ-globulins have been further elucidated both by column chromatography of tryptic digests[44] and by the technique of peptide mapping.[10, 89] The latter procedure has established that the Bence-Jones protein is equivalent to one portion of the autologous globulin and analogous to the L chains of the normal immunoglobulins. Composite peptide maps of Bence-Jones proteins and of the myeloma globulin from the same patient indicated that nearly all of the peptides of the Bence-Jones protein were present in the myeloma globulin.[89] However, the globulin had additional peptides characteristic of the H chains and also found in the F fragment. Additional support for the concept that Bence-Jones proteins are identical to the L chains of the myeloma globulin from the same patient was found by comparison of peptide maps of the reduced-alkylated proteins.[109] Type I and type II myeloma globulins, of course, have peptide maps that are similar in respect to the common H chain but differ because of the presence of L^I or L^{II} chains, respectively.[90] Since normal 7S γ-globulin contains both antigenic types, its peptide map is more like a composite of the two antigenic types of 7S γ pathological proteins (see figure 7).

Peptide maps of the Franklin proteins bear a close resemblance to those for the F fragments of normal and myeloma globulins of the 7S γ type. Approximately 20 tryptic peptides are shared by the F fragments of type I and II 7S γ myeloma globulins, the F fragment of normal 7S γ-globulin, and the two antigenic subtypes of the Franklin protein (the Cr and Zu types).[90] These peptides are designated by the stippled spots in figure 7.

The presence in normal 7S γ-globulin of the tryptic peptides of Bence-Jones proteins and myeloma globulins has thus far mainly been indicated by the technique of composite peptide mapping illustrated schematically in figure 7. However, several of the smaller peptides characteristic of type I Bence-Jones protein (B_1, B_{13}, B_{15}) have been isolated from normal γ-globulin and shown to have the same composition.[90]

c. β_{2A} *myeloma globulins.*—By comparison of the tryptic peptide maps of several β_{2A} myeloma globulins and the autologous Bence-Jones proteins, chemical confirmation of the antigenic relationships has been obtained similar to that

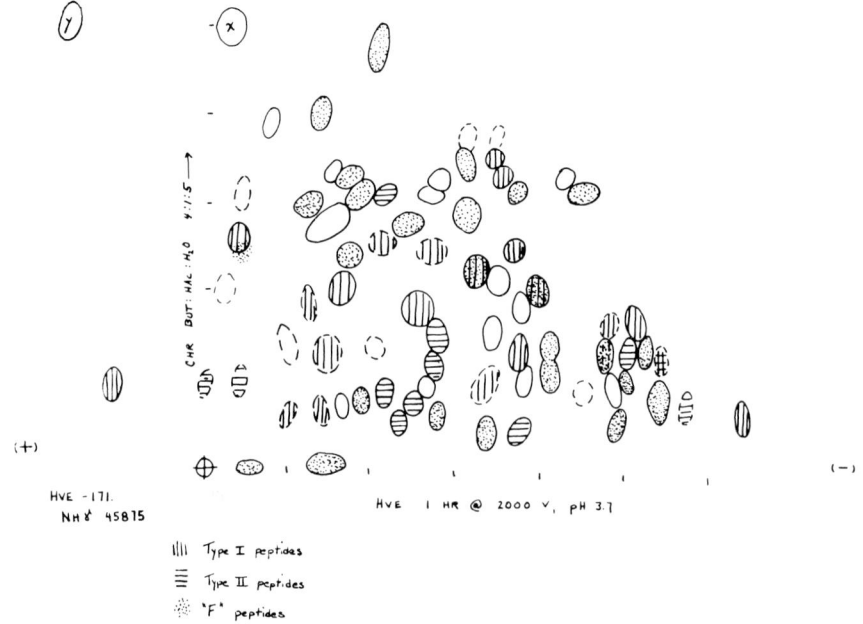

Fig. 7.—Tryptic peptide map of normal human 7S γ-globulin showing the overlap with peptides found in type I and type II Bence-Jones proteins. All peptide spots indicated by circling are found in normal 7S γ-globulin. Vertical and horizontal lines, respectively, indicate peptides characteristic of type I and type II Bence-Jones proteins. Those peptides confined to the F fragment of the $H^{7S\gamma}$ chain of normal 7S γ-globulin are identified by stippling.

described above for the 7S γ class.[8] The Bence-Jones proteins contain peptides characteristic of their antigenic class, and these peptides are also represented in the autologous pathological globulin. It thus appears that the β_{2A} myeloma globulins contain either L^I or L^{II} chains according to their antigenic type, and that these L chains are identical to the Bence-Jones protein of the same patient. In addition, the β_{2A} myeloma globulins have a structural moiety in common, as is indicated by the presence of a series of peptides that appear to represent the $H^{\beta_{2A}}$ chains. Structural comparison of the β_{2A} myeloma globulins to normal β_{2A}-globulin has not yet been accomplished because of the difficulty of purifying the normal protein.

d. *Macroglobulins.*—Peptide maps have not yet been reported either for normal β_{2M}-globulin or Waldenström macroglobulins. However, preliminary study[97] indicates that the chemical structure of the high molecular weight globulins is no more complex than for 7S γ-globulins. One type I Waldenström macroglobulin that was studied has many peptides characteristic of type I Bence-Jones proteins. This structural similarity of a part of the macroglobulin with Bence-Jones protein is in accord with the concept that the latter is equivalent to the L chains. It also explains why antisera with a high specificity for type I Bence-Jones protein may be prepared by use of an antigen consisting of a papain digest of a macroglobulin of type I.[74]

e. *Isolation and composition of the tryptic peptides.*—The structural study of human γ-globulin through the analysis of the tryptic peptides of Bence-Jones proteins may now be undertaken with some confidence because of the relationships established by peptide and antigenic mapping. However, just as peptide mapping of the abnormal hemoglobins has required confirmation by the isolation and sequence analysis of the normal and aberrant peptides, similar techniques will be needed for chemical confirmation of the structural relationships among the pathological proteins.

In the first report on the isolation and composition of tryptic peptides of Bence-Jones proteins, Putnam et al.[91] have given the amino acid composition of twelve of the 20 peptides of a type I protein (the B peptides). Eleven of these peptides have also been identified in different type I proteins by Hilschmann and Craig (personal communication). Most of these peptides are in the group that appears common to type I Bence-Jones proteins. The results thus far suggest that all Bence-Jones proteins of the same antigenic type share a fixed portion of their sequence and also have an individually characteristic part. Of special interest is the finding that the only methionine residue in the protein occurs in one peptide (designated B_3). In a type I Bence-Jones protein that lacks methionine, B_3 is replaced by a neighboring peptide (L_3). It will be important to ascertain whether all Bence-Jones proteins of the same antigenic type share a fixed portion of their sequence and also have a mutable part. This may aid in explaining the antigenic subgroup specificity, the chemical basis of the InV factors, and the possible involvement of the L chain in antibody specificity. In this connection, Smithies[111a] has proposed a genetic hypothesis explaining γ-globulin variability in terms of chromosomal rearrangements involving the structural genes affecting the Bence-Jones-like portions of the molecule.

Sequence analysis of the tryptic peptides of Bence-Jones proteins is now being undertaken in several laboratories. Since peptide mapping indicates certain peptides are shared in common by Bence-Jones proteins and normal γ-globulins, sequence determination for Bence-Jones proteins should aid in the structural study of normal human γ-globulin. The Franklin proteins may likewise serve as models for structural analysis of the H chains of 7S γ-globulin. In this way by study of the biosynthetic polypeptide chains (namely, the Bence-Jones proteins and Franklin proteins) and of F and S fragments, the sequence of the whole globulin may eventually be reconstructed. In like manner the structural features responsible for the genetic factors may be elucidated.

f. *Glycopeptides.*—At present most of the effort is concentrated on structural study of the protein moiety of the immunoglobulins. However, all the immunoglobulins with the exception of the Bence-Jones proteins also contain carbohydrate (see table II). The amount ranges from about 3 % in normal 7S γ-globulin to about 10 % in the $β_{2A}$- and $β_{2M}$-globulins. In molecular weight this corresponds to about 5,000 for 7S γ and 15,000 for $β_{2A}$- and $β_{2M}$-globulins. There is accumulating evidence that the carbohydrate is distributed among several similar or identical glycopeptides. Two such glycopeptides appear to be present in normal 7S γ-globulin. The carbohydrate content and composition differ for individual myeloma globulins. These differences may prove to be a major source of the specific antigenic determinants of the H chains of 7S γ-, $β_{2A}$-, and $γ_{2M}$-globulins.

7. *Biological Considerations*

a. *The Gm and InV factors.*—Demonstration of the presence of genetic determinants in γ-globulin by Grubb,[49] Grubb and Laurell,[50] Steinberg,[115] Ropartz,[105] and others has been of great practical and theoretical value. The factors
are demonstrated by incubation of the test serum with γ-globulin-coated red
blood cells and a rheumatoid arthritis serum which would otherwise agglutinate
the cells. Depending on the γ-globulin which is used to coat the cells (usually
anti-D antibody) and the specificity of the rheumatoid arthritis serum, certain
normal sera will inhibit the reaction while others will not. By extensive investigations, using many different rheumatoid sera and coated cell preparations, a
number of such inhibitory factors have been found in normal sera. The inhibitory
factors have been identified as γ-globulin molecules and are genetically determined.

The mode of inheritance of Gm (a, b, r, x) factors and InV (a, b) factors is
not entirely clear as yet, but Gm_a and Gm_b appear to be inherited as simple,
codominant, non-sex linked alleles.[104] As figure 8 indicates, the InV factors
(inherited independent of the Gm) are common to all classes of immunoglobulins,
but the Gm factors are confined to 7S γ-globulin.[32, 57] Furthermore, Waldenström macroglobulins, 7S γ and $β_{2A}$ myeloma globulins, and Bence-Jones proteins
of antigenic type I have been shown to be either InV (a+) or InV (b+); but
the macroglobulins, $β_{2A}$ myeloma proteins, and Bence-Jones proteins of type II
appear to be InV (a- b-). A clear-cut segregation of antigenic type and InV
activity has not been obtained in the case of 7S γ myeloma globulins.[52] The Gm
activity has been localized to the F fragment of papain-cleaved 7S γ-globulins
and the InV activity to the S fragment.[19, 40, 51]

Fudenberg, Heremans, and Franklin[45] have postulated a situation analogous
to the $α, β, γ$, and $δ$ chains of human hemoglobin, in which each serum immunoglobulin is the expression of two different genetic loci. One genetically determined
chain, analogous to the $α$ chain of hemoglobin, is present in each molecule (L
chain, dependent on InV locus) together with another genetically determined
chain (7S γ, $β_{2A}$, $β_{2M}$) analogous to the $β, γ$, and $δ$ chains of hemoglobin. These
authors have suggested a genetic mechanism for the hypogammaglobulinemias
based on the analogy.

Figure 8, which is based on our present knowledge and concepts, summarizes
the possible relationship between genes, genetic factors, and the polypeptide
chains of the immunoglobulins. If it should ultimately be the case that all type
II pathological proteins are InV (a- b-), the genetic findings will continue to
parallel the antigenic and structural typing. To extend the analogy with the
hemoglobins—in the latter case, a pair of one kind of chain ($α$) can combine with
a pair of another kind ($β, γ$, or $δ$) yielding three possible types of hemoglobins
(A, F, A_2), whereas in the immunoglobulins two totally different kinds of chains
exist (L^I and L^{II}), each capable of combining with any of three sets of H chains
to yield six combinations.

To investigate the site of synthesis of the H and L chains, Bernier and Cebra[5]
have recently stained normal lymphoid tissue with fluorescent antibodies of
different colors and specificities. Anti-type I Bence-Jones protein conjugated
with rhodamine was used in combination with anti-type II Bence-Jones protein

POSTULATED GENETIC CONTROL OF IMMUNOGLOBULIN SYNTHESIS

GENES	$H^{7S\gamma}$		$H^{\beta_{2A}}$		$H^{\beta_{2M}}$		L^I	L^{II}
GENETIC MARKERS	Gm (Gm$_1$) a,b,r,x		✦		✦		InV (Gm$_2$) a,b	✦
CHAIN COMBINATIONS##	$H^{7S\gamma}L^I$	$H^{7S\gamma}L^{II}$	$H^{\beta_{2A}}L^I$	$H^{\beta_{2A}}L^{II}$	$H^{\beta_{2M}}L^I$	$H^{\beta_{2M}}L^{II}$	L^I	L^{II}
PATHOLOGICAL PROTEINS	Myeloma Globulins				Macroglobulins		Bence-Jones Proteins	
	$7S\gamma \cdot I$	$7S\gamma \cdot II$	$\beta_{2A} \cdot I$	$\beta_{2A} \cdot II$	$\beta_{2M} \cdot I$	$\beta_{2M} \cdot II$	BJ · I	BJ · II
NORMAL COUNTERPARTS	7S γ-globulin		β_{2A}-globulin		β_{2M}-macroglobulin		γ_U	

✦ Genetic markers postulated, but not yet demonstrated

Number of chains unspecified

Fig. 8.—Schematic diagram partly summarizing the hypothetical relationship of genes, genetic factors, and polypeptide chains of the normal immunoglobulins and of the pathological proteins. The InV factors which are known to be associated with the L chains are here depicted as an expression of the L^I gene only, although this is not entirely consonant with all experimental findings (see text). Polypeptide chain combinations are represented for each of the normal and pathological immunoglobulins. The normal individual would have, e.g., β_2-macroglobulins of the $H^{\beta_{2M}} \cdot L^I$ and $H^{\beta_{2M}} \cdot L^{II}$ designations but a particular Waldenström's macroglobulin would be either $H^{\beta_{2M}} \cdot L^I$ or $H^{\beta_{2M}} \cdot L^{II}$. Bence-Jones proteins usually exist as dimers of L chains (of one or the other type). Normally occurring γ_U molecules appear to be in monomeric form usually.

coupled with fluorescein isothiocyanate. These investigators found that plasma cells stained specifically with one reagent or the other but rarely, if at all, with both. Conversely, they found a significant proportion of doubly-staining cells when they used conjugated antisera specific for the H chain of 7S γ-globulin in double-staining experiments with fluorescent antibody to Bence-Jones proteins of either type. Their results suggest that an individual cell may synthesize both the H and the L chains of a single 7S γ-globulin molecule. However, the cell is confined to the synthesis of either antigenic type I or type II molecules because it is capable of synthesizing only one kind of L chain at a given time. It remains to be established whether single cells can synthesize all three kinds of H chains (7S γ, β_{2A}, β_{2M}).

b. *Cellular aspects and etiologic considerations.*—It seems well established that the immune globulins are normally synthesized in cells of the plasmacytic-lymphocytic series. Multiple myeloma and macroglobulinemia are characterized by an abnormal proliferation of such cells, and studies with a variety of techniques have demonstrated that the pathological protein is synthesized in the abnormal cells. The results of tissue culture experiments[73] and immunohistological staining with fluorescent antibody[13, 18, 112] are consistent with the view that the abnormal cells are the source of the pathological protein(s).

By conventional histologic means, some degree of correlation between the morphology of the malignant cell and the class of pathological protein produced has been achieved. Thus, Olhagen et al.[75] found, in general, that in cases where only a Bence-Jones protein was produced, cells had a higher nucleo-cytoplasmic ratio, a more evenly distributed RNA, and a less well developed Golgi apparatus than in cases where a myeloma globulin was produced. Studies by Paraskevas et al.[79] have demonstrated that the so-called "flame cell" or "thesaurocyte" is relatively distinctive of β_{2A} myelomatosis. The "flame cell" is characterized by intra-cytoplasmic areas of P.A.S.-staining materials, which by electron microscopy[9] appear to represent dilated portions of the endoplasmic reticulum. Finally, rather large morphologic differences are seen to exist between the plasma cell of 7S γ or β_{2M} myelomatosis and the lymphocytoid cell of Waldenström's macroglobulinemia.[122] However, a continuum of cell types appears to be present in at least some cases of this disease, in which cells of both the lymphocytic type and plasma cell type appear to be involved in the synthesis of the abnormal protein.[112]

A series of recent histological investigations has dealt with possible etiologic factors in plasmacytoma and macroglobulinemia. With the use of chromosomal analysis, three separate groups[3, 12, 46] have demonstrated the presence of an extra, seemingly specific, chromosome in Waldenström's macroglobulinemia. In studies on multiple myeloma, however, conflicting results have been obtained.[11, 15, 98] Intracytoplasmic virus-like particles have been found in a single case of human myeloma[113] though they have been reported with frequency in the mouse myeloma system.[99]

In spite of these attempts, however, the etiology of myeloma and macroglobulinemia remains obscure, and it is yet to be established whether the synthesis of a pathological protein is incidental to or the basis of the cellular proliferation. In this regard it is interesting that Waldenström[123] has found that some myeloma proteins appear to possess antibody activity (antistreptolysin O), and it is tempting to speculate that other myeloma globulins may eventually be found to be antibody in nature.

It is difficult at present to conjecture as to whether the malignant cell of multiple myeloma and macroglobulinemia is at an arrested stage of synthesis. Indeed, little is really known regarding the modes and routes of cellular maturation in the normal immune response. The prime question is whether the three classes of immunoglobulins are all synthesized by the same cell at different stages of its maturation or whether a cell is committed to synthesis of a single kind of immunoglobulin by previous differentiation. There are, of course, several possible modes of this pre-differentiation, illustrated schematically for unitarian and trinitarian differentiation in figure 9. The knowledge that the appearance of β_{2M} antibody precedes 7S γ antibody and that the β_{2M}-, β_{2A}-, and 7S γ-globulins share chains in common makes attractive the possibility that one cell may synthesize each of the classes of immunoglobulin at a different stage of maturation (sequential or modified sequential differentiation as illustrated in figure 9). Some studies that bear on this point are those of Mellors and Korngold.[72]

8. *Conclusion*

In many ways the immunoglobulin family is an extraordinary collection of proteins. The intricacies of antibody specificity, antibody synthesis, and antibody structure are still enigmatic and thorny but, hopefully, closer to solution

FOUR POSSIBLE ROUTES OF IMMUNE CELLULAR MATURATION

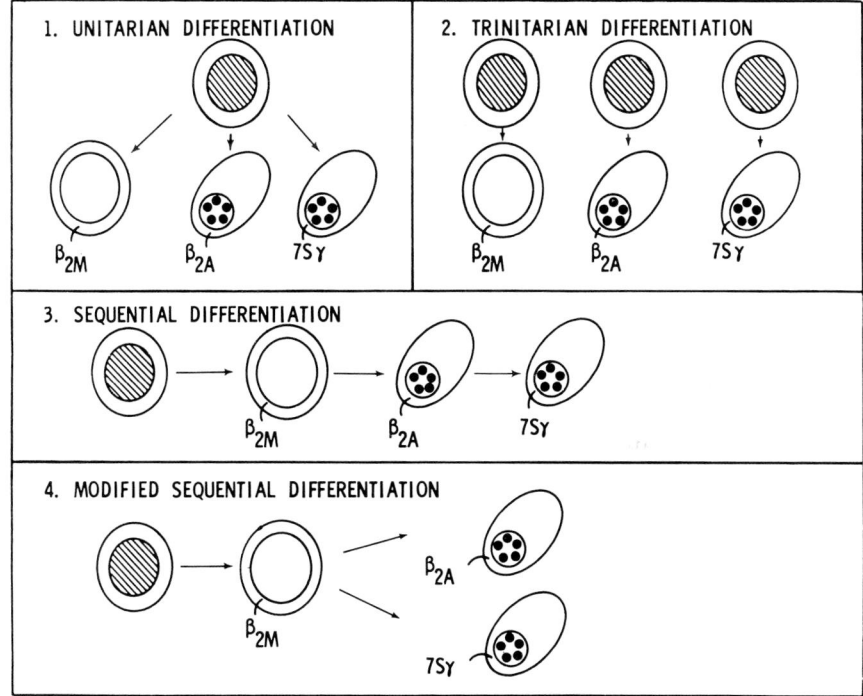

FIG. 9.—Four routes whereby cellular maturation and/or division can give rise to cells capable of synthesizing the various immunoglobulins. The trinitarian and unitarian hypotheses would involve a pre-differentiation and would regard each immunoglobulin-producing cell as a terminal stage. The two other routes are alternatives in which a single cell is capable of the synthesis of more than one immunoglobulin (at different times). A fifth possibility would be simultaneous synthesis of all three proteins.

as a result of the experiments recounted herein. Just as baffling as the problems of antibodies are the conditions of malignant over- and under-production of the immunoglobulins. It is remarkable that the β_{2A}-, β_{2M}-, and 7S γ-globulins may, in one kind of disease, reach serum concentrations greater than all other serum proteins combined, and in another kind of disease suffer from virtual agenesis.

As the biochemist breaks the genetic code, it seems likely that the myeloma proteins will be useful to him in the study of the *in vivo* biosynthetic relationship of DNA, RNA, and product. It seems equally probable that understanding of the relationship of genes and messengers and proteins can not help but contribute to an understanding of malignancies such as myeloma and macroglobulinemia.

REFERENCES

1. Bachmann, R., and Laurell, C.-B.: Electrophoretic and immunologic classification of M-components in serum. Scand. J. Clin. Lab. Invest. 15: 11–24, 1963.
2. Ballieux, R. E., Bernier, G. M., Tominaga, K. T., and Putnam, F. W.: Gamma globulin antigenic types defined by heavy (H) chain determinants. Science: in press.
3. Benirschke, K., Brownhill, L., and Ebaugh, F. G.: Chromosomal abnormalities in Waldenström's macroglobulinaemia. Lancet 1: 594–595, 1962.
4. Berggård, I., and Edelman, G. M.: Normal counterparts to Bence-Jones proteins: free L polypeptide chains of human γ-globulin. Proc. Nat. Acad. Sci. USA 49: 330–337, 1963.

5. Bernier, G. M., and Cebra, J. J.: Polypeptide chains of human γ-globulin: cellular localization by fluorescent antibody. Science: in press.
6. Bernier, G. M., and Putnam, F. W.: Monomer-dimer forms of Bence Jones proteins. Nature (London) 200: 223–225, 1963.
7. Bernier, G M., and Putnam, F. W.: Polymerism, polymorphism, and impurities in Bence-Jones proteins. Biochim. Biophys. Acta: 86: 295–308, 1964.
8. Bernier, G. M., Tominaga, K., Easley, C. W., and Putnam, F. W.: Studies of β_{2A} myeloma globulin structure. Fed. Proc.: 23, 558, 1964.
9. Bessis, M., Breton-Gorius, J., and Binet, J. L.: Étude comparée du plasmacytome et du syndrome de Waldenström. Nouv. Rev. Franc. Hemat. 3: 159–184, 1963.
10. Biserte, G., and Valdiguié, P.: Études sur l'hydrolyse enzymatique des protéines myélomateuses. Path. Biol. (Paris) 10: 1315–1326, 1962.
11. Bottura, C.: Chromosome abnormalities in multiple myeloma. Acta Haemat. (Basel) 30: 274–279, 1963.
12. Bottura, C., Ferrari, I., and Veiga, A. A.: Chromosome abnormalities in Waldenström's macroglobulinaemia. Lancet 1: 1170, 1961.
13. Burtin, P., and Buffe, D.: Immunofluorescent studies of human plasma cells in γ and β_{2A} myelomas. Proc. Soc. Exp. Biol. Med. 114: 171–175, 1963.
14. Burtin, P., Hartmann, L., Fauvert, R., and Grabar, P.: Études sur les protéines du myélome. I. Étude critique des techniques d'identification de la protéine de Bence-Jones et de leur valeur diagnostique. Rev. Franc. Etud. Clin. Biol. 1: 17–28, 1956.
15. Castoldi, G. L., Ricci, N., Punturieri, E., and Bosi, L.: Chromosomal imbalance in plasmacytoma. Lancet 1: 829, 1963.
16. Clamp, J. R., Bernier, G. M., and Putnam, F. W.: The source of the apparent carbohydrate content of Bence-Jones proteins. Biochim. Biophys. Acta: 86: 149–155, 1964.
17. Cohen, S.: Properties of the peptide chains of normal and pathological human γ-globulins. Biochem. J. 89: 334–341, 1963.
18. Curtain, C. C., and O'Dea, J. F.: Possible sites of macroglobulin synthesis: a study made with fluorescent antibody. Aust. Ann. Med. 8: 143–150, 1959.
19. Deicher, H.: Lokalisation der erblichen Determinante Gm(a) auf einem γ-Globulin-Fragment. Klin. Wschr. 40: 1008–1009, 1962.
20. Deutsch, H. F.: Molecular transformations of a γ_1-globulin of human serum. J. Molec. Biol. 7: 662–671, 1963.
21. Deutsch, H. F.: Crystalline low molecular weight γ-globulin from a human urine. Science 141: 435–436, 1963.
22. Deutsch, H. F., and Morton, J. I.: Dissociation of human serum macroglobulins. Science 125: 600–601, 1957.
23. Deutsch, H. F., Thorpe, N. O., and Fudenberg, H. H.: Some biological activities of papain-produced subunits of human 7S gamma globulins. Immunology 6: 539–550, 1963.
24. Edelman, G. M., and Gally, J. A.: The nature of Bence-Jones proteins; chemical similarities to polypeptide chains of myeloma globulins and normal γ-globulins. J. Exp. Med. 116: 207–227, 1962.
25. Edelman, G. M., and Poulik, M. D.: Studies on the structural units of the γ-globulins. J. Exp. Med. 113: 861–884, 1961.
26. Engle, R. L., Jr., Woods, K. R., and Pert, J. H.: Starch gel electrophoresis of serum proteins and urinary proteins from patients with multiple myeloma. J. Clin. Invest. 36: 888, 1957.
27. Fahey, J. L.: Immunochemical studies of twenty mouse myeloma proteins: evidence evidence for two groups of proteins similar to gamma and beta 2A globulins in man. J. Exp. Med. 114: 385–398, 1961.
28. Fahey, J. L.: Physicochemical characterization of mouse myeloma proteins: demonstration of heterogeneity for each myeloma globulin. J. Exp. Med. 114: 399–413, 1961.
29. Fahey, J. L.: Heterogeneity of myeloma proteins. J. Clin. Invest. 42: 111–123, 1962.
30. Fahey, J. L.: Two types of 6.6 S γ-globulins, β_{2A}-globulins and 18 S γ_1-macroglobulins in normal serum and γ-microglobulins in normal urine. J. Immun. 91: 438–447, 1963.
31. Fahey, J. L., and Goodman, H.: Antibody activity in six classes of human immunoglobulins. Science 143: 588–589, 1964.
32. Fahey, J. L., and Lawler, S. D.: Gm factors in normal γ-globulin fractions, myeloma proteins, and macroglobulins. J. Nat. Cancer Inst. 27: 973–981, 1961.
33. Fireman, P., Vannier, W. E., and Goodman, H. C.: The association of skin-sensitizing antibody with the β_{2A}-globulins in sera from ragweed-sensitive patients. J. Exp. Med. 117: 603–620, 1963.
34. Fleischman, J. B., Porter, R. R., and Press, E. M.: The arrangement of the peptide chains in γ-globulin. Biochem. J. 88: 220–239, 1963.
35. Flynn, F. V., and Stow, E. A.: Fractionation of Bence-Jones protein by starch gel electrophoresis. J. Clin. Path. 11: 334–338, 1958.
36. Franěk, F., and Nezlin, R. S.: Recovery of antibody combining activity by interaction of different peptide chains isolated from purified horse antitoxins. Folia Microbiol. (Praha) 8: 128–130, 1963.

37. Franklin, E. C.: Physicochemical and immunologic studies of gamma globulins of normal human urine. J. Clin. Invest. 38: 2159–2167, 1959.
38. Franklin, E. C.: Structural units of human 7S gamma globulin. J. Clin. Invest. 39: 1933–1941, 1960.
39. Franklin, E. C.: Two types of γ_{1A}-globulin in sera from normals and patients with multiple myeloma. Nature (London) 195: 393–394, 1962.
40. Franklin, E. C., Fudenberg, H., Meltzer, M., and Stanworth, D. R.: The structural basis for genetic variations of normal human γ-globulins. Proc. Nat. Acad. Sci. USA 48: 914–922, 1962.
41. Franklin, E. C., and Kunkel, H. G.: Comparative levels of high molecular weight (19S) gamma globulin in maternal and umbilical cord sera. J. Lab. Clin. Med. 52: 724–727, 1958.
42. Franklin, E. C., Meltzer, M., Guggenheim, F., and Lowenstein, J.: An unusual micro-gamma-globulin in the serum and urine of a patient. Fed. Proc. 22: 264, 1963.
43. Fried, M., and Putnam, F. W.: Comparative studies of partial hydrolysates of Bence-Jones proteins. J. Biol. Chem. 235: 3472–3477, 1960.
44. Fried, M., and Putnam, F. W.: Peptide chromatograms of normal human and myeloma γ-globulins. Biochemistry (Wash.) 1: 983–987, 1962.
45. Fudenberg, H. H., Heremans, J. F., and Franklin, E. C.: A hypothesis for the genetic control of synthesis of the gamma-globulins. Ann. Inst. Pasteur Lille 104: 155–168, 1963.
46. German, J. L., Biro, C. E., and Bearn, A. G.: Chromosomal abnormalities in Waldenström's macroglobulinaemia. Lancet 2: 48, 1961.
47. Grabar, P., and Williams, C. A.: Méthode permettant l'étude conjuguée des propriétés électrophorétiques et immunochimiques d'un mélange de protéines. Application au sérum sanguin. Biochim. Biophys. Acta 10: 193–194, 1953.
48. Gross, D., and Epstein, W. V.: Macroglobulinemia with Bence-Jones proteinuria: comparison of urinary protein and L chain of serum protein. J. Clin. Invest. 43: 83–93, 1964.
49. Grubb, R.: Agglutination of erythrocytes coated with "incomplete" anti-Rh by certain rheumatoid arthritic sera and some other sera. The existence of human serum groups. Acta Path. Microbiol. Scand. 39: 195–197, 1956.
50. Grubb, R., and Laurell, A. B.: Hereditary serological human serum groups. Acta Path. Microbiol. Scand. 39: 390–398, 1956.
51. Harboe, M., Osterland, C. K., and Kunkel, H. G.: Localization of two genetic factors to different areas of γ-globulin molecules. Science 136: 979–980, 1962.
52. Harboe, M., Osterland, C. K., Mannik, M., and Kunkel, H. G.: Genetic characters of human γ-globulins in myeloma proteins. J. Exp. Med. 116: 719–738, 1962.
53. Heimer, R., Schwartz, E. R., Engle, R. L., Jr., and Woods, K. R.: The relationship of structure to the thermal solubility characteristics of a Bence-Jones protein. Biochemistry (Wash.) 2: 1380–1386, 1963.
54. Hennemann, G., van Eijk, H. G., Witte, J. J., and Westenbrink, H. G. K.: On the variability of proteinuria in myelomatosis studied by means of starch gel electrophoresis. Proc. Kon. Nederl. Akad. Wet. (Biol. Med.) Series C, 66: 1–12, 1963.
55. Heremans, J. F.: Les globulines sériques du système gamma. Leur nature et leur pathologie. Bruxelles, Editions Arscia S. A., 1960.
56. Heremans, J. F., and Heremans, M.-Th.: Immunoelectrophoresis as a diagnostic tool for myeloma and macroglobulinemia. In Proceedings of the 7th Congress, International Society of Hematology, Rome, 1958, Vol. II, pp. 698–705. Rome, Il Pensiero Scientifico, 1958.
57. Heremans, J. F., Laurell, A. H. F., Mårtensson, L., Heremans, M.-Th., Laurell, C.-B., Sjöquist, J., and Waldenström, J.: Studies on "abnormal" serum globulins (M-components) in myeloma, macroglobulinemia and related diseases. Acta Med. Scand. Suppl. 367: 6–126, 1961.
58. Heremans, J. F., Vaerman, J.-P., Carbonara, A. O., Rodhain, J. A., and Heremans, M.-Th.: γ_{1A}-Globulin (β_{2A}-globulin): its isolation, properties, functions, and pathology. In Peeters, H. (Ed.): Protides of the Biological Fluids, Proceedings of the Tenth Colloquium, pp. 108–121. Amsterdam, Elsevier, 1963.
59. Heremans, J. F., Vaerman, J.-P., and Vaerman, C.: Studies on the immune globulins of human serum. II. A study of the distribution of anti-brucella and anti-diphtheria antibody activities among γ_{SS^-}, γ_{1M^-}, and γ_{1A}-globulin fractions. J. Immun. 91: 11–17, 1963.
60. Imhof, J. W., and Ballieux, R. E.: Atypical β_{2A}-myeloma. Acta Med. Scand. 170: 449–459, 1961.
61. Imhof, J. W., and Ballieux, R. E.: Mono-, di-, and tri-clonal gammopathies. In Proceedings of the 9th Congress of the European Society of Haematology, Lisbon, 1963. Basel, S. Karger, in press.
62. Ingram, V. M.: A specific chemical difference between the globins of normal human and sickle-cell anaemia haemoglobin. Nature (London) 178: 792–794, 1956.
63. Jaquet, H., Bloom, B., and Cebra, J. J.: The reductive dissociation of rabbit immune globulin in sodium dodecylsulfate. J. Immun.: in press.

64. Jones, H. Bence: Papers on chemical pathology; prefaced by the Galstonian Lectures, read at the Royal College of Physicians, 1846, Lecture 3. Lancet 2: 88–92, 1847.
65. Korngold, L.: The antigenic relationship of two human γ_2-globulins to the γ_2-myeloma globulins. Int. Arch. Allerg. 23: 9–22, 1963.
66. Korngold, L., and Lipari, R.: Multiple-myeloma proteins. III. The antigenic relationship of Bence Jones proteins to normal gamma-globulin and multiple-myeloma serum proteins. Cancer 9: 262–272, 1956.
67. Kuijpers, E. W., Niemeijer, J. A., and Westenbrink, H. G. K.: Some observations on the relationship of Bence-Jones proteins to γ-globulin. Proc. Kon. Nederl. Akad. Wet. (Biol. Med.), Series C, 66: 363–370, 1963.
68. Kunkel, H. G.: Macroglobulins and high molecular weight antibodies. In Putnam, F. W. (Ed.): The Plasma Proteins. Vol. I, Isolation, Characterization, and Function, pp. 279–307. New York, Academic Press, 1960.
69. Mannik, M., and Kunkel, H. G.: Classification of myeloma proteins, Bence Jones proteins, and macroglobulins into two groups on the basis of common antigenic characters. J. Exp. Med. 116: 859–877, 1962.
70. Mannik, M., and Kunkel, H. G.: Antigenic specificity of individual "monoclonal" γ-globulins. Fed. Proc. 22: 264, 1963.
71. Mannik, M., and Kunkel, H. G.: Two major types of normal 7S γ-globulin. J. Exp. Med. 117: 213–230, 1963.
72. Mellors, R. C., and Korngold, L.: The cellular origin of human immunoglobulins (γ_2, γ_{1M}, γ_{1A}). J. Exp. Med. 118: 387–396, 1963.
73. Meyer, F.: In vitro incorporation of C^{14}-lysine into Bence-Jones protein. Proc. Soc. Exp. Biol. Med. 110: 106–109, 1962.
74. Migita, S., and Putnam, F. W.: Antigenic relationships of Bence Jones proteins, myeloma globulins, and normal human γ-globulin. J. Exp. Med. 117: 81–104, 1963.
75. Olhagen, B., Thorell, B., and Wising, P.: The endocellular nucleic acid distribution and plasma protein formation in myelomatosis. Scand. J. Clin. Lab. Invest. 1: 49–59, 1949.
76. Osserman, E. F., and Takatsuki, K.: Plasma cell myeloma: gamma globulin synthesis and structure. Medicine (Balt.) 42: 357–384, 1963.
77. Osserman, E. F., and Takatsuki, K.: Clinical and immunochemical studies of four cases of $H_{\gamma 2}$ chain (Franklin's) disease. Am. J. Med.: in press.
78. Palmer, J. L., Mandy, W. J., and Nisonoff, A.: Heterogeneity of rabbit antibody and its subunits. Proc. Nat. Acad. Sci. USA 48: 49–53, 1962.
79. Paraskevas, F., Heremans, J., and Waldenström, J.: Cytology and electrophoretic pattern in γ1A (β2A) myeloma. Acta Med. Scand. 170: 575–589, 1961.
80. Peetoom, F., and Kramer, E.: Development and anomalies of 7S gammaglobulin (γ_{SS}) investigated with monkey anti-human serum. In Proceedings of the 9th Congress of the European Society of Haematology, Lisbon, 1963. Basel, S. Karger, in press.
81. Porter, R. R.: The hydrolysis of rabbit γ-globulin and antibodies with crystalline papain. Biochem. J. 73: 119–126, 1959.
82. Porter, R. R : The structure of gamma-globulin and antibodies. In Gellhorn, A., and Hirschberg, E. (Eds.): Basic Problems in Neoplastic Disease, pp. 177–194. New York, Columbia University Press, 1962.
83. Potter, M., Dreyer, W. J., Kuff, E. L., and McIntire, K. R.: Heritable variation in Bence Jones protein structure in BALB/c mice: relation to gamma globulin. J. Molec. Biol.: in press.
84. Potter, M., and Fahey, J. L.: Studies on eight transplantable plasma-cell neoplasms of mice. J. Nat. Cancer Inst. 24: 1153–1164, 1960.
85. Putnam, F. W.: Abnormal human serum globulins. Science 122: 275–277, 1955.
86. Putnam, F. W.: Aberrations of protein metabolism in multiple myeloma. Interrelationships of abnormal serum globulins and Bence-Jones proteins. Physiol. Rev. 37: 512–538, 1957.
87. Putnam, F. W.: Plasma-cell myeloma and macroglobulinemia. I. Physicochemical, immunochemical and isotopic turnover studies of the abnormal serum and urinary proteins. New Eng. J. Med. 261: 902–908, 1959.
88. Putnam, F. W.: Abnormal serum globulins. In Putnam, F. W. (Ed.): The Plasma Proteins. Vol. II, Biosynthesis, Metabolism, Alterations in Disease, pp. 345–406. New York, Academic Press, 1960.
89. Putnam, F. W.: Structural relationships among normal human γ-globulin, myeloma globulins, and Bence-Jones proteins. Biochim. Biophys. Acta 63: 539–541, 1962.
90. Putnam, F. W., Bernier, G. M., Tominaga, K., and Easley, C. W.: Unpublished observations.
91. Putnam, F. W., Easley, C. W., and Helling, J. W.: Structural study of human γ-globulin through the analysis of the tryptic peptides of Bence-Jones proteins. Biochim. Biophys. Acta 78: 231–233, 1963.
92. Putnam, F. W., Easley, C. W., and Lynn, L. T.: Site of cleavage of γ-globulins by papain. Biochim. Biophys. Acta 58: 279–290, 1962.
93. Putnam, F. W., Easley, C. W., Lynn, L. T., Ritchie, A. E., and Phelps, R. A.: The heat precipitation of Bence-Jones proteins. Arch. Biochem. 83: 115–130, 1959.

94. Putnam, F. W., Migita, S., and Easley, C. W.: Structural and immunochemical relationships among Bence-Jones proteins. *In* Peeters, H. (Ed.): Protides of the Biological Fluids, Proceedings of the Tenth Colloquium, pp. 93–107. Amsterdam, Elsevier, 1963.
95. Putnam, F. W., and Miyake, A.: Proteins in multiple myeloma. VIII. Biosynthesis of abnormal proteins. J. Biol. Chem. 231: 671–684, 1958.
96. Putnam, F. W., and Stelos, P.: Proteins in multiple myeloma. II. Bence-Jones proteins. J. Biol. Chem. 203: 347–358, 1953.
97. Putnam, F. W., Tominaga, K., and Easley, C. W.: Unpublished observations.
98. Richmond, H. G., Ohnuki, Y., Awa, A., and Pomerat, C. M.: Multiple myeloma—an *in vitro* study. Brit. J. Cancer 15: 692–700, 1961.
99. Rifkind, R. A., Osserman, E. F., Hsu, K. C., and Morgan, C.: The intracellular distribution of gamma globulin in a mouse plasma cell tumor (X5563) as revealed by fluorescence and electron microscopy. J. Exp. Med. 116: 423–432, 1962.
100. Ritzmann, S. E., Coleman, S. L., and Levin, W. C.: The effect of some mercaptanes upon a macrocryogelglobulin; modifications induced by cysteamine, penicillamine and penicillin. J. Clin. Invest. 39: 1320–1329, 1960.
101. Rockey, J. H., and Kunkel, H. G.: Unusual sedimentation and sulfhydryl sensitivity of certain isohemagglutinins and skin-sensitizing antibody. Proc. Soc. Exp. Biol. Med. 110: 101–105, 1962.
102. Roholt, O. A., Onoue, K., and Pressman, D.: Specific combination of H and L chains of rabbit γ-globulins. Proc. Nat. Acad. Sci. USA 51: 173–178, 1964.
103. Roholt, O. A., Radzimski, G., and Pressman, D.: Antibody combining site: the B polypeptide chain. Science 141: 726–727, 1963.
104. Ropartz, C.: Serum groups defined by agglutination inhibition tests: Gm groups and InV groups. Vox Sang. 7: 385–393, 1962.
105. Ropartz, C., Lenoir, J., and Rivat, L.: A new inheritable property of human sera: the InV factor. Nature (London) 189: 586, 1961.
106. Ropartz, C., Rivat, L., and Lenoir, J.: Fréquence des facteurs Gm^a, Gm^b, Gm^x, Gm-like et InV chez quartre cents Noirs Africains. Rev. Franc. Etud. Clin. Biol. 5: 814–816, 1960.
107. Scheurlen, P. G.: Plasmozytom mit mehrfacher Proteinanomalie. Deutsch. Med. Wschr. 89: 42–45, 1964.
108. Schultze, H. E.: The synthesis of antibodies and proteins. Clin. Chim. Acta 4: 610–626, 1959.
109. Schwartz, J. H., and Edelman, G. M.: Comparisons of Bence-Jones proteins and L polypeptide chains of myeloma globulins after hydrolysis with trypsin. J. Exp. Med. 118: 41–54, 1963.
110. Sela, M., Givol, D., and Mozes, E.: Resolution of rabbit γ-globulin into two fractions by chromatography on diethylaminoethyl-Sephadex. Biochim. Biophys. Acta 78: 649–657, 1963.
111. Smith, R. T.: Response to active immunization of human infants during the neonatal period. *In* Wolstenholme, G. E. W., and O'Connor, M. (Eds.): Ciba Foundation Symposium on Cellular Aspects of Immunity, pp. 348–371. Boston, Little, Brown and Co., 1960.
111a. Smithies, O.: Gamma-globulin variability: a genetic hypothesis. Nature (London) 199: 1231–1236, 1963.
112. Solomon, A., Fahey, J. L., and Malmgren, R. A.: Immunohistologic localization of gamma-1-macroglobulins, beta-2A myeloma proteins, 6.6S gamma-myeloma proteins, and Bence Jones proteins. Blood 21: 403–423, 1963.
113. Sorenson, G. D.: Electron microscopic observations of viral particles within myeloma cells of man. Exp. Cell. Res. 25: 219–221, 1961.
114. Stein, S., Nachman, R. L. and Engle, R. L., Jr.: Individual and sub-group antigenic specificity of Bence-Jones protein. Nature (London) 200: 1180–1184, 1963.
115. Steinberg, A. G., Giles, B. D., and Stauffer, R.: A Gm-like factor present in Negroes and absent in whites: its relation to Gm^a and Gm^x. Amer. J. Hum. Genet. 12: 44–51, 1960.
116. Steinberg, A. G., Stauffer, R., Blumberg, B. S., and Fudenberg, H.: Gm phenotypes and genotypes in U.S. whites and Negroes; in American Indians and Eskimos; in Africans; and in Micronesians. Amer. J. Hum. Genet. 13: 205–213, 1961.
117. Stevenson, G. T.: Detection in normal urine of protein resembling Bence-Jones protein. J. Clin. Invest. 39: 1192–1200, 1960.
118. Svehag, S.-E., and Mandel, B.: The formation and properties of poliovirus-neutralizing antibody. I. 19S and 7S antibody formation: differences in kinetics and antigen dose requirement for induction. J. Exp. Med. 119: 1–19, 1964.
119. Takatsuki, K., and Osserman, E. F.: Demonstration of two types of low molecular weight γ-globulin in normal human urine. J. Immun. 92: 100–107, 1964.
120. van Eijk, H. G., Monfoort, C. H., and Westenbrink, H. G. K.: Purification, analysis and properties of some Bence-Jones proteins. Proc. Kon. Nederl. Akad. Wet. (Biol. Med.), Series C, 66: 345–362, 1963.
121. van Eijk, H. G., Monfoort, C. H., Witte, J. J., and Westenbrink, H. G. K.: Isolation

and characterization of some Bence-Jones proteins. Biochim. Biophys. Acta 63: 537–539, 1962.

122. Waldenström, J.: Incipient myelomatosis or "essential" hyperglobulinemia with fibrinogenopenia—a new syndrome. Acta Med. Scand. 117: 216–247, 1944.

123. Waldenström, J.: Studies on conditions associated with disturbed gamma globulin formation (gammopathies). Harvey Lect., Series 56: 211–231, 1960–61.

124. Waldenström, J.: Hypergammaglobulinemia as a clinical hematological problem: a study in the gammopathies. *In* Tocantins, L. M. (Ed.): Progress in Hematology. Vol. III, pp. 266–293. New York, Grune and Stratton, 1962.

125. Webb, T., Rose, B., and Sehon, A. H.: Biocolloids in normal human urine. II. Physicochemical and immunochemical characteristics. Canad. J. Biochem. 36: 1167–1175, 1958.

126. Weicker, H., and Huhnstock, K.: Characterization of some urinary protein fractions in patients with multiple myeloma. Nature (London) 196: 480–481, 1962.

127. Williams, C. A.: Immunoelectrophoresis: a new method for the analysis of complex antigen and antibody mixtures. Application to human serum antigens and hyperimmune horse serum. Thesis, New Brunswick, New Jersey, Rutgers University, 1954.

Recent Advances In Acute Leukemia

————EMIL J FREIREICH and EMIL FREI, III————

THE diagnostic term "acute leukemia" has historically been applied to the type of leukemia associated with a brief and rapidly progressive clinical course. However, since the introduction of chemotherapy in 1947, the duration of the disease has been substantially prolonged, particularly for children with acute lymphocytic leukemia. As a result, there is considerable overlap between duration of disease for acute and chronic leukemias. For children, acute leukemia has become a major form of chronic illness with a duration of over a year for more than half of the patients. The term "acute leukemia", therefore, is used for patients in whom the predominant leukemic cell is of the immature form most closely resembling the normal blast or stem cell, rather than for duration of disease.

The etiology of human leukemia remains unknown. In recent years an increasing number of experimental leukemias have been found to be induced by viruses. Recently, particles resembling the mouse leukemogenic viruses have been found in blood of patients with leukemia by several investigators[72, 10]. These findings make the virus etiology of human leukemia an important working hypothesis. Studies of the relationship between exposure to ionizing radiation and increased frequency of leukemia, as well as between Down's syndrome and leukemia also provide leads for further investigation. The etiology and pathogenesis of the disease as well as other aspects of acute leukemia have been discussed[19, 86]. It is the purpose of this paper to concentrate on recent advances in our knowledge of the clinical disease and its management. The work performed at the National Cancer Institute and by the Leukemia Group B receive major emphasis, because of the intimate association of the authors with these programs. Thus, this is not a comprehensive review and no attempt will be made to include all of the important advances in leukemia research that have occurred in the recent past.

The rapid and complete regression of the leukemic process induced by chemotherapy is the most important event in acute leukemia. Such complete clinical and hematological remissions occur in over 90% of patients with acute lymphocytic leukemia under age 20[33, 81]. During periods of remission the patients are free from the risks of both morbidity and mortality from their disease. Patients who have hematological remission have a similar overall duration of active disease to those who fail to respond to chemotherapy as well as to those patients studied prior to the introduction of chemotherapy. Therefore, improved survival for patients responding to therapy can be accounted for almost entirely by the time spent in remission (Figure 1)[33, 5]. Thus, the major objective of therapy is "induction" of remission and the "maintenance" of patients in a state of remission for the longest possible time. These parameters will be discussed separately.

From the National Cancer Institute, Bethesda, Maryland.

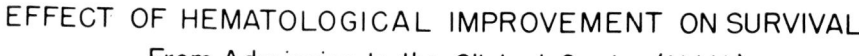

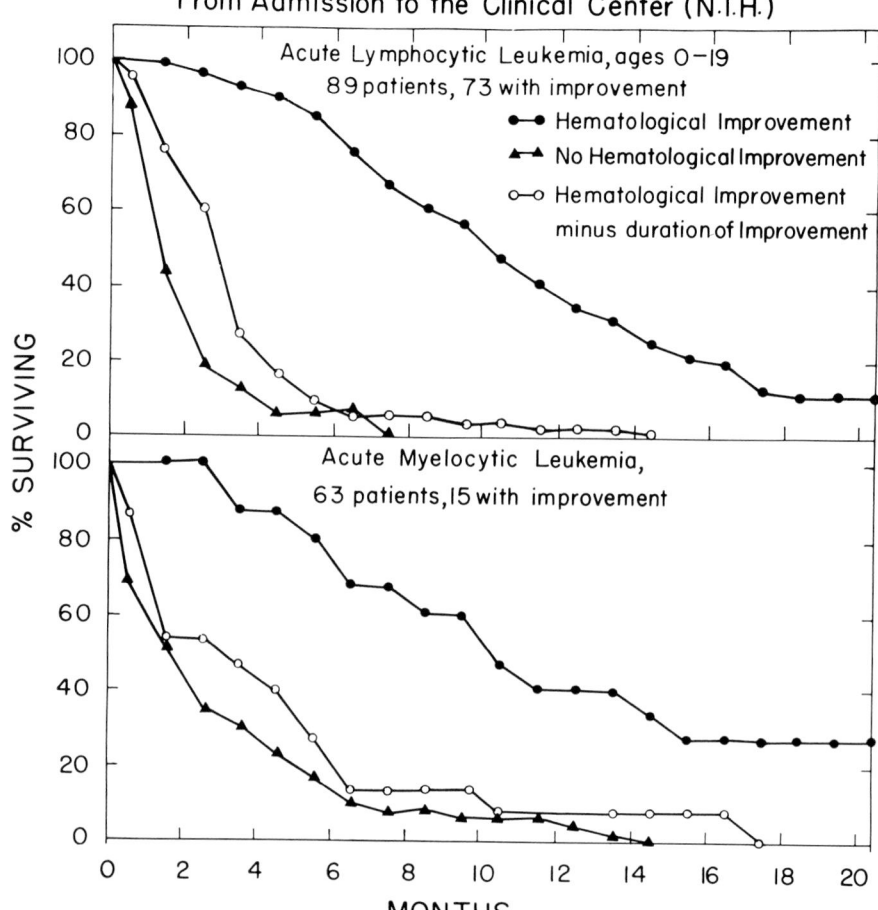

Fig. 1.—Prognosis for survival is much better for patients showing hematological improvement than for those who have no improvement. The difference can be accounted for almost entirely by the duration of improvement. Hematological improvement is observed more frequently in childhood ALL than in AML which is responsible for the poorer overall survival in the latter group. (Reprinted by permission of Freireich et al. Journal of Chronic Diseases 14: 593, 1961.)

Remission Induction Therapy

For remission induction there are five classes of agents of established effectiveness: The folic acid antagonists of which methotrexate (MTX) is most commonly used[16]; the purine analogs, such as 6-mercaptopurine (6-MP)[8]; the adrenal corticosteroids, such as prednisone (Pred.)[18, 71]; the alkaloid, vincristine (VCR)[51, 52]; and the alkylating agent, cyclophosphamide (CTX)[87, 20]. The frequency of induction of complete remission for each of these agents is shown in Table I for patients with acute lymphocytic leukemia (ALL) under 20 years of age (childhood ALL). They are ranked in order of effectiveness. All agents are less effective in adult ALL. 6-MP induces complete re-

TABLE I.—*Compounds Capable of Inducing Complete Remission (C.R.) Childhood Acute Lymphocytic Leukemia*

	No. of Patients	% C.R.	Reference
1. Prednisone	72	57	(31)
2. Vincristine	119	55	(32)
3. 6-mercaptopurine	43	27	(27)
4. Methotrexate	48	21	(27)
5. Cyclophosphamide	44	18	(20)

mission in approximately 15% of patients with acute myelocytic leukemia (AML). The remaining compounds have low activity (less than 10%) in acute myelocytic leukemia. Another compound, methyl glyoxal bis-guanylhydrazone (Methyl GAG) is capable of inducing complete remission in about 25% of patients with AML. This compound, however, because of serious toxicity to skin, gastrointestinal tract and neuromuscular organs is only of limited practical value[30, 56, 75].

The effects of the five remission-inducing agents on the leukemic process are independent. Thus, the response or lack of response of a given patient's disease to any one of the five agents does not effect response to another. For example, if patients with childhood ALL receive 6-MP therapy, 27% will have a complete remission. When MTX is subsequently used, the frequency of remission for those who failed to respond to 6-MP is the same as for the patients who did respond. Moreover, patients who receive MTX after 6-MP therapy is completed show the same frequency of response as patients who receive MTX as their initial therapy. For these two agents, therefore, the sequence of therapy does not affect frequency of induced remission[27]. Available data indicate that this is also true for VCR, Pred., and CTX. These considerations might suggest that sequential use of the five independently active agents would be optimal. However, patients who fail to respond to a given agent have a probability of death from complications, so that the chance of surviving to receive the next compound diminishes progressively with each therapeutic regimen. This, as well as the possibility of drug synergism or potentiation, led to the study of these agents in combination.

For combination chemotherapy, the nature of the acute toxicity of the compounds must be considered (Table II). The severity of the acute toxicity

TABLE II.—*Acute Toxicity of Active Agents*

	Severity at Therapeutic Dose	Major Toxic Effects
1. Prednisone	±	Hypertension, electrolyte imbalance, osteoporosis
2. Vincristine	+	Peripheral neuropathy
3. 6-mercaptopurine	++	Marrow depression and nausea and vomiting
4. Methotrexate	+++	Stomatitis and marrow depression
5. Cyclophosphamide	++++	Marrow depression

TABLE III.—*Effects of Combination Chemotherapy on Remission Induction in Acute Lymphocytic Leukemia of Childhood*

Combination	No. of Patients	Frequency of Remission	Predicted from Independent Action	Reference
VCR + Pred.	66	85%	82	(81)
Pred. + 6-MP	158	81%	69	(29)
MTX + 6-MP	39	45%	42	(27)
VCR + MTX + 6-MP + Pred.	17	94%	90	(35)

Abbreviation of drugs: VCR = vincristine; Pred. = prednisone; 6-MP = 6-mercaptopurine; MTX = methotrexate.

observed at therapeutic doses of each of these agents is inversely related to the remission-inducing effectiveness of the compound. The effectiveness of the compound for inducing remission, therefore, may be a function of the therapeutic index of the compounds. A major reason that all of the patients do not respond to therapy is that toxic effects limit the amount of drug that can be administered. Thus, one possible way to select agents for combination therapy would be to combine agents with high toxicity with those of low toxicity. Another factor to be considered is the qualitative nature of the toxicity. The first two agents, Prednisone and Vincristine, have little or no marrow depressing effects and their dose limiting toxicity is different. Thus, combination of these two with each other or with one of the other three should permit full dosage of each compound to be given simultaneously. Because the last three agents all cause marrow depression as a limiting toxic effect, combinations of these might require lower doses. These speculations are largely supported by available data.

The combinations which have been studied are shown in Table III. The frequency of remission for the combination is always higher than from use of any one agent. Thus, for the combination of Prednisone (60%, when given alone) and VCR (55%), the rate is 85%. If one computes the expected response rate "predicted from independent action," then 60% would respond to Prednisone and 55% of the remaining 40%, an additional 22%, would respond to VCR, giving a predicted rate of 82%. Likewise, for Prednisone and 6-MP and for MTX and 6-MP, the observed response rates correspond with those predicted. These observations have recently led to study of four agents in combination; VCR, MTX, 6-MP and Pred. This treatment produced complete marrow remissions in 16 of 17 consecutive patients. Thus, combinations offer an advantage in getting the highest proportion of patients into remission. The question of which is the best choice for over-all survival will be discussed after consideration of techniques for prolonging remission and of resistance to therapy.

Remission Maintenance Therapy

The influence of various types of maintenance therapy on remission duration is presented in Table IV. With Pred. or VCR remission induction followed by no maintenance therapy, the median duration of remission is 5–9 weeks. Maintenance therapy of such remissions with VCR or Pred. is relatively in-

TABLE IV.—*Effect of Treatment on Remission Duration in Acute Lymphocytic Leukemia of Childhood*

Drug Used for Remission Induction	Remission Maintenance	Median Duration of Remission (Wks.)	Reference
Pred.	None	9	(31)
VCR	None	5	(32)
Pred.	Pred.	9–12	(30)
VCR	VCR	8	(32)
Pred. or 6-MP	6-MP	33	(31 & 27)
MTX	MTX	28	(16)
Pred.	CTX	12	(47)
CTX	CTX	14	(20)
Pred. + 6-MP	MTX + 6-MP	27	(29)
Pred. + 6-MP	MTX alternated with 6-MP	26	(29)

Abbreviations of drugs: Pred. = prednisone; VCR = vincristine; 6-MP = 6-mercapto-purine; MTX = methotrexate; CTX = cyclophosphamide.

effective in prolonging remission. This is due in considerable part to dose limitation imposed by toxicity associated with the chronic administration of these agents. 6-MP or MTX maintenance therapy will prolong remissions significantly. In general, there is an inverse correlation between an agent's ability to induce and to maintain remissions (compare Tables I and IV). It is conceivable that agents exist which are highly effective in maintaining remissions but are inactive in inducing remissions. Such agents would not be detected by the usual procedure of evaluating new agents in patients with active disease. Short duration of unmaintained remissions and the significant prolongation produced by some active agents serve as a framework for the testing of new agents as remission maintainers. The new agent hydroxyurea has recently been studied using such an experimental design. It was inactive[23, 85].

Even with active agents relapse eventually occurs and the patient is refractory to further conventional treatment with the same agent. Since the effect of further treatment on the host tissues remains the same it has been inferred that relapse results from the development or selection of drug resistant leukemic cells. This problem has been intensively studied in experimental systems, and biochemical mechanisms of resistance for 6-MP and MTX have been elucidated[93]. Evidence to date indicates that the mechanism of resistance of human leukemic cells to these agents may differ from those in animals[2, 12]. Prevention or delay in the development of such resistance is a major objective of current research. Combinations of antileukemic agents may delay the development of resistance in experimental systems[91] and combinations of antimicrobial agents are particularly effective in delaying the emergence of resistant mycobacteria[6]. This, plus the evidence that combinations of active agents produce an additive increase in the remission induction rate, led to a study of remission maintenance with combinations (Table IV). Remission duration was not prolonged by these or other combinations[46]. Drug resistance to antimetabolites probably results from the selection of those few cells in the initial leukemic cell population which are drug resistant. Since it takes a period of time, at least four weeks, for such cells to reach relapse levels, it is reasonable to hypothesize that alternating therapy would successfully prevent the ascendance of resistant cells and prolong remission. For 6-MP and MTX given for four week periods, the alternating sequence was not superior to 6-MP alone[29]. However, Zuelzer[92, 91] and Brubaker[7] have recently reported promising results with this type of therapy.

Drug Schedule

The schedule of drug administration has been shown to be of importance for MTX in animal tumor systems[43]. The use of MTX in man by an every four day, parenteral schedule, has given a complete remission rate of 70% in 23 patients with childhood ALL[78]. This contrasts to the rate of 21% for MTX given daily orally. The intermittent schedule allows for larger doses of drug (30 mgm/square meter surface area/twice a week; total dose of 60 mgm/sq. m/wk.) as compared to the daily schedule (3 mgm/sq. m/day; total dose of 21 mgm/sq. m/wk.). Perhaps even more important than the increased effectiveness for remission induction, is the recent demonstration that an intermittent parenteral schedule is much more effective for prolonging remissions than the daily oral treatment[81].

Consideration of past and future advances in chemotherapy generally involves the discovery of new agents active against the disease. It is clear, however, that study of sequence of drug administration, route and schedule of drug administration, drug combinations and remission induction as opposed to maintenance chemotherapy have, in the past, and should, in the future, be areas of major importance.

Supportive Therapy

As already emphasized, the ability to induce remissions of disease depends on supporting the patients through the periods of active disease. The major fatal complications result from hemorrhage and infection[5, 33]. The primary factor responsible for the hemorrhagic diathesis associated with acute leukemia is thrombocytopenia. The potential threat of hemorrhage is quantitatively estimated by the platelet count[41]. Platelet transfusion for replacement therapy has proven useful for management of this complication[17, 36, 13]. Use of a plasmapheresis technique can greatly increase the available supply of fresh platelets for transfusion[54]. A single donor can donate a liter of plasma, equivalent of four 500 cc units of whole blood per week, without significant depletion[53]. A single adult donor consequently can donate the major portion of the platelets required for maintaining the platelet level of a child with leukemia at satisfactory levels. Platelet transfusion has proven to be repeatedly effective in elevating the platelet count in over 80% of children studied[36]. When patients do form antibodies to platelets, selection of appropriate compatible donors occasionally can overcome this problem[1]. The use of the complement fixation technique and other *in vitro* tests for platelet antibodies can be helpful for selection of appropriate donors[57]. Because no effective storage technique is known for platelets, freshly drawn blood or plasma offers the best source of supply. However, blood stored for 24 hours at 4°C. in ACD anticoagulant is still approximately 50% as effective as fresh platelets in elevating the platelet count and may be useful for emergency situations[58]. Transfusion of platelets as platelet concentrates obviates the necessity for transfusing large quantities of plasma. However, such preparations are only approximately 50% as effective as platelet rich plasma transfusions[61, 13]. Nonetheless, for adult patients and for patients with large requirements for platelets, a single donor cannot supply all the platelets for transfusion. Pooled preparations from several donors, either as platelet rich plasma or concentrates, are as effective as single donor transfusions[61]. While platelet transfusion in its present state is very useful for reducing morbidity from hemorrhage, improvement in techniques of preparation and concentration of platelets, development of effective storage techniques and more effective *in vitro* techniques for predicting compatibility of platelet transfusions will be needed to make this form of therapy as effective and useful as red blood cell transfusion.

The advances in our knowledge of antibiotic and chemotherapeutic control of infection have been of major importance for control of bacterial infection. Infections caused by staphylococcus, pneumococcus, meningococcus, hemophilus, tuberculosis and other organisms, which were invariably fatal to the patient with leukemia, can be regularly cured. Particularly important has been the development of the penicillinase resistant compounds which have largely controlled the resistant staphylococcus infections which were a major cause of death in patients with leukemia. However, the usually saprophytic organisms such as the gram negative bacilli of which pseudomonas is the most prevalent, the fungi of which monilia and aspergillus are the most common offenders, and virus diseases such as disseminated cytomegalic inclusion disease and disseminated varicella, have become the major causes of death in patients with leukemia[28]. In a recent survey, over 80% of the deaths observed in a group of patients with leukemia could be ascribed primarily to such infections. The mechanism of the collapse of host resistance to these normally saprophytic organisms is only partially understood. The loss of the circulating granulocyte, like the loss of circulating red blood cells and platelets is one important feature. Replacement of the granulocytes by transfusion of cells from normal donors, however, has not been successful. While there are undoubtedly many reasons for this, the lack of effective techniques for the collection of large numbers of granulocytes is an important limitation. Because patients with uncontrolled chronic myelocytic leukemia (CML) may have levels of circulating granulocytes 30–50 times those of normal individuals, they may serve as donors for large numbers of granulocytes. Using a plasmapheresis technique and patients with CML as donors, transfusion of 10^{11} granulocytes per square meter body surface area of leukopenic recipients with acute leukemia has resulted in increments of circulating granulocytes of over 1,000 per cu. mm. These transfusions have been associated with dramatic temporary control of clinical infections, particularly pseudomonas septicemia[67, 37]. Studies indicate that inadequate dosage of granulocytes is probably a major cause for failure of granulocyte transfusion. If doses of 10^{11} granulocytes are needed, then all of the granulocytes in the circulating blood volume of two adult donors would be required for a single dose. Evidently, the techniques for collecting leukocytes will have to be greatly improved to achieve such a result. It is possible that some biomechanical equipment such as the ADL Cohn fractionator or a continuous flow leukocyte separator will provide a technique of leukopheresis capable of collecting these quantities of granulocytes[34].

The loss of granulocyte function is only part of the reason for the sharply reduced host defense. The loss of immunological apparatus in the host is another part. Although patients with acute leukemia show adequate concentrations of gamma globulins[15], unimpaired delayed hypersensitivity and fairly good response to antigenic stimulation[83], the chemotherapeutic agents used for suppression of the leukemic process also result in suppression of immune response[60]. These drugs can suppress completely development of delayed hypersensitivity and circulating antibody production following primary antigenic stimulation. In addition, they result in marked destruction of the lymphoid tissue. Finally, study of the inflammatory response by the skin window technique has shown that the chemotherapeutic agents used for treatment of acute leukemia can markedly suppress the mononuclear cell infiltration seen in 24 hour skin windows. This suppression occurs in the presence of normal peripheral blood cytologic values, and indicates another aspect of the suppressed host defense resulting from chemotherapy[44]. Techniques for repairing these deficits are presently matters of speculation only. It is conceivable that some form of replacement therapy can be developed. But for this, as well as for granulocyte replacement, much more knowledge of histocompatibility and immune function will be required.

Another area of supportive therapy of importance for management of acute leukemia is therapy of renal failure associated with hyperuricemia[25]. This type of renal failure occurs most commonly following institution of chemotherapy for acute leukemia. The rapid dissolution of leukemic tissue results in a great increase in urate production, and urate load for the kidney. It can also be observed during periods of active disease in the absence of chemotherapy. The pathogenesis of the renal disease is consistent with renal tubular obstruction resulting from intraluminal precipitation of urate[77]. Most effective therapy of this complication is prophylaxis. Prior to institution of therapy, the maintenance of high rates of urine flow can permit the excretion of enormous quantities of urate without renal failure. This result is most readily achieved by water diuresis, although mannitol-induced diuresis may be necessary to increase urine flow in patients with established renal failure. Adequate renal function is of great importance for patients receiving chemotherapy; it is particularly important for drugs primarily excreted by the kidney, such as MTX. Renal failure during MTX therapy can result in greatly increased toxicity.

Prognosis in Acute Leukemia

Of the many clinical features of acute leukemia which have prognostic significance, the morphological diagnosis is perhaps the most important. For patients with acute myelocytic leukemia (AML) the overall prognosis for survival is still poor. Median survival from diagnosis is only 2–4 months, and has not changed significantly since 1948[5, 14, 33]. The poor prognosis results primarily from the low frequency of remission induction in these patients. The patients with AML who do respond to therapy have a prognosis comparable to that for patients with childhood acute lymphocytic leukemia (Figure 1). Since only a small minority of patients with AML achieve remission, such improvement does not affect the median. The problem for the future is to increase the fraction of patients that respond to therapy. For patients with AML, the morphological appearance of the leukemic cells in the marrow is also of prognostic importance. Patients who show some evidence of cellular maturation (i.e., granules and Auer rods) have a better prognosis than those with less well differentiated leukemic cells because the remission rate is higher and the duration of remission is longer (59). For patients with ALL, age is of prognostic importance. Most frequent response to therapy and longest survival are observed in young children, age 3–5. Prognosis is not as good for infants (< 2 years), and survival decreases with increasing age, over 10[33, 5]. The period from onset of symptoms to diagnosis is also of importance for patients under 20. Those patients with short intervals between symptoms and diagnosis have less frequent remissions, shorter duration of remission and shorter survival[31].

The degree of leukocytosis is a clinical feature of great prognostic importance in acute leukemia. Patients with extreme degrees of leukocytosis (peripheral white blood cell counts of over 300,000 per cu. mm.) have a very high frequency of fatal intracerebral hemorrhage[40]. This complication is associated with leukostasis in intracerebral vessels and the formation of intracerebral leukemic nodules, around which massive hemorrhage occurs. This sudden clinical event can occur in the presence of normal platelet levels and appears to be a direct result of leukemic cell proliferation[38]. In addition to the association of fatality with high white blood cell counts, there is a correlation in overall survival with degree of leukocytosis at the time of diagnosis[33, 5, 64]. Patients with high counts have shorter survival time after diagnosis, in part because of a lower frequency of remission induction and shorter duration of remission[31].

These prognostic parameters in leukemia are reminiscent of the classical parameters of malignancy for other tumors. The more extensive the disease at diagnosis (the height of the white blood cell count), the shorter the duration from symptoms to diagnosis, and the less differentiated the tumor cells, the poorer the prognosis.

Leukemic Meningeal Infiltration

Another manifestation of leukemia, meningeal involvement, is becoming increasingly important. This clinical syndrome includes all of the manifestations associated with chronically increased cerebrospinal fluid pressure[82]. It results from leukemic cell infiltration of the subarachnoid and perivascular spaces[66], can occur in patients with active disease, but also occurs commonly in patients whose leukemic disease is under control elsewhere as a result of chemotherapy. Patients having bone marrow remission can develop recurrent nausea and vomiting, cranial nerve palsies (7th nerve palsy is most common), headaches and seizures. Lumbar puncture reveals increased pressure and pleocytosis of mononuclear cells which can often be recognized as leukemic cells. Prompt recognition of this syndrome is important because of the irreversible cranial nerve palsies and hydrocephalus which can result from long-standing disease. The proliferation of leukemic cells in the subarachnoid space in the face of adequate chemotherapeutic control elsewhere apparently results because of the relative exclusion of the drugs from the cerebrospinal fluid by the "blood-brain barrier" [73]. Only corticosteroids have activity against meningeal leukemia when given systemically. However, the clinical control of meningeal leukemia can be regularly accomplished by intrathecal injection of MTX or aminopterin. Intrathecal administration is effective even when the disease is resistant to systemic therapy, because of the enormous drug concentrations which can be achieved in the small volume of the cerebrospinal fluid. The therapeutic advantage can be further increased by the use of concomitant citrovorum factor given systemically to protect the other organ systems, permitting even larger doses to be given intrathecally[79]. Unfortunately, this form of therapy is only palliative as evidenced by the high recurrence rate in patients who have meningeal leukemia[89]. Thus, once the diagnosis of meningeal leukemic involvement is made regular prophylactic therapy at 3–4 week intervals is indicated, and effective in preventing morbidity.

The Failure of Therapy

Despite the advances in chemotherapy, supportive therapy and knowledge of natural history of acute leukemia, the disease is still uniformly fatal. It seems reasonable to inquire into the reasons for this failure. The agents effective in producing complete remission of the disease evidently have a high degree of specificity, as is indicated by the extensive destruction of leukemic tissue which occurs while the normal cellular elements of the marrow undergo regeneration and recovery to their normal state. One possible interpretation of these findings is that the morphological aspect of the cells which permits recognition of the leukemia is only a peripheral manifestation of the disease process. It is possible that the apparently normal cells which appear in the marrow are still leukemic cells. A situation resembling this state of affairs has been observed in patients with chronic myelocytic leukemia (CML). A high proportion of these patients have a specific cytogenetic abnormality in the myeloid cells of the marrow: deletion of a portion of a chromosome in group 21-22, the Philadelphia (Ph[1]) chromosome[69]. When a patient with CML is treated effectively and enters a state of complete hematological remission as manifested by normal bone marrow and peripheral blood cytology, normal leukocyte alkaline phosphatase and no clinical evidence of leukemic infiltrations, the apparently normal appearing marrow cells still contain the Ph[1] chromosome[11, 4]. Thus, for such patients, a major abnormality persists despite effective control of the disease. Leukocytes of patients with acute leukemia, however, have shown no *specific* chromosomal abnormality. Many patients with acute leukemia do show chromosome abnormalities which tend to be characteristic for a given patient, but many different types of abnormalities are found in different patients[48, 49, 70, 76]. When abnormalities are found in patients with acute leukemia, these abnormalities disappear when a complete remission occurs following chemotherapy, and the chromosome pattern in the marrow returns to normal. When the patient has recurrence of leukemia, a chromosome abnormality which resembles that found prior to remission is again observed[70, 76]. This finding supports the concept that the chemotherapy has resulted in destruction of the leukemic cells and that recurrence stems from incomplete eradication of the malignant cell line. This may be followed by development of resistance to the chemotherapeutic agent, with recurrence of the leukemia.

The concept of incomplete eradication of leukemic cells receives considerable support from transplantable rodent leukemia L-1210. In this model system eradication of all cells results in cure, while inadequate therapy of advanced disease results only in control of leukemia with prolongation of survival[84, 39]. We have recently studied 15 patients who died from causes other than leukemia while in bone marrow remission. In 10 of the 15, microscopic infiltrates of leukemic cells were found in organs such as liver, kidney, central nervous system, and lungs, even though the bone marrow was histologically normal[68]. These findings also support the concept that recurrence results from incomplete eradication of leukemic cells. Why should the chemotherapy fail to eradicate the leukemic cells? One reason may be the existence of "pharmacological hideouts". As already emphasized in the preceding discussion of meningeal leukemic infiltration, the subarachnoid space of the brain is one such "hideout". Here, the leukemic cells are protected from high drug concentrations by the blood-cerebrospinal fluid barrier. Moreover, in this milieu of low drug concentration, the opportunities for developing resistance to the drugs is optimal[73]. Spread from such a site would result in recurrent disease. The fact that patients who develop frank meningeal leukemia can rarely have the infiltration eliminated also supports the concept that persistence of leukemic cells in the subarachnoid space may be a major reason for failure to eradicate the disease with chemotherapy[89]. The subarachnoid space need not be the only "pharmacological hideout". Studies in rodents have demonstrated that in large tumor nodules the drug concentrations achieved in the center of such nodules are much lower than at the periphery and can allow for survival of such cells[42, 3]. In leukemic human subjects, we have observed recurrent leukemia in testicles, lymph nodes and skin at times when the bone marrow remains histologically normal. It is possible that persistence of focal collections of leukemic cells in these sites was responsible for the recurrent disease. Search for agents which can cross the blood-cerebrospinal fluid and other pharmacological barriers is an important area of current study. The recent discovery that certain nitrosourea compounds can eradicate the meningeal infiltration in experimental animals[80] led to clinical investigation of bis-beta-chloroethyl nitrosourea in man. In 4 of 5 patients control of meningeal leukemic infiltration was observed. However, delayed toxicity to the liver and bone marrow makes this compound difficult to use[74]. Hopefully, discovery of new agents capable of penetrating such pharmacological barriers may bring the chemotherapist closer to his goal.

The discovery that choriocarcinoma in women can be eradicated with MTX therapy is a very important finding in human cancer research[63, 45]. In this disease treatment with MTX can result in prompt regression of all clinical evidence of tumor. Yet at this phase of clinical complete remission, many women have persistence of elevated chorionic gonadotrophin excretion indicating persistence of malignant cells. If chemotherapy is continued until gonadotrophin excretion returns to normal, then vitually all women remain free of disease for years. In leukemia, unfortunately, no such sensitive indicator of persistent tumor has been recognized. Studies of patients in complete remission fail to show any abnormality which might be ascribed to persistent tumor. Yet because of the above considerations it seems that repeated courses of intensive therapy early in the course of the disease should be investigated for the possibility of eradication of the leukemic cells[35, 24, 46a].

Another approach to eradication of disease is by intense therapy combined with transplantation of homologous bone marrow[88]. By use of chemotherapy or total body radiation, sufficient suppression of immune response occurs to permit marrow homografts to survive at least temporarily[62]. Such bone marrow homografts may exploit the graft versus host reaction to accomplish eradication of persistent leukemic cells. A recent report from Mathé indicates that this approach offers promise. Control of acute leukemia for more than 10 months has been observed in a patient with a surviving marrow homograft[65]. It is possible that advances in organ homografting will permit much more intensive treatment to the point of eradicating a patient's marrow and will allow replacement of this organ with normal homologous marrow.

Finally, it is possible that eradication of all leukemic cells would also fail to "cure" the disease. If the carcinogenic agent responsible for induction of the disease persists, then recurrence might be due to re-induction of the malignant process. If a viral agent is such a carcinogen, then treatment designed to eradicate the virus or to prevent its action will be required. Certainly, for the patient with acute leukemia, eradication of the leukemic cells will still be necessary.

This brief survey of the rapidly expanding knowledge of human acute leukemia points to the many promising areas for investigation of the disease. There are many "hot leads" to pursue and many disappointments to face. The progress to date permits the investigator an optimistic view. Moreover, many hopefully feel that control of this malignant disease will be the key to unlocking the mystery of the control of other malignant diseases in man.

REFERENCES

1. Aster, R. H., Levin, R. H., Cooper, H. E., Freireich, E. J., Morse, E. E., and Singer, D. L.: Correlation of complement-fixing antibodies with platelet survival in thrombocytopenic patients. Clin. Res. 10: 195, 1962.
2. Bertino, J. R., Donohue, D. M., Simmons, B., Gabrio, B. W., Silber, R., and Huennekens, F. M.: The "induction" of dihydrofolic reductase activity in leukocytes and erythrocytes of patients treated with amethopterin. J. Clin. Invest. 42: 466–475, 1963.
3. Block, J. H., Millar, S. K., Harris, A. R., Berlin, N. I., and White, J.: Water exchange in animal and human tumors. J. Appl. Physiol. 16: 181–185, 1961.
4. Block, J. B., Carbone, P. P., Oppenheim, J. J., and Frei, E., III: The effect of treatment in patients with chronic myelogenous leukemia. Ann. Intern. Med. 59: 629–635, 1963.
5. Boggs, D. R., Wintrobe, M. M., and Cartwright, C. E.: The acute leukemias. Analysis of 322 cases and review of the literature. Medicine 41: 163–225, 1962.
6. Report to the British Medical Research Council by their tuberculosis chemotherapy trials committee: Various combinations of isoniazid with streptomycin or with P. A. S. in the treatment of pulmonary tuberculosis. Brit. Med. J. 1: 435, 1955.
7. Brubaker, C. A., Wheeler, H. E., Sonley, M. J., Hyman, C. B., Williams, K. O., and Hammond, D.: Cyclic chemotherapy for acute leukemia in children. Blood 22: 820, 1963.
8. Burchenal, J. H., Murphy, M. L., Ellison, R. R., Sykes, M. P., Tan, T. C., Leone, L. A.,

Karnofsky, D. A., Carver, L. F., Dargeon, H. W., and Rhoads, C. P.: Clinical evaluation of a new antimetabolite, 6-mercaptopurine, in the treatment of leukemia and allied disease. Blood 8: 965–999, 1953.

9. Burchenal, J. H., Murphy, M. L., Tan, C. T., and Dargeon, H. D.: Chemotherapy of neoplastic disease in children. Advances Pediat. 12: 189–226, 1962.

10. Burger, C. L., Harris, W. W., Anderson, N. G., Hartlett, T. W., and Kniseley, R. M.: Virus-like particles in human leukemic plasma. Proc. Soc. Exper. Biol. Med. 115: 151–156, 1964.

11. Carbone, P. P., Tjio, J. H., Whang, J., Block, J. B., Kremer, W. B., and Frei, E., III: The effect of treatment in patients with chronic myelogenous leukemia. Ann. Intern. Med. 59: 622–628, 1963.

12. Davidson, J. D., and Winter, T. S.: Purine nucleotide pyrophosphorylases in 6-mercaptopurine sensitive and resistant human leukemias. Cancer Res. 24: 261–268, 1964.

13. Djerassi, I., Farber, S., and Evans, A. E.: Transfusions of fresh platelet concentrates to patients with secondary thrombocytopenia. New Eng. J. Med., 258: 211, 1963.

14. Ellison, R. R., Silver, R. T., and Engle, R. L., Jr.: Comparative study of 6-chloropurine and 6-mercaptopurine in acute leukemia in adults. Ann. Intern. Med., 51: 322, 1959.

15. Fahey, J. L., and Boggs, D. R.: Serum protein changes in malignant diseases I. The acute leukemias. Blood 16: 1479, 1960.

16. Farber, S., Diamond, L. K., Mercer, R. D., Sylvester, R. F., Jr., and Wolff, J. A.: Temporary remissions in acute leukemia in children produced by folic acid antagonist 4-aminopteroyl-glutamic acid (Aminopterin). New Eng. J. Med. 238: 787–793, 1948.

17. Farber, S., and Klein, E.: The nature and control of bleeding in acute leukemia and other thrombocytopenic states. Ann. Paediat. 3: 348, 1957.

18. Farber, S., Schwachman, H., Toch, R., Downing, V., Kennedy, B. H., and Hyde, J.: The effect of ACTH in acute leukemia in childhood. In Proc. First Clinical ACTH Conference, Philadelphia, Blakiston, 1950, p. 328, Mote, J. R. (Ed.)

19. Farber, S., Toch, R., Sears, E. M., and Pinkel, D.: Advances in cancer chemotherapy in man. Advances Cancer Res. 4: 1–72, 1956.

20. Fernbach, D. J., Sutow, W. W., Thurman, W. G., and Vietti, T. J.: Clinical evaluation of cyclophosphamide. A new agent for the treatment of children with acute leukemia. J. A. M. A. 182: 30–37, 1962.

21. Fessas, P., Wintrobe, M. M., Thompson, R. B., and Cartwright, G. E.: Treatment of actue leukemia with cortisone and corticotrophin. A.M.A. Arch. Intern. Med. 94: 384–401, 1954.

22. Finch, S. C.: Transmission of leukemia. Progress in Hematology. Vol 2. Tocantins, L. M. (Ed.) Grune and Stratton, New York, 1959. p. 192–205.

23. Fishbein, W. N., Carbone, P. P., Freireich, E. J., Misra, D., and Frei, E., III: Clinical trials of hydroxyurea in patients with cancer and leukemia. Manuscript in preparation.

24. Frei, E., III: Potential for eliminating leukemic cells in childhood acute leukemia. Proc. Amer. Ass. Cancer Res. 5: 20, 1964.

25. Frei, E., III, Bentzel, C. J., Rieselbach, R., Block, J. B.: Renal complications of leukemic disease. J. Chronic Dis. 16: 757, 1963.

26. Frei, E., III, Freireich, E. J.: Leukemia. Sci. Amer. In press, May 1964.

27. Frei, E., III, Freireich, E. J., Gehan, E., Pinkel, D., Holland, J. F., Selawry, O., Haurani, F., Spurr, C. L., Hayes, D. M., James G. W., Rothberg, H., Sodee, D. B., Rundles, R. W., Schroeder, L. R., Hoogstraten, B., Wolman, I. J., Traggis, D. G., Cooper, T., Gendel, B. R., Ebaugh, F., and Taylor, R.: Studies of sequential and combination antimetabolite therapy in acute leukemia: 6-mercaptopurine and methotrexate, from the Acute Leukemia Group B. Blood 18: 431–454, 1961.

28. Frei, E., III, Levin, R. H., Bodey, G. P., Morse, E. E., and Freireich, E. J.: The nature and control of infections in patients with acute leukemia. Proceedings of conference on obstacles to control of acute leukemia. Cancer Res. In press.

29. Frei, E., III, and Taylor, R. J.: The effect of continuous alternating intrathecal chemotherapy on the duration of remissions in acute leukemia. Proc. Amer. Ass. Cancer. Res. 4: 20, 1963.

30. Freireich, E. J., Frei, E., III, and Karon, M.: Methylglyoxal bis (guanylhydrazone): A new agent active against acute myelocytic leukemia. Cancer Chemother. Rep. 16: 183–186, 1961.

31. Freireich, E. J., Gehan, E., Frei, E., III, Schroeder, L. R., Wolman, I. J., Anbari, R., Burgert, E. O., Mills, S. D., Pinkel, D., Salawry, O. S., Moon, J. H., Gendel, B. R., Spurr, C. L., Storrs, R., Haurani, F., Hoogstraten, B., and Lee, S.: The effect of 6-mercaptopurine on the duration of steroid-induced remissions in acute leukemia: A model for evaluation of other potentially useful therapy. Blood 21: 699–716, 1963.

32. Karon, M.: Preliminary report on Vincristine (Oncovin®) from Acute Leukemia Group B. Proc. Amer. Ass. Cancer Res. 4: 33, 1963.

33. Freireich, E. J., Gehan, E. A., Sulman, D., Boggs, D. R., and Frei, E., III: The effects of chemotherapy on acute leukemia in the human. J. Chronic Dis. 14: 593–608, 1961.

34. Freireich, E. J., Judson, G., Levin, R. H.: Separation and collection of leukocytes. Proceedings of conference on obstacles to control of acute leukemia. Cancer Res. In Press.

35. Freireich, E. J., Karon, M., and Frei, E., III.: Quadruple combination therapy (VAMP) for acute lymphocytic leukemia of childhood. Proc. Amer. Ass. Cancer Res. 5: 20, 1964.

36. Freireich, E. J., Kliman, A., Gaydos, L. A., Mantel, N., and Frei, E., III: Response to repeated platelet transfusion from the same donor. Ann. Intern. Med. 59: 277–287, 1963.
37. Freireich, E. J., Levin, R. H., Whang, J., Carbone, P. P., Bronson, W., Morse, E. E.: The function and fate of transfused leukocytes from donors with chronic myelocytic leukemia in leukopenic recipients. Ann. N. Y. Acad. Sci. 113: 1081–1089, 1964.
38. Freireich, E. J., Thomas, L. B., Frei, E., III, Fritz, R. D., and Forkner, C. E., Jr.: A distinctive type of intracerebral hemorrhage associated with "blastic crisis" in patients with leukemia. Cancer 13: 146–154, 1960.
39. Friedkin, M., and Goldin, A.: The use of dihydrofolate reductase in studies of mixed populations of sensitive and resistant leukemic cells. Cancer Res. 22: 607–616, 1962.
40. Fritz, R. D., Forkner, C. E., Jr., Freireich, E. J., Frei, E., III, and Thomas, L. B.: The association of fatal intracranial hemorrhage and "blastic crisis" in patients with acute leukemia. New Eng. J. Med. 261: 59–64, 1959.
41. Gaydos, L. A., Freireich, E. J., and Mantel, N.: The quantitative relation between platelet count and hemorrhage in patients with acute leukemia. New Eng. J. Med. 266: 905–909, 1962.
42. Goldacre, R. J., and Sylven, B.: On the access of blood-borne dyes to various tumour regions. Brit. J. Cancer 16: 306–322, 1962.
43. Goldin, A., Venditti, J. M., Humphreys, S. R., Mantel, N.: Modification of treatment schedules in the management of advanced mouse leukemia with amethopterin. J. Nat. Cancer Inst. 17: 203, 1956.
44. Hersh, E. M., Levin, R. H., Wong, V., and Freireich, E. J.: Inhibtion of the local inflammatory response in man by antimetabolites. Clin. Res. 11: 399, 1963.
45. Hertz, R., Lewis, J., Jr., Lipsett, M. B.: Five years' experience with the chemotherapy of metastatic choriocarcinoma and related trophoblastic tumors in women. Amer. J. Obst. Gynec. 82: 631–640, 1961.
46. Heyn, R. M., Brubaker, C. A., Burchenal, J. H., Cramblett, H. G., and Wolff, J. A.: The comparison of 6-mercaptopurine with the combination of 6-mercaptopurine and azaserine in the treatment of acute leukemia in children: Results of a cooperative study. Blood 15: 350–359, 1960.
46a. Holland, J. F. and Hananian, J.: Unpublished data from Acute Leukemia Group B. Protocol №6313.
47. Hoogstraten, B.: Cyclophosphamide (Cytoxan) in acute leukemia. Cancer Chemother. Rep. 16: 167–171, 1962.
48. Hungerford, D. A.: Chromosome studies in human leukemia. I. Acute leukemia in children. J. Nat. Cancer Inst. 27: 983–1011, 1961.
49. Hungerford, D. A., Nowell, P. C.: Chromosome studies in human leukemia. III. Acute granulocytic leukemia. J. Nat. Cancer Inst. 29: 545, 1962.
50. Hyman, C. B., Borda, E., Brubaker, C., Hammond, D., and Sturgeon, P.: Prednisone in childhood leukemia: Comparison of interrupted with continuous therapy. Pediatrics 24: 1005–1008, 1959.
51. Johnson, I. A., Armstrong, J. G., Gorman, M., and Burnett, J. P., Jr.: The vinca alkaloids: A new class of oncolytic agents. Cancer Res. 23: 1390–1427, 1963.
52. Karon, M. R., Freireich, E. J., and Frei, E., III.: A preliminary report on vincristine sulfate—a new active agent for the treatment of acute leukemia. Pediatrics 30: 791–796, 1962.
53. Kliman, A., Carbone, P. P., Gaydos, L. A., and Freireich, E. J.: Effects of intensive plasmapheresis on normal blood donors. Blood 23: 647–656, 1964.
54. Kliman, A., Gaydos, L. A., Schroeder, L. R., and Freireich, E. J.: Repeated plasmapheresis of blood donors as a source of platelets. Blood 18: 303–309, 1961.
55. Law, L. W., Taormina, V., and Boyle, P. J.: Response of acute lymphocytic leukemias to the purine antagonist 6-mercaptopurine. Ann. N.Y. Acad. Sci. 60: 244–250, 1954.
56. Levin, R. H., Brittin, G. M., Freireich, E. J.: Different patterns of remission in acute myelocytic leukemia. A comparison of the effects of methyl-glyoxal-bis-guanylhydrazone and 6-mercaptopurine. Blood 21: 689–698, 1963.
57. Levin, R. H., Cooper, H. E., Aster, R. H., and Freireich, E. J.: Usefulness of complement (C′) fixation studies in predicting response to platelet transfusions. Clin. Res. 11: 33, 1963.
58. Levin, R. H., Freireich, E. J., and Chapell, W.: Effect of storage up to 48 hours on response to transfusions of platelet rich plasma. Transfusion, In press.
59. Levin, R. H., and Kundel, D.: Prognostic implications of bone marrow morphology in acute myelocytic leukemia. Proc. Amer. Ass. Cancer Res. 5: 40, 1964.
60. Levin, R. H., Landy, M., and Frei, E., III: The effect of 6-mercaptopurine of immune response in man. New Eng. J. Med. In press.
61. Levin, R. H., Pert, J. H., and Freireich, E. J.: Effect of in vitro manipulations of platelet viability. Manuscript in preparation.
62. Levin, R. H., Whang, J., Tjio, J. H., Carbone, P. P., Frei, E., III, Freireich, E. J.: Persistent mitosis of transfused homologous leukocytes in children receiving antileukemic therapy. Science 142: 1305–1311, 1963.
63. Li, M. C., Hertx, R., and Spencer, D. B.: Effect of methotrexate therapy upon choriocarcinoma and chorioadenoma. Proc. Soc. Exp. Biol. Med. 93: 361, 1956.

64. MacMahon, B., and Forman, D.: Variation in the duration of survival of patients with acute leukemia. Blood 12: 683, 1957.
65. Mathé, G., Amiel, J. L., Schwarzenberg, L., Cattan, A., Schneider, M.: Haematopoietic chimera in man after allogenic (homologous) bone-marrow transplantation. Control of the secondary syndrome. Specific tolerance due to the chimerism. Brit. Med. J. 2: 1633–1635, 1963.
66. Moore, E. W., Thomas, L. B., Shaw, R. K., and Freireich, E. J.: The central nervous system in acute leukemia: A postmortem study of 117 consecutive cases, with particular reference to hemorrhage, leukemic infiltrations, and the syndrome of meningeal leukemia. A.M.A. Arch. Intern. Med. 105: 451–468, 1960.
67. Morse, E. E., Bronson, W., Carbone, P. P., and Freireich, E. J.: Effectiveness of granulocyte transfusion from donors with chronic myelocytic leukemia to patients with leukopenia. Clin. Res. 9: 332, 1961.
68. Nies, B. A., and Bodey, G.: Persistence of leukemia infiltrates in patients with acute leukemia dying in bone marrow remission. Manuscript in preparation.
69. Nowell, P. C., and Hungerford, D. A.: Minute chromosome in human chronic granulocytic leukemia. Science 132: 1497, 1960.
70. Oppenheim, J. J., Whang, J., Tjio, J. H., and Frei, E., III.: Chromosome studies in acute leukemia. Manuscript in Preparation.
71. Pearson, O. H., Eliel, L. P., Rawson, R. W., Dobrinen, K., and Rhoads, C. P.: ACTH- and cortisone-induced regression of lymphoid tumors in man: A preliminary report. Cancer 2: 943, 1949.
72. Porter, G. H., III., Dalton, A. J., Moloney, J. B., and Mitchell, E. Z.: The association of electron-dense particles with human acute leukemia. J. Nat. Cancer Institute. In press.
73. Rall, D. P.: Experimental studies of the blood-brain barrier. Proceedings of conference on obstacles to control of acute leukemia. Cancer Res. In Press.
74. Rall, D. P., Ben, M., and McCarthy, D. M.: 1,3-bis-β-chloroethyl-1-nitrosourea (BCNU): Toxicity and initial clinical trial. Proc. Amer. Ass. Cancer Res. 4: 55, 1963.
75. Regelson, W., and Holland, J. F.: Clinical experience with methylglyoxal bis (guanylhydrozone) dihydrochloride: a new agent with clinical activity in acute myelocytic leukemia and the lymphomas. Cancer Chemother. Rep. 27: 15–26, 1963.
76. Reisman, L. E., Mitani, M., and Zuelzer, W. W.: Chromosome studies in leukemia. I. Evidence for the origin of leukemic stem lines from aneuploid mutants. New Eng. J. Med. 270: 590–597, 1964.
77. Rieselbach, R. E., Bentzel, C. J., Cotlove, E., Frei, E., III., and Freireich, E. J.: The pathogenesis and therapy of acute renal insufficiency associated with secondary hyperuricemia. Amer. J. Med. In press.
78. Rieselbach, R. E., Morse, E., Freireich, E. J., and Frei, E., III.: An intermittent dose schedule of folic acid antagonsists for treatment of acute lymphocytic leukemia. Manuscript in preparation.
79. Rieselbach, R. E., Morse, E. E., Rall, D. P., Frei, E., III., and Freireich, E. J.: Intrathecal aminopterin therapy of meningeal leukemia. Arch. Intern. Med. 111: 620–630, 1963.
80. Schabel, F. M., Jr., Johnston, T. P., McCaleb, G. S., Montgomery, J. A., Laster, W. R., Jr., and Skipper, H. E.: Experimental evaluation of potential anticancer agents. VIII. Effects of certain nitrosoureas on intracerebral L1210 leukemia. Cancer Res. 23: 725–733, 1963.
81. Selawry, O. S., and Frei, E., III: Prolongation of remission in acute lymphocytic leukemia by alteration in dose schedule and route of administration of methotrexate. Clin. Res. 12: 231, 1964.
82. Shaw, R. K., Moore, E. W., Freireich, E. J., and Thomas, L. B.: Meningeal leukemia: A syndrome resulting from increased intracranial pressure in patients with acute leukemia. Neurology 10: 823–833, 1960.
83. Silver, R. T., Utz, J. P., Fahey, J., and Frei, E., III.: Antibody response in patients with acute leukemia. J. Lab. Clin. Med. 56: 634, 1960.
84. Skipper, H. E., Schabel, F. M., Jr., Wilcox, W. S.: Experimental evaluation of potential anticancer agents. XIII. On the criteria and kinetics associated with "curability" of experimental leukemia. Cancer Chemoth. Rep. 35: 1–111, 1964.
85. Storrs, R., Chairman, Unpublished data, Acute Leukemia Group B, Protocol #6306.
86. Sutow, W. W., Sullivan, M. P., and Taylor, G.: Status of present treatment of acute leukemia. Proceedings of conference on obstacles to control of acute leukemia. Cancer Res. In press.
87. Tan, C. T. C., Phoa, J., Lyman, M., Murphy, M. L., Dargeon, H. W., and Burchenal, J. H.: Hematological remissions in acute leukemia with cyclophosphamide. Blood 18: 808, 1961.
88. Thomas, E. D., and Epstein, R. B.: Bone marrow transplantation in acute leukemia. Proceedings of conference on obstacles to control of acute leukemia. Cancer Res. In press.
89. Thomas, L. B.: Pathology of leukemia in the brain and meninges: Postmortem studies of patients with acute leukemia and of mice inoculated with L1210 leukemia. Proceedings of conference on obstacles to control of acute leukemia. Cancer Res. In press.

90. Vendetti, J. M., and Goldin, A.: Drug synergism in antineoplastic chemotherapy. Advances Chemother. Vol. 1, Academic Press. To be published.
91. Zuelzer, W. W.: Proceedings of conference on obstacles to control of acute leukemia. Cancer Res. In press.
92. Zuelzer, W. W. and Flatz, G.: Acute childhood leukemia: A ten year study. Amer. J. Dis. Child. 100: 886–907, 1960.
93. Welch, A. D.: The problem of drug resistance in cancer chemotherapy. Cancer Res. 19: 359–371, 1959.

Von Willebrand's Disease

—————EMILY M. BARROW and JOHN B. GRAHAM—————

HISTORICAL SURVEY

PROF. ERIK VON WILLEBRAND of the University of Helsinki, Finland became acquainted with the inhabitants of the islands of Åland in the Gulf of Bothnia in the late 1890's. Von Willebrand observed a high frequency of "bleeders" which led him to discover the hemorrhagic diathesis which now is designated von Willebrand's disease (v.W.d.). He became conscious of the malady through a family in which five of seven daughters had bled to death at early ages. His recorded studies began in 1924 with re-examination of one survivor from this kindred, both of whose parents belonged to "bleeder" families. On investigating sixty-six of the members of the kindred, he discovered twenty-three additional persons who bled excessively[72]. Both males and females were affected and Federly, a geneticist from the University of Helsinki, decided that the trait was dominantly inherited.

The only laboratory test which von Willebrand found consistently abnormal was the bleeding time. Some, but not all, of his patients had positive tourniquet tests. Their platelets were normal in number and appearance and samples of their blood clotted in the usual time. After comparing his cases with other hemorrhagic states, notably Glanzmann's description of "thromboasthenia", he concluded that the Åland islanders had a distinctive condition which he designated "pseudohemophilia" [73].

In the early 1930's, von Willebrand and R. Jürgens re-investigated the original patients. They concluded that the disease resulted from a qualitative platelet disorder manifested by poor clot retraction and impaired platelet agglutination. These observations led to a new designation: "die Konstitutionelle Thrombopathie (von Willebrand-Jürgens)" [74].

During the period between 1930 and the end of World War II, many reports appeared of persons resembling the patients of von Willebrand. Estren et al. in 1946[21] reviewed sixty-two cases described after 1900 and added eleven patients of their own. They stressed the unusual finding of prolonged bleeding time accompanied by normal platelet count, clot retraction and clotting time. Revol et al.[61] reviewed 88 cases described between 1921 and 1949 and added three of their own. Soulier and Larrieu[67] reviewed all cases published between 1913 and 1953 which might represent either von Willebrand's disease or one of the "thrombopathies" and attempted to classify them. Buchanan and Leavell[14] reviewed 113 cases published between 1946 and 1956 and described 13 new ones. Thus more than 200 patients had been described by 1957.

The general point of view of all reviewers was that a hemorrhagic disorder existed which affected both males and females, was characterized by a pro-

Supported by a research grant (HE-03140) from the Public Health Service.

From the Department of Pathology, University of North Carolina School of Medicine, Chapel Hill, North Carolina.

longed bleeding time, and had variable effects on other tests of platelet function, including prothrombin consumption and whole blood clotting time. It was not clear whether the diathesis was caused by a vascular defect, platelet dysfunction or a combination of these defects.

Important new understanding was achieved in 1953 when Alexander and Goldstein demonstrated that the plasma antihemophilic factor (AHF) level is reduced in v.W.d.[2]. Since then Nilsson et al.[47, 48] and van Creveld[69] have shown that the prolonged bleeding time is probably related to a plasma factor other than AHF, rather than an abnormality of platelets or of the vascular wall. More recently, appreciation that AHF synthesis is under the control of genes on different chromosomes has revived interest in v.W.d.[4, 27, 28, 44]. Intensive study of v.W.d. during the next few years promises to increase greatly our understanding of AHF synthesis in normal persons and throw new light on the essential nature of hemophilia.

Clinical Aspects

The hemorrhagic tendency in v.W.d. is generally evident at an early age. In the aggregate, the patients seem to have fewer and less severe complications than men with hemophilia A. The condition usually is manifested as epistaxis, hematuria, gingival bleeding, "easy bruising", gastro-intestinal bleeding, or prolonged oozing of blood from a surface injury or site of operation. Tooth extraction presents a serious problem in some patients. In contrast to hemophilia A, bleeding rarely occurs into joints, Biggs[7] having noted joint involvement in only 8% of published cases. The complications of the bleeding tendency decrease strikingly with increasinge age.

The most frequent and disabling complication in women is menorrhagia which has led frequently to production of artificial menopause by surgery or irradiation. Nilsson[51] reported severe menstrual bleeding in 15 of 27 mildly affected women. Interestingly, 22 had borne children and only 8 had experienced abnormal bleeding during and after delivery. Pregnancy clearly has had a beneficial effect in some instances. The AHF level of one pregnant patient increased progressively to more than 100 per cent of normal by time of delivery[51] and van Creveld[70] has described a woman with a resting AHF level of less than 1 per cent whose plasma level had increased to 30 per cent by the middle of the seventh month.

Treatment of bleeding episodes can be difficult in v.W.d. Plasma fractions rich in AHF are probably best, but suitable AHF-rich human fractions are not readily available in the U.S. Nilsson and Blombäck[51] listed thirty-nine surgical procedures performed successfully on v.W.d. patients treated before and after operation with the Swedish Fraction I-O. Interestingly, they achieved periods of normalization of the bleeding time as well as increased plasma AHF levels. Biggs and Matthews[8] believe the maintenance of a sufficiently high AHF level to be more important for hemostasis than normalization of the bleeding time. This appears to have been our experience also, but may be a result of the type of the bleeding time test. Cornu et al.[19] have noted that shortening of the Duke[20] bleeding time is associated with the hemostasis during and after surgical procedures, while the Ivy bleeding time[32] (the method used by Biggs and ourselves) may remain prolonged. Fresh-frozen plasma is effective in v.W.d. but bank-blood appears less so. We have treated the menorrhagia of v.W.d. quite satisfactorily by menstrual suppression with the commercial hormonal preparation, Enovid, containing norethynodrel and mestranol.

PHYSIOLOGICAL ASPECTS

A. *The Vascular Wall*

There were few laboratory aids when von Willebrand first studied his patients. He performed bleeding times, platelet counts, whole blood clotting times and the Rumpel-Leede tourniquet test. As new techniques have become available, further observations have been made. In 1941, Macfarlane[42] described five patients in whom bleeding times were prolonged despite adequate numbers of platelets which appeared normal in size and shape. He suggested that a capillary defect was responsible for the prolonged bleeding times, since he was able to demonstrate nail-bed capillaries which were abnormal in shape and failed to contract after puncture. Similar capillary abnormalities have been described in v.W.d. by others[2, 30, 39, 40, 43, 52, 55, 61, 63]. Jamra et al.[33] concluded that the response of the capillaries to injury was not significantly different between a group of persons with v.W.d. and a group of normal individuals.

The bleeding time test is used extensively in studying abnormalities of the "vascular wall". There is great variability in the results between different persons with v.W.d. and even within a single individual at different times. Roskam[62] obtained a value of 3 minutes (normal) in one ear and 48 minutes (grossly abnormal) in the other using the Duke bleeding time method. Buchanan and Leavell[14] described a patient with Duke bleeding times of 17 minutes and 180 minutes in opposite ear lobes. Pitney[56] performed Duke bleeding times monthly on a patient during an entire year. This man's values fluctuated between 3 minutes and greater than 30 minutes.

The tourniquet test[58] is another means for evaluating the "vascular wall". In scurvy, for example, it is strikingly abnormal. Patients with v.W.d. vary markedly in their response to this test also. In Buchanan and Leavell's analysis of cases published prior to 1956, positive results were reported in 54.3% of the patients on whom the test was performed. It is probably equally significant that the results were normal in 45.7%.

The results obtained with all of the tests for integrity of the "vascular wall" suggest that hemostasis is abnormal in v.W.d. The crudeness and lack of specificity of the tests and the variability of the results throw considerable uncertainty, however, on an hypothesis suggesting that v.W.d. is due primarily to a defect of the vascular wall.

B. *The Platelets*

It was suggested early that the bleeding time abnormality in v.W.d. was the expression of a "qualitative" platelet defect. This has been elaborated on by Jürgens et al.[35] and Johnson et al.[34] and specified as a deficiency of "platelet factor 3"[29]. Others[9, 48, 67] have stated that the concentration of "platelet factor 3" is quite normal in v.W.d. In 1933, von Willebrand and Jürgens[74] tested the blood of some of the Åland islanders with a "capillary thrombometer". Their results led them to believe that the disease resulted from poor agglutination of platelets. Others have commented on defective platelet agglutination but most workers consider this to be a variable and inconstant phenomenon in v.W.d.

Borchgrevink[12] devised a test for measuring platelet adhesiveness *in vivo* and described five persons with v.W.d. whose platelet adhesiveness was abnormal. Cornu et al.[19] have also stated that the *in vivo* platelet adhesiveness is abnormal in v.W.d. Caen[15] has reported abnormally high levels of platelet ATP and a disturbance of the platelet ADP/ATP ratio in his patients. He believes that these changes in high energy phosphate are the cause of the poor adhesiveness of the platelets.

Rapport et al.[59] demonstrated that platelets liberate a powerful vasoconstricting substance which they called serotonin and was later shown to be 5-hydroxytryptamine. Zucker and Borrelli[78] tested the sera of 11 patients with "pseudohemophilia"; serotonin was reduced in two. Bigelow[5], Reid[60] and Nilsson et al.[47] have tested serum or platelets from patients with v.W.d. and have reported that the liberation of serotonin from their platelets is normal. Ingram[31] described a patient, probably having von Willebrand's disease, whose platelets were apparently defective in liberation of serotonin.

The evidence suggesting that v.W.d. results primarily from a defect of the platelets is far from conclusive. One problem has been the unsatisfactory state of the art of studying platelets. Another has been an uncritical approach by some investigators who have drawn sweeping conclusions after using methods with large built-in errors on small population samples. It is possible that a primary platelet defect may yet be demonstrated to be of pathogenetic importance in v.W.d., but we are increasingly skeptical.

C. *Plasma Antihemophilic Factor*

Two papers published in 1953 described patients with prolonged bleeding times and normal platelet function[2, 38] whose plasma, but not serum, was abnormal in the thromboplastin generation test (TGT) of Biggs and Douglas[6]. This is the typical finding in classic hemophilia A, and it was shown [38, 57] that the plasma of such persons did not correct the coagulation defect of persons with hemophilia A. It was then proposed that a "new" disease existed. This disorder was called "pseudo-hemophilia B" by Singer and Ramot[65], "angio-hemophilia" by Achenbach[1] and "vascular hemophilia" by Schulman et al.[63]. More recently the identity of this condition with v.W.d. has been established by re-study of the Åland islanders.

Reports from Sweden in 1956 and 1957[46, 48, 49] described 13 patients with prolonged bleeding times, Factor VIII (AHF) deficiency, normal platelet function and an autosomal dominant mode of inheritance. The same investigators later visited the Åland islands and tested 15 individuals with classic "von Willebrand's disease". All proved to have moderately decreased levels of AHF and normal platelet factor 3 activity. The Swedish group concluded that the defect in the Swedish and Åland island patients was the same as that

TABLE 1

Type of Plasma	Partial Thromboplastin Time, secs.
1. Normal	76
2. Hemophilia A	356
3. Hemophilia B	372
4. Normal + Hemophilia A	94
5. Normal + Hemophilia B	87
6. Hemophilia A + Hemophilia B	90
7. Normal	72
8. Hemophilia A	200
9. v.W.d.	106
10. Normal + Hemophilia A	89
11. Normal + v.W.d.	73
12. Hemophilia A + v.W.d.	129

Comparison of the relations of hemophilias A and B and of hemophilia A to v.W.d. The clotting test was the partial thromboplastin time (PTT) and the mixtures consisted of equal parts of the respective plasmas.

described by Singer, Achenbach, and Schulman and suggested naming the disorder von Willebrand's disease.

At about the same time, Jürgens[36] retested some of the Åland islanders and confirmed reduced values for AHF in 7 of the 14 patients studied. In contrast to Nilsson et al., however, he thought he had also demonstrated a platelet abnormality in the thromboplastin generation test. Scrutiny of his results leaves us skeptical that he has established his claim. The data are not extensive, controls are unclear, and his ranges of variation for normal and abnormal populations are not shown.

Since the original report of reduced plasma AHF levels in v.W.d. in 1953, more than 200 patients have been described with documented plasma AHF reductions accompanied by prolonged bleeding times, normal platelet counts, and good clot retraction. As discussed below, family studies have revealed that not all genotypically abnormal persons show both abnormalities at all times. It is useful and sometimes even necessary to find a relative with the full-blown syndrome in order to establish the diagnosis in an individual patient.

Table 1 illustrates the difference between X-linked hemophilias A and B on the one hand and hemophilia A and v.W.d. on the other. In the upper portion a type of test tube "complementation" is noted between the two forms of X-linked hemophilia (Line 6). This "complementation" is the basic evidence for the *non-identity* of the mutant phenotypes. The lower portion of the table illustrates that the clotting time of v.W.d. plasma is not improved by addition of hemophilia A plasma (cp. Lines 9 and 12). This absence of *in vitro* "complementation" is the evidence of *identity* between the defects in the two types of plasma. If AHF (F. VIII) is abnormal in hemophilia A, Table 1 argues that it must also be abnormal in v.W.d.

This lack of "complementation" *in vitro* plus the obviously different location of the genes responsible for v.W.d. and hemophilia A has led to new speculation about control of AHF synthesis, a matter which will be discussed at length below.

D. *The "von Willebrand Factor"*

Both of the defects encountered in v.W.d. have been studied intensively since Nilsson and Blombäck[50] demonstrated in 1959 that the prolonged bleeding time in these patients could be shortened by Cohn's Fraction I-O prepared from either normal or hemophilia A plasma. The Swedish workers concluded that a *plasma*, not a *vascular* or *platelet*, factor was responsible for the maintenance of a normal bleeding time, and they now designate this plasma substance the "von Willebrand factor" [11]. It has also been referred to as "vascular factor" by our group[4, 27, 28, 44].

The Swedish workers[11] reported improvement in both AHF level and bleeding time when either their fraction I-O or the AHF-rich subfraction I-1-A was infused, provided the latter was given in large quantities. Whole blood appeared less effective than carefully prepared plasma or plasma fractions in correcting the bleeding time[51], but this may have been a quantitative matter. Infusion of fresh platelets apparently has no effect on the bleeding time in v.W.d.[19]. Biggs[8], and Fantl[22] have transfused normal serum into affected individuals and have demonstrated increased AHF activity without normalization of the bleeding times. We have observed that increased AHF activity after transfusions of plasma is sometimes but not always accompanied by shortening of the Ivy bleeding time.

The evidence suggests that v.W.d. plasma lacks a non-cellular component ("vascular factor", "von Willebrand's factor"). Transfusion of normal or hemophilia A plasma replaces the deficit and normalizes the prolonged bleeding time. The substance is labile, being destroyed by prolonged storage, contact with "non-wettable" surfaces, heating and clotting of blood (i.e., it is not present in serum). It is not known whether the active factor is dialyzable, because it is difficult to dialyze plasma or fractions and maintain the sterility required for I.V. infusion in humans. The relationship of the "bleeding time" factor to the "AHF stimulator" is obscure.

E. *Conversion of Prothrombin During Clotting:*

Prothrombin disappears so quickly from clotting normal blood that little or none can be found in the serum 60 minutes later. In 1939, Brinkhous[13] demonstrated that prothrombin persists in hemophilic blood after clotting has occurred, being converted to thrombin only very slowly. Delayed prothrombin conversion is recognized as a hallmark of hemophilia, and it is thought that one of the "activators" necessary for the conversion of prothrombin to thrombin is the antihemophilic factor, a factor which is also "consumed" in the clotting process[23]. If AHF is reduced in v.W.d., the rate of prothrombin consumption should be reduced. This was shown to be the case even before the AHF reduction was clearly demonstrated[35, 38, 57].

There is not complete agreement on the rate and extent of conversion of prothrombin in patients with v.W.d.[3, 7, 16, 35, 39, 67]. Experience with hemophilia A would lead to the expectation that any person with a low AHF level ($<$ 5%) would not convert prothrombin completely in one hour. Therefore, it is

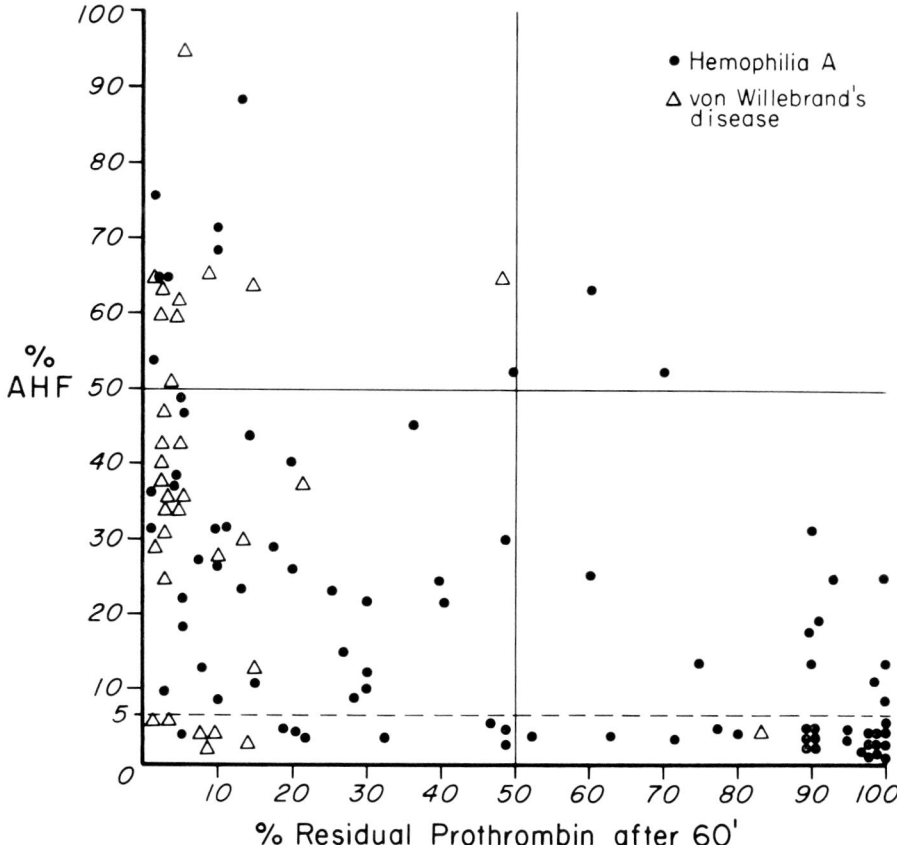

Fig. 1.—Assays for AHF and one-hour residual prothrombin values on 84 persons with hemophilia A and 33 with v.W.d. The AHF assays were performed by the method of Langdell et al.[37] and prothrombin consumption by the method of Graham et al.[24]

surprising that some observers have described complete prothrombin conversion in v.W.d. despite low AHF levels.

We have located in our patient files AHF assay and prothrombin utilization data on 84 hemophilia A patients and 33 patients with v.W.d. The determinations were made on the same diagnostic blood samples and had been collected one-by-one during the past 7 years. Figure 1 is a plot of plasma AHF level against the one hour residual prothrombin. The AHF assays were performed by the method of Langdell et al.[37] using hemophilia A plasma as test substrate, and the residual prothrombins were determined by the Iowa 2-stage method[75]. Inspection suggests that at any level of AHF more prothrombin is converted in v.W.d. than in hemophilia A. This difference is statistically significant for all AHF values less than 50%, but is most highly significant at very low AHF levels. A total of 40 persons had AHF levels of 5% or less. Seven had v.W.d. and 33 had hemophilia A. Six of seven with v.W.d. had residual prothrombin values less than 50%, while 25 of 33 with hemophilia A had residual prothrombin levels greater than 50%. In a 2 × 2 table, this is a statistically highly significant observation ($X^2 = 9.13$; p < .001).

Our results showing the more rapid consumption of prothrombin in v.W.d.

than hemophilia A are consistent with the clinical impression that patients with v.W.d. are less apt to bleed. The obvious conclusion is that the rate of prothrombin consumption is more nearly a reflection of hemostasis than is the corrective clotting effect on a hemophilia A substrate. It should be remembered that the v.W.d. plasma has been shown to be defective in three types of clotting tests, each operating at a different level in the clotting mechanism. The TGT is a reflection of early stages of clotting; prothrombin consumption is a reflection of early and intermediate phases of clotting; and the Langdell type of AHF assay is a summation of all stages of coagulation. The dissociation between hemophilia A and v.W.d. as regards prothrombin conversion and the Langdell type assay may imply some as yet unsuspected role of AHF in the last stages of clotting. The results seem to say that the AHF of v.W.d. is more effective in the early and intermediate phases of clotting than in the later phases. Whatever the meaning, there is something very interesting responsible for this discrepancy.

TRANSFUSIONS

Alexander and Goldstein reported in 1953[2] that the prolonged clotting time, but not the bleeding time, of their female patient was improved by "transfusions" without giving details. Schulman stated in 1955[63] that fresh-frozen plasma administered to one of his patients produced "striking improvement in the bleeding time, prothrombin consumption and thromboplastin generation". Van Creveld[69] demonstrated reduction of the clotting time after administering either lyophilized Fraction I or heparinzed plasma to one of his patients. Thus, the general response of v.W.d. patients to transfusions appeared similar to that of patients with hemophilia A.

In 1956 the Blombäcks[10] began testing an AHF-rich plasma fraction, prepared by using Cohn's Fraction I[17] as starting material. This fraction, designated I-O, contained 96% of the original fibrinogen and 100% of the AHF. Nilsson et al.[46] described a patient with v.W.d. with an AHF level of 5% and a bleeding time of more than an hour who was operated upon successfully after administration of the Blombäck's Fraction I-O. This was not unanticipated, but the effective duration of the transfusional effect was quite unexpected. Instead of a return to the pre-infusion level of AHF within 18–24 hours, as occurs in hemophilia A, the plasma AHF did not revert for five days. Also, the bleeding time which had been reduced to nearly normal values, remained normal for almost two days.

During the experimental period of preparing human fraction I-O, the Blombäcks had used bacterial filters. Filtration had removed most of the AHF activity but not the bleeding time factor[48]. They then prepared fraction I-O from patients with severe hemophilia A. The hemophilic fraction without measurable AHF activity, also brought the prolonged bleeding times of two patients with v.W.d. to normal. The astonishing thing was that the AHF levels of these patients also slowly and progressively increased. Fraction I-O prepared from the plasma of one v.W.d. patient and given to another failed to stimulate a rise in AHF, establishing that the AHF rise did not result from a by-product of the fractionation procedure. The authors concluded that the "von Willebrand factor" found in both normal and hemophilia A plasma and associated with the normalization of the bleeding time is also concerned either with the production or activation of AHF.

Since the original observation, the Swedish group has given fraction I-O to more than 30 patients with v.W.d. and many patients with hemophilia A. Most of the v.W.d. patients have responded like Nilsson's first patient, i.e., with an increase in plasma AHF which has been greater and maintained longer than in hemophilia A patients.

Reciprocal whole blood transfusions were made by Cornu[18] between a patient with hemophilia A and one with v.W.d. The v.W.d. patient responded with a rise in AHF which persisted for more than forty hours. The hemophilia A patient showed neither a rise in AHF nor improvement in other clotting tests.

Several investigators[8, 18, 41, 76] have demonstrated that patients with v.W.d. give an unexpected increase in AHF when transfused with plasma or plasma fractions prepared from hemophilia A. We have confirmed these results also by transfusion of fresh-frozen hemophilia A plasma[4]. In each of our patients the peak level of plasma AHF was reached at about 24 hours after transfusion. The broken curve (A) in Figure 2 is such a result. Here a rise from 8% before transfusion to 52% at 36 hours was achieved with hemophilia A plasma

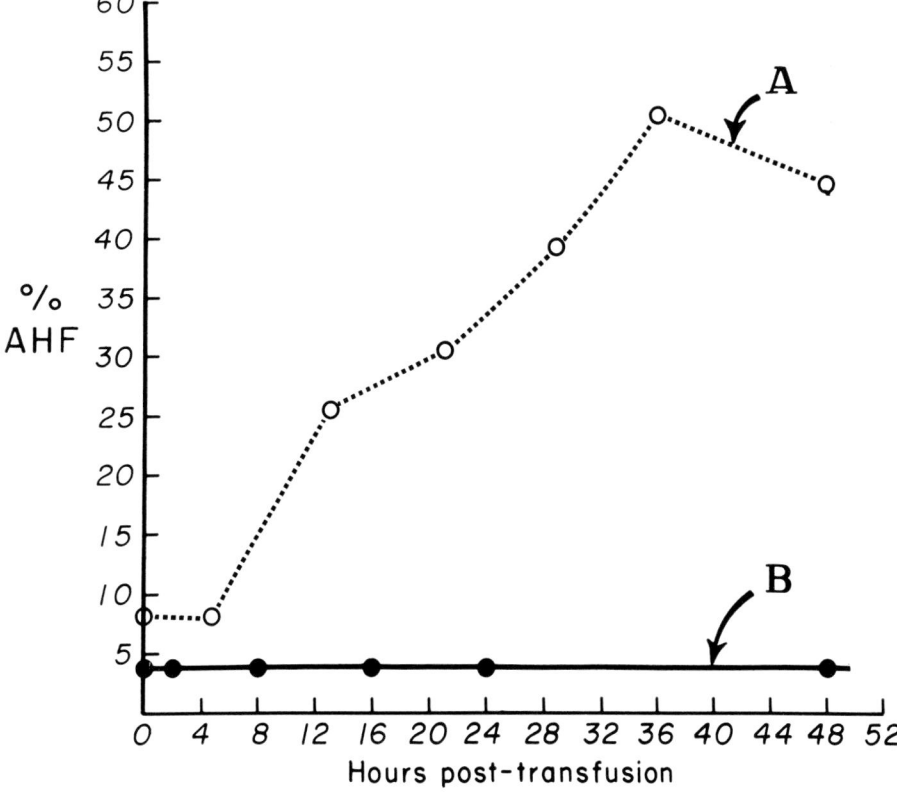

FIG. 2—Reciprocal compatible plasma transfusions between a person with v.W.d. and one with hemophilia A. Donations were obtained from each recipient *before* transfusion. Each was then transfused with the other's plasma. Curve A = v.W.d. recipient. Curve B = hemophilia A recipient.

TABLE 2

Recipient	AHF Circulating Before Transfusion ml%	AHF Transfused ml%	AHF Expected ml%	AHF Observed at Peak of Rise, ml%	"Newly Synthesized" AHF, ml%
J.F. (mild v.W.d.)	94,500 (2700 × 35%)	*2995 (599 × 5%)	97,495	213,840 (2970 × 72%)	116,345
P.C. (mild v.W.d.)	75,264 (2352 × 32%)	*2500 (500 × 5%)	77,764	169,680 (2424 × 70%)	91,916
C.Ch. (mod. v.W.d.)	20,416 (2552 × 8%)	*3425 (685 × 5%)	23,841	123,939 (2637 × 47%)	100,098
F.Mar. (mild v.W.d.)	86,163 (2611 × 33%)	**169,785 (539 × 315%)	255,948	395,500 (2825 × 140%)	139,552
J.H.M. (Severe Hem. A)	9490 (1898 × 5%)	***16,422 (714 × 23%)	25,912	10,145 (2029 × 5%)	−15,767
J.D. (mod. Hem. A)	10,055 (2011 × 5%)	***24,000 (600 × 40%)	34,055	38,800 (2160 × 18%)	4745

Plasma transfused:

     * = Hemophilia A.

    ** = Normal.

   *** = v.W.d.

Expected and observed AHF in persons with v.W.d. and Hemophilia A. The value for "new synthesis" is conservative; neither destruction nor diffusion into other compartments has been taken into account in calculating "expected AHF".

assaying at less than 5%. The solid line marked B shows that when the hemophilia A donor was transfused with plasma from the v.W.d. recipient there was no alteration in his plasma AHF. This non-reciprocity with transfusion must be highly significant.

It has been possible to estimate approximately the amount of "newly synthesized" AHF produced in experiments like those of Figure 2. This is done by calculating the total amount of plasma AHF circulating before transfusion, adding the amount of AHF passively transfused, and subtracting the sum from the total amount of plasma AHF circulating at the peak of the rise. The data required for the calculation are the appropriate AHF levels and the volumes of distribution. Several such calculations are shown in Table 2. The total amount of AHF is expressed as ml%, the product of the AHF level by the plasma volume in ml. The first three lines are the results on 3 patients with v.W.d. given approximately the same amounts of hemophilia A plasma. "New synthesis" was between 91,000 and 116,000 ml% in each instance. The fourth line contains results when a v.W.d. patient received normal plasma containing much preformed AHF. "New synthesis" is seen to total 139,000 ml% when appropriate arithmetic is carried out. Thus, "new synthesis" was approximately equal whether the transfused material came from hemophilia A or normal donors. The last two lines show that "new synthesis" essentially does not occur when hemophilia A patients receive plasma from patients with v.W.d. These data aruge that the "AHF stimulator" is present in normal and hemophilia A plasmas in equal amounts.

An interesting question is whether the AHF newly synthesized in v.W.d. is structurally normal. We have tried to determine this by examining the AHF of 4 persons with v.W.d. after transfusion[4]. Our tests of pH and heat stability, and activity in the thromboplastin generation test did not distinguish between the AHF of normal plasmas and post-transfusional v.W.d. plasmas.

The nature of the substance responsible for stimulating AHF production in patients with v.W.d. is an enigma. The original experiments suggested that the "von Willebrand's factor" served this function. Many observers, however, have noted the AHF stimulation without bleeding time correction. Biggs and Matthews[8] have recently found that tricalcium phosphate-adsorbed serum from normal persons strongly stimulates AHF production when given to a person with v.W.d. Thus, the "stimulator" is not consumed during clotting of blood nor associated with any of the presently-known coagulation factors. Biggs and Matthews obtained important negative results when they infused large quantities of human albumin and gamma globulin into persons with v.W.d. without stimulating AHF production. We have suggested several possible theoretical models to explain the AHF stimulatory effects in v.W.d.[27, 28, 44]. It is not an exaggeration to say that speculation has greatly outstripped the acquiring of hard evidence bearing on these matters.

GENETIC ASPECTS

A. *Formal Genetics*

The evidence that v.W.d. is an hereditary disturbance of hemostasis was reviewed by Graham in 1959[26]. He suggested in the body of his paper that double heterozygosity at two abnormal genetic loci might be responsible for the complex features of v.W.d., then pointed out in an addendum why this was unlikely. Evidence at hand at that time indicated that the gene which mutates to produce v.W.d. must be located on a chromosome other than the X. The critical evidence consisted of several clear examples of father-to-son transmission in matings where the mother was very probably genotypically normal. A location on the y chromosome was similarly excluded by numerous examples of mother-daughter transmission. The autosomal chromosome bearing the v.W.d. locus is as yet unidentified. The trait has not yet been linked to another autosomal trait nor has a chromosomal aberration been described in association with a v.W.d. kindred which might lead to the localization of the gene by cytogenetic analysis.

A dominant hereditary trait may be regarded as one manifested in heterozygotes. Most persons affected with v.W.d. appear to be heterozygous because their parents appear to constitute an affected-by-normal mating. Assays have shown that some persons, presumably heterozygous, have levels of AHF as low as 1–10% of normal (see Fig. 2). On *a priori* grounds, the level of a plasma protein, if it is the primary product of m-RNA, would be expected to be reduced to approximately 50% of normal in heterozygotes; this seems to be

TABLE 3

	Progeny								Total
	Males				Females				
	Affected	Normal	Unk.	T	Affected	Normal	Unk.	T.	
Including Probands	21	20	3	44	34	22	7	63	107
Excluding Probands	18	20	3	41	26	22	7	55	96

Distribution of progeny from 21 affected by normal matings for v.W.d.[47, 56, 71].

true for most of the clotting factors. The fact that some heterozygotes for v.W.d. may have levels in the 1-10% range makes this a genetically unique disorder. Until an indubitable homozygote for v.W.d. is described, the v.W.d. trait must be considered formally to be a "conditional dominant".

The mutant gene is expressed in both males and females to about the same extent. A possible excess of affected females reported in the literature very likely results from under-reporting of affected males, a bias probably growing out of less critical examination of males on the assumption that "hemophilic males" have the X-linked disorder.

Table 3 shows the distribution of children produced from 21 matings of affected parents with normal parents in 12 families as recorded by three authors[47, 56, 71]. The sex ratios are approximately equal as are the numbers of affected and normal progeny of both sexes. It must be emphasized that these ratios were obtained by scoring persons as "abnormal" on the basis of either prolonged bleeding time or reduced AHF level.

A very interesting aspect of this dominant trait is its pleiotropy, the presence of both reduced AHF and prolonged bleeding time. Many observers have recorded the fact that these abnormal laboratory tests may be observed together or separately at different times in the same person or in different members of the same family. As pointed out above, the clear results of Table 3 are produced only by taking pleiotropy into account and scoring the children as genotypically abnormal when showing either abnormality. Pitney and Arnold[56] have documented that each abnormality, particularly the prolonged bleeding time, may fluctuate widely within a single individual.

Figure 3 is a kindred studied in our laboratory which illustrates the variability of expression of the gene and the difficulties of family studies in v.W.d. The proband is the v.W.d. patient of Figure 2 and C. Ch. of Table 2. She is quite clearly abnormal both for bleeding time and AHF level, and shows the paradoxical transfusion response. If her relatives are scored for bleeding time and AHF level as indicated in Figure 3, only two other persons (II-5 and III-30) are doubly abnormal. Five others show only reduced AHF level while 6 others show only prolonged bleeding time, many being barely abnormal by the standards indicated. Most of her affected relatives are in the maternal line, on her grandfather's side, and consanguinity could not be established. It is assumed that she received a single mutant gene for v.W.d. from her mother via the grandfather. Her father was not available for testing, but II-9, the grandmother who should have been normal, scored mildly abnormal for bleeding

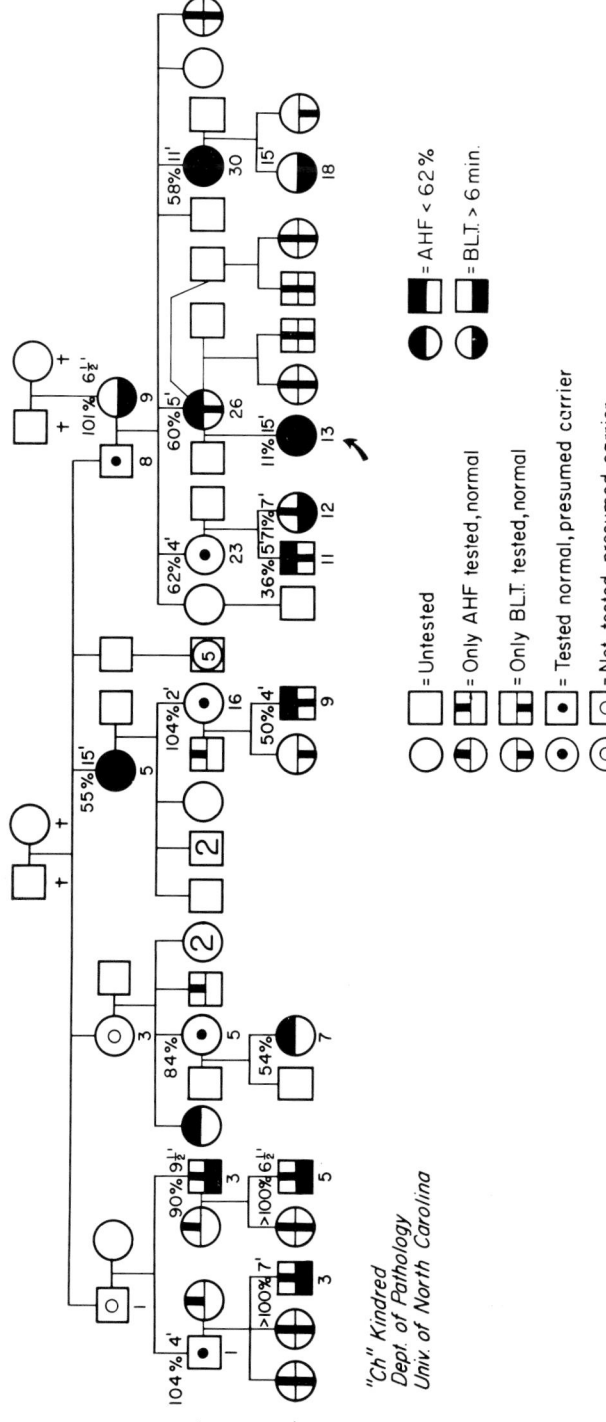

FIG. 3.—A kindred in which the v.W.d. gene is segregating. The choice of AHF level less than 62% and bleeding time greater than 6½ minutes as the discriminators is explained in reference 26.

time. This kindred is fairly typical. We believe that each member, normal on first study, should be re-studied several times before the conclusion is reached that he is in fact normal. In one instance in another kindred, nine bleeding times were normal and only the tenth proved to be prolonged and established the fact that a "female hemophiliac" was in fact suffering from v.W.d.

If it is assumed that all persons scored as "affected" in this kindred are heterozygous for the v.W.d. allele, the variable expressivity of the gene is very apparent. AHF levels among those assumed to be heterozygous range from 15% to 60%, and bleeding times from 6½ min. to more than 15 min. Only 3 of the 8 with low AHF levels have prolonged bleeding times. Only 3 of the 9 with prolonged bleeding times have reduced AHF levels.

Genetic carriers of the v.W.d. trait may be symptomatic or asymptomatic. In the kindred above, as is usually the case, the proband is the most severely affected person. It is clear, however, from this and other kindred that the mutant gene is being carried by many persons who are completely asymptomatic.

Penetrance, the statistical yardstick relating expected numbers of abnormal phenotypes to observed numbers, is usually difficult to gauge with a highly variable trait such as v.W.d. It is somewhat surprising, therefore, that the data in Table 3 suggest no excess of normal children in affected-by-normal matings. This outcome is undoubtedly related to our decision to accept *either* prolonged bleeding time or reduced AHF level as evidence of expression of the gene. Furthermore, some evidence of an abnormal genome can usually be found if the search is sufficiently intensive or if the observations are repeated frequently. Unfortunately, the kindred were not studied for many generations in great depth, hence clear evidence of "skipping" was not expected to be encountered.

The frequency of the v.W.d. allele has not yet been determined in any population. Because of the variable expression, it is a poor gene to use for such studies. Nevertheless, the fact that its effects are mild but expressed in heterozygotes suggests that it may be present in fairly high frequency and may account for a significant proportion of the otherwise unexplained "bleeders" encountered by physicians. The gene is widely distributed in humans. The disease was originally described in Scandinavians[45, 72] and has usually been studied in a population of Western European origin. It has been described in America in both Caucasians and Negroes, in Australia[56], South America[54], and Japan[77]. This last observation is particularly important because the gene in American Negroes may have been introduced by West Europeans. The presence in Japanese undoubtedly represents separate mutation.

B. *Implications of Genetics for Ideas About AHF Biosynthesis*

One of the interesting recent outgrowths of the study of v.W.d. has been the impact which it has had upon ideas of AHF biosynthesis. It was pointed out several years ago[26] that the existence of autosomal v.W.d. and x-linked hemophilia A imply that plasma AHF level is controlled in normal persons by two clearly separable genes. This is not an unprecedented situation for a mammalian protein (which AHF is thought to be) because human hemoglobin[66] and rabbit lactic dehydrogenase[64] are both clearly under dual genetic control. The mode of operation of the dual control raises interesting questions about the synthesis of AHF. The dominance of the v.W.d. mutant and the recessiveness of the hemophilia A mutant plus the non-reciprocal transfusion between the mutant phenotypes suggested to McLester and Graham[27, 28, 44] that the v.W.d. locus might be occupied by a regulatory gene and the hemophilia A locus by a structural gene. A consequence of this idea is that the AHF produced in v.W.d. after transfusion of hemophilia A plasma will be structurally normal. If the AHF produced in v.W.d. proved to be structurally *abnormal*, it *might* be distinguishable from wild-type AHF, which would exclude the hypothesis. In recent experiments, Barrow et al. examined the newly synthesized AHF in v.W.d. persons[4, 28] and were unable to distinguish this AHF from the normal type. This does not *prove* that the hypothesis about the nature of the v.W.d. locus is correct; the results are merely consistent with the hypothesis. The authors emphasize that although this regulatory model suggests that v.W.d. *homozygotes* should be more severely affected than *heterozygotes*, the transfusion of hemophilia A plasma should stimulate AHF synthesis equally well in the two abnormal v.W.d. genotypes. Location of a v.W.d. homozygote followed by transfusion studies should provide a critical test of the regulatory hypothesis. The absence of evidence that the Jacob and Monod type of regulation operates in humans makes us suspect that the regulatory model will not be sustained.

Graham et al.[28] have proposed that a combining subunit model of AHF biosynthesis is a leading possibility because of the analogies with hemoglobin and lactic dehydrogenase and the evidence of Thelin and Wagner[68] that AHF is a polymer. Owen[53] has recently suggested that double exponential decay of AHF activity in stored plasma suggests that two types of AHF exist in plasma. If Owen's results are confirmed, AHF may prove to be a polymer whose chains disintegrate at different rates, one chain coded at the v.W.d. and the other at the hemophilia A locus. It is possible that the AHF level-prothrombin consumption dissociation is related in some way to separate structural mutations. The ultimate test would be amino acid sequencing of the AHF from normal and v.W.d. persons. This approach has handicaps.

One of the serious problems in studying the synthesis of AHF is lack of knowledge of the cell in which it is synthesized. The evidence summarized by Graham[25] suggested synthesis in a cell type not localized to a single organ and certainly not the liver parenchymal cell, lymphocyte, or spleen. This excludes many possible and obvious experimental approaches. A possible attack would be study of the *in vitro* conditions which might result in "complementation" between v.W.d. and hemophilia A plasmas. Another approach would be an immunologic study of the nature of the products in v.W.d., hemophilia A and normal persons.

In all the recent speculation it has generally been overlooked that the ultimate genetic hypothesis for v.W.d. must also account for the "von Willebrand factor". It seems very clear that the presence of a single mutant gene at the v.W.d. locus affects both aspects of hemostasis while mutation of the X-located gene does not. It is still not apparent whether the two products which characterize v.W.d. are produced in sequence or in parallel and whether one affects the synthesis of the other. Thus, continued study of the molecular biological aspects of v.W.d. promises to provide a number of important insights into several aspects of hemostasis.

SUMMARY

Von Willebrand's disease (v.W.d.) is an hereditary hemorrhagic diathesis characterized by prolonged bleeding time and reduction in plasma antihemophilic factor (AHF, Factor VIII). Both males and females are equally affected and it is inherited as an autosomal dominant trait with highly variable expression within and between affected persons and kindred. The gene is widely distributed in the human race although its frequency is unknown.

Professor Erik von Willebrand first described this disorder in 1926. He observed it in several kindred living on the islands of Åland in the Gulf of Bothnia off the coast of Finland where it is present in high frequency. Since the original publication, more than 200 well-documented cases have been described. For 30 years the bleeding disorder was attributed to a platelet dysfunction, a vascular defect, or a combination of these. The evidence supporting platelet or vascular wall defects leaves something to be desired. In 1953, it was recognized that those affected not only had prolonged bleeding times but also deficiency of a plasma factor, apparently the same one abnormal in classical X-linked hemophilia A. This is the factor usually designated antihemophilic factor (AHF, Factor VIII), and one which is believed to be a protein circulating in plasma as a polymer.

Clinically, v.W.d. differs from hemophilia A in several respects. Bleeding into the joints rarely occurs and internal bleeding is unusual. The major sites of bleeding are the surface areas of the body. In women, menorrhagia is the most common complaint. The severity of the bleeding tendency appears to diminish with age.

Patients with v.W.d. respond differently to transfusions of normal blood or plasma than patients with hemophilia A. In the classic hemophiliac, the rise in circulating AHF can be anticipated accurately by assaying the plasma to be transfused; also AHF disappears from the circulation in 24 hours or less in hemophilia A. In v.W.d., there is a slow and progressive increase in circulating AHF which sometimes reaches a peak in 48 hours and persists for 72 hours or more.

Paradoxically, the v.W.d. patient shows the same rise in AHF after transfusion of substances lacking measurable AHF. Whole blood, plasma, or plasma fractions prepared from persons with hemophilia A result in "new synthesis" of AHF when transfused into v.W.d. patients. The amount of "newly synthesized AHF" is approximately the same whether the donor is normal or has hemophilia A. Transfusions of v.W.d. plasma into persons with hemophilia A do not result in "new synthesis". Serum, after adsorption with tricalcium phosphate, stimulates AHF production, indicating that the "AHF-synthesizing-stimulating substance" is not associated with any of the known clotting factors, all of which are either destroyed during clotting or are adsorbable. Also, AHF-stimulation may occur without shortening of the bleeding time.

Correction of the prolonged bleeding time in v.W.d. patients is more difficult to achieve and maintain than increase in plasma AHF. It is, however, fairly well established that normalization of the bleeding time depends upon a non-cellular plasma factor.

Thus, a disease clearly observed first on islands near Finland, where it is present in relatively high frequency, has proved to be hereditary, widespread, and of very considerable clinical interest. Its greatest significance may prove to be the challenge it poses to blood clotting theory.

REFERENCES

1. Achenbach, W.: Angiohemophilia. *In* Brinkhous, K. M. (Ed.): Hemophilia and Other Hemorrhagic States. Chapel Hill, The University of North Carolina Press, 1959.
2. Alexander, B., and Goldstein, R.: Dual hemostatic defect in pseudohemophilia. J. Clin. Invest. 32: 551, 1953.
3. Andre, A.: Contribution a l'etude de la thrombasthenie. Le Sang. 23: 54–60, 1952.
4. Barrow, E. M., Roberts, H. R., Pons, K., and Graham, J. B.: Studies of the antihemophilic factor (AHF, Factor VIII) produced in von Willebrand's disease. Proc. Soc. Exp. Biol. Med. 115: 760–763, 1964.
5. Bigelow, F. S.: Serotonin activity in blood. Measurements in normal subjects and in patients with thrombocythemia hemorrhagica and other hemorrhagic states. J. Lab. Clin. Med. 43: 759–773, 1954.
6. Biggs, R., and Douglas, A. S.: The thromboplastin generation test. J. Clin. Path. 6: 23–29, 1953.
7. Biggs, R., and Macfarlane, R. G.: Human Blood Coagulation and its Disorders. Philadelphia, F. A. Davis, 3rd edition, 1962.
8. Biggs, R., and Matthews, J. M.: The treatment of haemorrhage in von Willebrand's disease and the blood level of factor VIII (AHG). Brit. J. Haemat. 9: 203–214, 1963.
9. Blackburn, E. K.: Primary capillary hemorrhage (including von Willebrand's disease). Brit. J. Haemat. 7: 239–249, 1961.
10. Blombäck, B. and Blombäck, M.: Purification of human and bovine fibrinogen. Ark. Kemi 10: 415–443, 1956.
11. Blombäck, M. and Blombäck, B.: Response to fractions in von Willebrand's disease. *In* Brinkhous, K. M. (Ed.): The Hemophilias, Third International Symposium. Chapel Hill, The University of North Carolina Press, In press.
12. Borchgrevink, C. F.: Platelet adhesion *in vivo* in patients with bleeding disorders. Acta Med. Scand. 170: 231–243, 1961.
13. Brinkhous, K. M.: A study of the clotting time in hemophilia: the delayed formation of thrombin. Amer. J. Med. Sci. 198: 509–516, 1939.
14. Buchanan, J. C. and Leavell, B. S.: Pseudohemophilia: Report of 13 new cases and statistical review of previously reported cases. Ann. Intern. Med. 44: 241–256, 1956.
15. Caen, J., and Cousin, C.: Le trouble d'adhesivite "in vivo" des plaquettes dans la maladie de Willebrand et les thrombasthenies de Glanzmann. Nouv. Rev. Franc. Hemat. 2: 685–694, 1962.
16. Cazal, P., and Izarn, P.: Consideration sur la pseudohemophilie de Willebrand, a propos de deux nouveaux cas. Acta Haemat. 4: 357–362, 1950.
17. Cohn, E. J., Strong, L. E., Hughes, W. L., Jr., Mulford, D. J., Ashworth, J. N., Melin, M., and Taylor, H. L.: Preparation and properties of serum and plasma proteins. IV. A system for the separation into fractions of proteins and lipoprotein components of biological tissues and fluids. J. Am. Chem. Soc. 68: 459–475, 1946.
18. Cornu, P., Larrieu, M. J., Caen, J., and Bernard, J.: Maladie de Willebrand: etude clinique, genetique et biologique. Nouv. Rev. Franc. Hemat. 1: 231–262, 1961.
19. Cornu, P., Larrieu, M. J., Caen, J., and Bernard, J.: Transfusion studies in von Willebrand's disease: effect on bleeding time and factor VIII. Brit. J. Haemat. 9: 189–202, 1963.
20. Duke, W. W.: Relation of blood platelets to hemorrhagic disease: description of method for determining bleeding time and coagulation time and report of three cases of hemorrhagic disease relieved by transfusion. J.A.M.A. 55: 1185–1192, 1910.
21. Estren, S., Sanchez-Medal, L., and Dameshek, W.: Pseudohemophilia. Blood. 1: 504–533, 1946.
22. Fantl, P., and Sawers, R. J.: Stimulation of factor VIII (antihemophilic) activity by transfused serum. Nature. 200: 1214–1215, 1963.
23. Graham, J. B., Penick, G. D., and Brinkhous, K. M.: Utilization of the antihemophilic factor during clotting of canine blood and plasma. Am. J. Physiol. 164: 710–715, 1951.
24. Graham, J. B., Langdell, R. D., and Brinkhous, K. M.: Estimation of the rate of prothrombin utilization. *In* Tocantins, L. M. (Ed.): The Coagulation of Blood: Methods of Study. New York, Grune & Stratton, 1955.

25. Graham, J. B.: Biochemical genetics of blood coagulation. Am. J. Human Genet. 8: 63–79, 1956.
26. Graham, J. B.: The inheritance of "vascular hemophilia", a new and interesting problem in human genetics. J. Med. Ed. 34: 385–396, 1959.
27. Graham, J. B.: Biochemical genetic speculations provoked by considering the enigma of von Willebrand's disease. Thromb. Diath. Haemorrh. 9, Suppl. 2: 119–125, 1963.
28. Graham, J. B., McLester, W. D., Pons, K., Roberts, H. R., and Barrow, E. M.: Genetics of vascular hemophilia and biosynthesis of the plasma antihemophilic factor (AHF, Factor VIII). In Brinkhous, K. M. (Ed.): The Hemophilias, Third International Symposium. Chapel Hill, The University of North Carolina Press, In press.
29. Hecht, E. R., Cho, M. H., and Seegers, W. H.: Thromboplastin: nomenclature and preparation of protein-free material different from platelet factor 3 or lipid activator. Am. J. Physiol. 193: 584–592, 1958.
30. Imerslund, O.: Familial haemorrhagic diatheses with prolonged bleeding time (thrombopathias). Acta Paediat. 34: 315–333, 1947.
31. Ingram, G. I. C.: Observations in a case of multiple haemostatic defect. Brit. J. Haemat. 2: 180–193, 1956.
32. Ivy, A. C., Shapiro, P. F., and Melnick, P.: The bleeding tendency in jaundice. Surg. Gynec. Obst. 60: 781–784, 1935.
33. Jamra, M. M., Lichtenstein, R., Vieira, C. B., and Ribiero Leite, M. O.: Capilaropatia constitutional: forma de von Willebrand e forma capilar simples. Rev. Hosp. Clin. 7: 12–32, 1952.
34. Johnson, S. A., Monto, R. W., and Rebuck, J. W.: The nature of the coagulation defect in pseudohemophilia B. Clin. Res. Proc. 5: 291, 1957.
35. Jürgens, R., and Ferlin, A.: Uber den sog. prothrombin-konsumptionstest bei hämophilie (hämophilie, konduktorinnen) und bei konstitutioneller thrombopathie (v. Willebrand-Jürgens). Schweiz. Med. Wschr. 80: 1098–1101, 1950.
36. Jürgens, R., Lehmann, W., Wegelius, O., Eriksson, A. W., and Hiepler, E.: Mitteilung über den mangel an antihämophilem globulin (factor VIII) bei der Åaländischen thrombopathie (v. Willebrand-Jürgens). Thromb. Diath. Haemorrh. 1: 257–260, 1957.
37. Langdell, R. D., Wagner, R. H., and Brinkhous, K. M.: Effect of antihemophilic factor on one-stage clotting tests. J. Lab. Clin. Med. 41: 637–647, 1953.
38. Larrieu, M. J., and Soulier, J. P.: Deficit en facteur antihemophilique A chez une fille associe a un trouble du saignement. Rev. Hemat. 8: 361–370, 1953.
39. Lelong, M., et Soulier, J. P.: Sur une maladie hemorrhagique constitutionelle caracterisee par l'allongement isole du temps de saignement. Rev. Hemat. 5: 13–23, 1950.
40. Levy, L., II: Non-hemophilic hereditary hemorrhagic diathesis: report of family of bleeders. Ann. Intern. Med. 27: 96–102, 1947.
41. Lewis, J. H.: Synthesis of AHF in von Willebrand's disease. Blood. 23: 233–238, 1964.
42. Macfarlane, R. G.: Critical review: the mechanism of hemostasis. Quart. J. Med. 10: 1–29, 1941.
43. Macfarlane, J. C. W., and Simpkiss, M. J.: The investigation of a large family affected with von Willebrand's disease. Arch. Dis. Child. 29: 483–497, 1954.
44. McLester, W. D., and Graham, J. B.: Synthesis of plasma antihemophilic factor. Nature. 197: 708, 1963.
45. Nevanlinna, H. R., Ikkala, E., and Vuopio, P.: von Willebrand's disease. Acta Haemat. 27: 65–77, 1962.
46. Nilsson, I. M., Blombäck, B., Blombäck, M., and Svennerud, S.: Kvinnlig hämofili och dess behandling med humant antihämofiliglobulin. Nord. Med. 56: 1654–1656, 1956.
47. Nilsson, I. M., Blombäck, M., and von Francken, I.: On an inherited autosomal hemorrhagic diathesis with antihemophilic globulin (AHG) deficiency and prolonged bleeding time. Acta Med. Scand. 159: 37–57, 1957.
48. Nilsson, I. M., Blombäck, M., Jorpes, E., Blombäck, B., and Johansson, S. A.: von Willebrand's disease and its correction with human plasma fraction I-O. Acta Med. Scand. 159: 179–188, 1957.
49. Nilsson, I. M., Blombäck, M., and von Francken, I.: In an inherited autosomal hemorrhagic diathesis with antihemophilic globulin deficiency and prolonged bleeding time. In VI Congr. Soc. Europ. Hematol., Copenhagen, Communication 177: 629–636, 1957.
50. Nilsson, I. M., and Blombäck, M.: The pathogenesis and treatment of von Willebrand's disease. In Brinkhous, K. M. (Ed.): Hemophilia and Other Hemorrhagic States. Chapel Hill, The University of North Carolina Press, 1959.
51. Nilsson, I. M., and Blombäck, M.: von Willebrand's disease in Sweden—occurrence, pathogenesis and treatment. Thromb. Diath. Haemorrh. 9, Suppl. 2: 103–118, 1963.
52. O'Brien, J. R.: Familial capillary fragility (diffuse capillary telangiectasia). In Moore, C. V. (Ed.): Proceedings of the Third International Congress of the International Society of Hematology. New York, Grune & Stratton, 1951.
53. Owen, C. A.: Discussion on von Willebrand's disease. In Brinkhous, K. M. (Ed.): The Hemophilias, Third International Symposium. Chapel Hill, The University of North Carolina Press, In press.
54. Pavlovsky, A.: Behavior of several therapeutical measures in the treatment of von Willebrand's disease. Thromb. Diath. Haemorrh. 9: 143–145, 1963.

55. Perkins, W.: Pseudohemophilia. Blood. 1: 497–503, 1946.
56. Pitney, W. R., and Arnold, B. J.: Laboratory findings in families of patients suffering with von Willebrand's disease. Brit. J. Haemat. 6: 81–87, 1960.
57. Quick, A. J., and Hussey, C. V.: Hemophilic condition in the female. J. Lab. Clin. Med. 42: 929–930, 1953.
58. Quick, A. J.: Hemorrhagic Diseases. Philadelphia, Lea & Febiger, 1957.
59. Rapport, M. M., Green, A. A., and Page, I. H.: Crystalline serotonin. Science. 108: 329–330, 1948.
60. Reid, G.: A preliminary note on the relationship of the blood platelets to the mechanism of haemostasis. Med. J. Australia. 2: 244, 1943.
61. Revol, L., Favre-Gilly, L., and Ollagnier, Ch.: La maladie de Willebrand (thrombopathie constitutionnelle ou pseudo-hemophilie). Rev. Hemat. 5: 24–39, 1950.
62. Roskam, J.: Arrest of Bleeding. Springfield, Illinois, Charles C. Thomas, 1954.
63. Schulman, I., Smith, C. H., Erlandson, M., and Fort, E.: A familial hemorrhagic disease in males and females characterized by combined antihemophilic globulin deficiency and vascular abnormality. Amer. J. Dis. Child. 90: 526, 1955.
64. Shaw, C. R., and Barto, E.: Genetic evidence for the subunit structure of lactate dehydrogenase isozymes. Proc. Nat. Acad. Sci (U.S.). 50: 211, 1963.
65. Singer, K., and Ramot, B.: Pseudohemophilia type B. Hereditary hemorrhagic diathesis characterized by prolonged bleeding time and decrease in antihemophilic factor. Arch. Intern. Med. 97: 715–725, 1956.
66. Smith, E. W., and Torbert, J. V.: Study of two abnormal hemoglobins with evidence for a new genetic locus for hemoglobin formation. Bull. J. Hopkins Hosp. 102: 38–45, 1958.
67. Soulier, J. P., and Larrieu, M. J.: Syndrome de Willebrand-Jürgens et thrombopathies. Etude de 65 cas. Essai de classification. Rev. Hemat. 9: 77–122, 1954.
68. Thelin, G. M., and Wagner, R. H.: Sedimentation of plasma antihemophilic factor. Arch. Biochem. Biophysics. 95: 70–76, 1961.
69. van Creveld, S., Jordan, F. L. J., Punt, K., and Veder, H. A.: Deficiency of antihemophilic factor in a woman combined with a disturbance in vascular function. Acta Med Scand. 151: 382–389, 1955.
70. van Creveld, S., Kloosterman, G. J., Mochtar, I. A., and Koppe, J. G.: Interchange between blood of mother and fetus in vascular hemophilia. Biol. Neonat. 4: 379–382, 1962.
71. Verstraete, M.: The hereditary pattern in angiohemophilia. Thromb. Diath. Haemorrh. 9: 133–140, 1963.
72. von Willebrand, E. A.: Hereditär pseudohämofili. Finsk. Lakaresallsk. Handl. 68: 87–112, 1926.
73. von Willebrand, E. A.: Uber hereditäre pseudo-hämophilie. Acta Med. Scand. 76: 521–550, 1931.
74. von Willebrand, E. A., and Jürgens, R.: Uber ein neues vererbbares blutungsübel: die konstitutionelle thrombopathie. Deutsch. Arch. Klin. Med. 175: 453–483, 1933.
75. Warner, E. D., Brinkhous, K. M., and Smith, H. P.: Titration of prothrombin in certain plasmas. Arch. Pathol. 18: 587, 1934.
76. Weiss, H. J.: The use of Cohn fraction I from diverse sources in the therapy of von Willebrand's disease. Vox Sang. 7: 97–99, 1962.
77. Yoshida, K.: Coagulation difficulties in babies with haemophilia and similar hemorrhagic diseases. Abstract No. 1762, Abst. Jap. Med. 2: 590–591, 1962.
78. Zucker, M. B., and Borrelli, J.: Concentration of serotonin in thrombocytopathia, pseudohemophilia and thrombocytosis. Amer. J. Clin. Path. 26: 13–20, 1956.

Platelet and Leukocyte Isoantigens and Their Antibodies: Serologic, Physiologic and Clinical Studies

N. RAPHAEL SHULMAN, VICTOR J. MARDER,
————————MERILYN C. HILLER and————————
ELLEN M. COLLIER

INTRODUCTION

Early Work

DURING the period 1953 to 1959, much evidence was accumulated to indicate that fetal cells entering the maternal circulation or transfused blood can stimulate antibodies against platelet and leukocyte isoantigens. The existence of platelet isoantigens unrelated to erythrocyte isoantigens was suggested in 1953 by Harrington et al.[1] and by Stefanini et al.[2] on the basis of finding platelet agglutinins in the serum of normal mothers whose infants had neonatal purpura and in the serum of repeatedly transfused patients in whom survival of homologous platelets was shortened. Several years later, Payne[3, 4] and van Loghem et al.[5] showed a correlation between frequency of blood transfusion and development of leukocyte agglutinins, and Brittingham and Chaplin[6] documented the induction of leukoagglutinins by transfusion and showed their causative relationship to febrile transfusion reactions. In 1958, Payne and Rolfs,[7] and in 1959, van Rood et al.[8] detected leukoagglutinins in the sera of approximately 10 per cent of multiparous women who had never received transfusions. The leukocyte and platelet agglutination tests that were used in the work from 1953 to 1959, although adequate for delineating some of the clinical causes and effects of isoimmunization, were insufficiently sensitive and reproducible to define group specificity of isoantigens with the usual isoantibodies that were detected. However, Moulinier[9] in 1957, using an exceptional antibody from a mother whose infant had neonatal purpura, was able to obtain positive anti-globulin consumption tests with 22 per cent of 82 platelet suspensions and named the reactive antigen, DUZO[a]. Dausset[10] in 1958, on the basis of finding that seven different antisera from transfused individuals gave a similar pattern of agglutination with 20 leukocyte suspensions, named the antigen that appeared to be present on 12 of the leukocytes, MAC.

A number of investigators in the period 1954 to 1959 concluded that platelets and leukocytes possess many of the antigens present on erythrocytes, e.g., A, B,[11, 12, 13, 14, 15] C, D, E,[15, 16, 17] M, N, Tj[a],[14, 15] and others,[14, 15] but there were some reports to the contrary, e.g., C, D, E.[14, 18] More recent reports strongly suggest that the presence of contaminating erythrocyte stroma,[19, 20, 21] or soluble

From the Clinical Hematology Branch, National Institute of Arthritis & Metabolic Diseases, National Institutes of Health, Bethesda, Maryland.

A or B substances adsorbed on platelets[22] may have caused false-positive reactions with the agglutination and adsorption technics that were used. The work by Bakemeier and Swisher,[21] in particular, points out the difficulties of interpreting leukoagglutination by serologic methods that might result in nonspecific "mixed agglutination" of leukocytes with intact or lysed erythrocytes. In view of conflicting reports and the fact that technics used were susceptible to false-positive reactions, it seems likely that erythrocyte isoantigens either are not present on leukocytes and platelets or are present in relatively insignificant amounts.

Monographs by Walford[23] and by Killmann[24] comprehensively review the literature up to 1959 on leukocyte isoantibodies and technics used to study them; and an article by van de Wiel et al.[25] in 1961 reviews the serology of platelet isoantibodies.

Recent Work

In the past few years, several investigators have taken advantage of the simplified agglutination technic of Dausset and Malinvaud[26] to identify platelet isoantigens with strong platelet agglutinins that occasionally arise after transfusion. The technic is insensitive, but gives unequivocally reproducible results with the rare agglutinins that are discovered by screening hundreds of sera from transfused individuals. With this technic, van Loghem et al.[27] and van der Weerdt et al.[28] found two antibodies that recognized allelic antigens they called Zw[a] and Zw[b]; and van der Weerdt et al.,[29] and Dausset and Berg,[30] using the same technic, found an agglutinin against a third platelet antigen that was named Ko. Van Rood and van Leeuwen,[31] in a formidable undertaking with a leukoagglutination procedure that was subject to several technical snares, selected from 66 reactive maternal sera those that appeared to recognize allelic antigens by statistical analysis with a computer and designated the alleles, 4[a] and 4[b].

We have used mainly complement (C′) fixation technics in defining platelet and leukocyte isoantigens for a number of reasons. The usual isoantibodies encountered clinically could be measured more sensitively, reliably and conveniently by C′ fixation than by agglutination procedures. Cell suspensions could be stored for months or obtained by mail, and still give reproducible results, and incomplete antibodies undetectable by other methods could be measured.

Using C′ fixation technics with sera from two patients who had developed thrombocytopenia after blood transfusion, we identified a platelet isoantigen that was called Pl[A1].[32] Anti-Pl[A1] proved to be identical with anti-Zw[a] of van Loghem when serum samples were exchanged between laboratories. With antibodies from mothers whose infants had neonatal purpura and with sera from transfused patients, we subsequently identified the antigens PlGrLy[B1] [33, 34, 35] and PlGrLy[C1] [34, 35] which are shared by platelets, granulocytes and lymphocytes, the antigen Ly[D1] [34] that is present only on lymphocytes; and recently the allelic platelet antigens, Pl[E1] and Pl[E2].

Well defined isoantibodies against antigens present on platelets or leukocytes have been uniquely suited for studying the pathophysiology of immune blood cell destruction. Platelet isoantibodies have been used to calculate the number of antibody molecules attached per cell when cellular destruction occurs in vivo[36] and to determine the mechanisms and organs involved in destruction of immunologically altered cells.[37, 38, 39] In vivo and in vitro reactions of well characterized platelet isoantibodies have been used as models for defining the nature of the thrombocytopenic factor associated with idiopathic purpura[39, 40] and for evaluating the effects of splenectomy and adrenocortical steroid therapy on immunologic thrombocytopenia.[39] Specific isoantibodies have also been used in obtaining information on platelet and leukocyte production and reserve[34, 39] and at the same time on factors of significance in the development of febrile transfusion reactions. Quantitative studies of the antigen-antibody reactions responsible for the remarkable syndrome of post-transfusion purpura in which isosensitization results in destruction of the sensitized individual's own cells, have provided some insight into possible mechanisms of autoimmunity.[32, 36, 37, 38] Finally, correlation of immunologic and serologic findings and results of experimental therapy in isoimmune neonatal thrombocytopenia have established a firmer basis for diagnosis and evaluating therapy of this disorder.[35]

The purpose of this communication is (1) to describe the serology of antibodies against the known specific platelet and leukocyte isoantigens with emphasis on principles that can be used to define new ones, (2) to present examples of the usefulness of some of these specific isoantibodies in pathophysiologic studies, and (3) to relate recent experimental studies to problems of clinical medicine.

SEROLOGY

Outlines of serologic technics and methods of preparing and storing cells that have been found to be most useful are provided in the Appendix.

The Zw or Pl^A System

In 1959 van Loghem and co-workers[27] reported on serological and genetical studies of a platelet isoantigen that was identified with an agglutinin present in the serum of a thrombocytopenic patient who had received several blood transfusions. The antibody agglutinated 97.6 per cent of 287 platelet suspensions and the antigen, named Zw, was inherited as a dominant character. That same year we studied two patients who developed severe thrombocytopenia approximately one week after blood transfusion and found them to have an isoantibody in their sera that fixed complement with 98.5 per cent of the platelet preparations tested.[32] The antigen, which was inherited as a dominant character, was called Pl^A1 in an attempt to follow the recommendations of Ford[41] for systematic notation of blood groups. We subsequently sent anti-Pl^A1 to Dr. van Loghem who found that it reacted with Zw-positive platelets, but not with Zw-negative platelets. The antigen Pl^A1 is therefore the same as Zw, or Zw^a, as it was called when the allelic antigen was recognized.[28] By precedence, the antigen should be referred to as Zw^a. However, with prospects of many new antigens being defined in the near future, some system of nomenclature should be applied. We will therefore use the designation Pl^A1, and have used the same system in naming a number of other platelet and leukocyte isoantigens.

The anti-Pl^A1 antibody was unusual in several respects. Development of antibody in patients after transfusion was heralded by clinical purpura (the probable reasons for this will be discussed under the section on Clinical Observations) and the antibody not only fixed complement, but also agglutinated platelets, gave a positive anti-globulin consumption test, inhibited clot retraction, and could be used to determine the gene-dose of cellular antigens.

Gene Dosage Effects

In the course of phenotyping platelets by complement fixation, it was found that reactive platelets formed two groups based on differences in the amount of complement fixed per platelet,[31] as shown in figure 1. Of a total of 75 different platelet preparations tested quantitatively in this way, 73 per cent (55 individuals) fixed approximately twice as much complement per platelet as did the remaining 27 per cent. Moreover in studies of family groups containing a non-reactive parent and reactive children (e.g., families 4 and 5 in fig. 2) the high-activity platelets adsorbed approximately twice as much antibody per platelet as did the children's low-activity platelets (fig. 3). Of 18 children tested (including 11 previously reported)[32] all had low-activity platelets. Qualitative

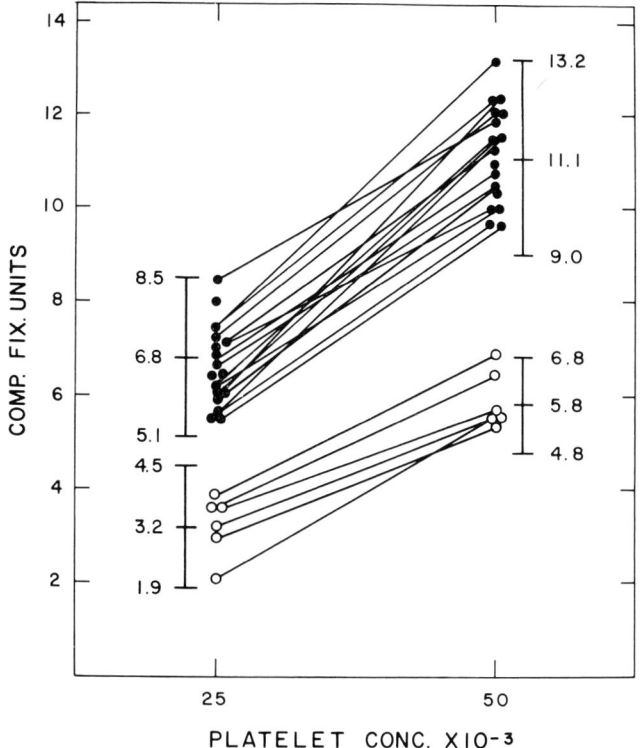

Fɪɢ. 1—Quantitative activity of platelets from random donors. The two final platelet concentrations used were 25,000/mm.³ and 50,000/mm.³ in reaction mixtures containing excess antibody. The brackets delimit 2 standard deviations from the mean for each group. The graph is a composite of results obtained with different donors on different days. The spread of values within each group was less than that shown here when all assays were performed on the same day and platelet suspensions were standardized on the basis of nitrogen content. This figure is from Ref. 32, courtesy of the publisher.

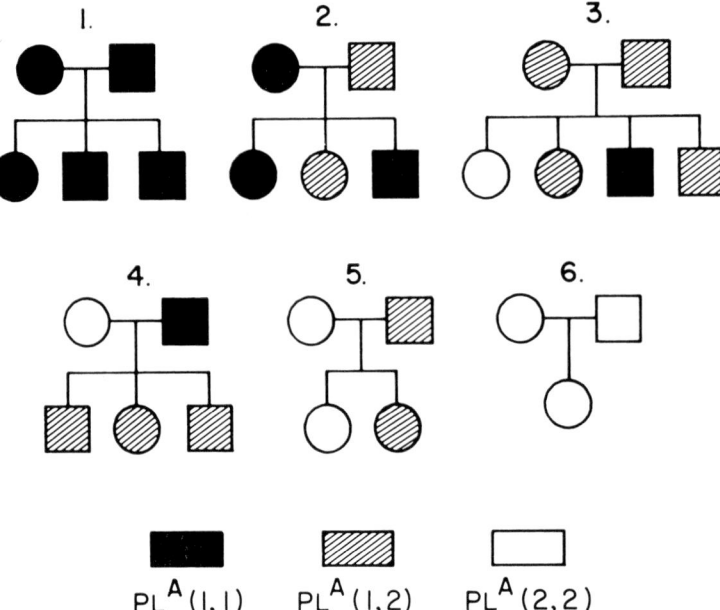

FIG. 2—Quantitative activity of platelets from family groups. Individuals whose plate-lets, at a final concentration of 50,000/mm.³, fixed less than 5.8 U of C′ in the presence of excess antibody are represented by hatched symbols and those whose platelets fixed greater than 9.2 U of C′ under the same conditions are represented by solid symbols (see fig. 1). No values for C′ fixation were obtained in the range of 5.8 to 9.2 U. Open symbols represent individuals whose platelets did not react. Squares are males; circles, females. Other family studies are in Ref. 32.

tests on an additional 203 children in 62 families were all consistent with dom-inant inheritance of the reactive character. It therefore appeared that inheritance of the antigen was controlled by a pair of alleles, and that high-reactive platelets had a homozygous or double dose of antigen, and low-reactive platelets a hetero-zygous or single dose of antigen.

The relative amounts of C′ that were fixed with homozygous and heterozy-gous cells are shown in figures 4 and 5. In figure 4, the concentration of cells is kept constant and antibody concentration is varied, and in figure 5 antibody concentration is kept constant and cell concentration is varied.

Of a total of 452 random donors tested, 97 per cent were positive reactors. Assuming that non-reactors (3 per cent of the population) represented individuals homozygous for the antigen allelic to Pl^{A1} then, in accordance with the Hardy-Weinburg Law,[*][42] the frequency of the gene controlling the allelic antigen

* The Hardy-Weinburg Law states essentially that if there are two allelic genes, p and q, at a particular locus, then the interaction of these genes will produce the genotypes, $(p + q)^2$ or $p^2 + 2pq + q^2$. The relative proportions of the three types of individuals in the popula-tion will be determined by the frequency of the genes p and q. If an antibody reacts with an antigen determined by the gene, p, then reactors in the general population would be either type p^2 or pq, but nonreactors would be only type q^2. Therefore, given an antibody that reacts with the product of a single gene (p), the frequency of the gene controlling the allelic antigen (q) will be equivalent to the square root of the frequency of non-reactors,

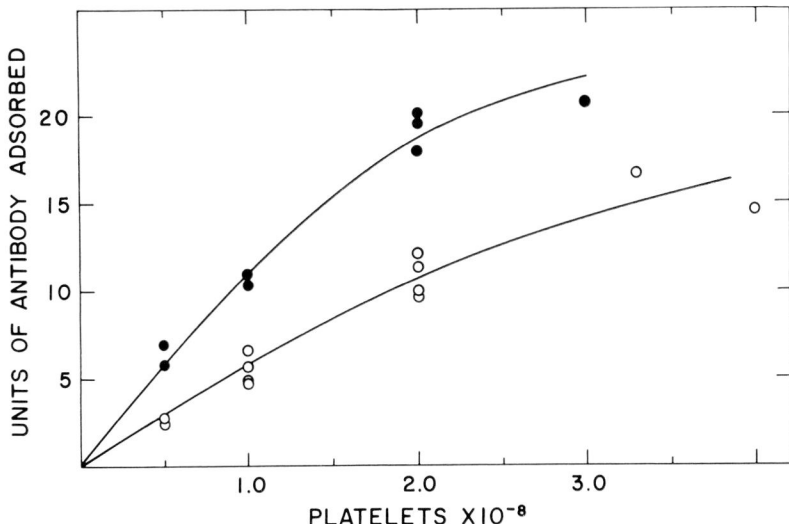

FIG. 3—Adsorption of antibody by high-activity and low-activity platelets. Buttons prepared from suspensions of high-activity and low-activity platelets were resuspended in 0.25 ml. serum containing anti-Pl^{A1}. The mixtures were incubated for 90 minutes at 37°C., centrifuged at 15,000 g for 15 minutes, and antibody remaining in the supernatant serum was titered using a standard curve to relate the amount of C′ fixed to the concentration of antibody, as described in the Appendix. Individual points for each concentration of platelets used were obtained with platelets from a different donor. The C′-fixing activity of the platelets (● high-activity, ○ low-activity) was determined as described in figure 1. This figure is from Ref. 32, courtesy of the publisher.

(Pl^{A2}) would be equal to $\sqrt{.03}$ or .17, and the gene frequency of Pl^{A1} therefore would be .83. The distribution of the three genotypes in the general population would be $(Pl^{A1})^2 + 2 \times Pl^{A1} \times Pl^{A2} + (Pl^{A2})^2$ which, on substituting values for gene frequencies, would be $(.83)^2 + 2 \times .83 \times .17 + (.17)^2$. Therefore 69 per cent of the population would be homozygous reactors, $Pl^{A}(1,1)$, 28 per cent heterozygous reactors, $Pl^{A}(1,2)$, and 3 per cent nonreactors, $Pl^{A}(2,2)$. The experimental finding that platelets from 73 per cent of reactors had almost double the antigenic content of the remaining reactors was consistent with the theoretical calculations. It was therefore concluded that two alleles were present in the Pl^{A} system and that the antigenic dose per platelet was proportional to the genetic composition of the individual.[32] This was an unusual and informative dividend of the C′ fixing procedure.

In 1963 van der Weerdt et al.[28] found an agglutinin that did indeed recognize the antigen allelic to Zw (Pl^{A1}) and at this point the symbol, Zw, was changed to Zw^a and the allelic was called Zw^b. A sample of anti-Zw^b, sent to us by Dr. van

i.e., $\sqrt{q^2}$. The frequency of the gene controlling the reactive antigen would be $(1 - \sqrt{q^2})$. By substituting values for the frequencies of the two genes in the equation, $p^2 + 2pq + q^2$, the expected frequency of individuals homozygous for each gene and heterozygous individuals can be calculated. Such calculations are usually valid for blood group antigens because a locus most often has two alleles and the genes express themselves in a co-dominant manner. The results, however, are not always those one would intuitively feel they should be (see values in table 6).

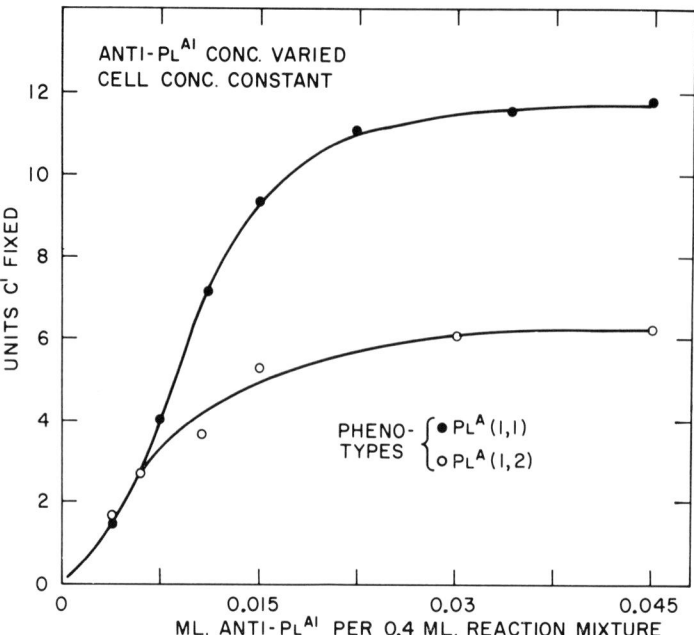

Fig. 4—Complement fixation with various concentrations of anti-Pl[A1] and a fixed concentration of homozygous Pl[A](1,1) or heterozygous Pl[A](1,2), platelets. C' fixation was carried out in a 0.4 ml. volume as described in the Appendix. Final platelet concentration was kept constant at 50,000/mm.[3] in all tubes. Amounts of serum containing anti-Pl[A1] are shown on the abscissa. In other reports,[32, 33] we have defined a unit of antibody activity to permit comparison of sera containing different concentrations of antibody.

der Weerdt, reacted not only with cells of the few available individuals who were Pl[A1]-negative, but also with cells of 15 individuals who had been designated as heterozygous Pl[A](1,2) on the basis of their low activity with anti-Pl[A1]. Anti-Zw[b] did not react with 55 individuals whose cells had high activity with anti-Pl[A1]. Van der Weerdt et al. found that anti-Zw[b] reacted with 26 per cent of 435 individuals tested, and with the sample they sent us, we found 27 per cent positive reactors among 75 individuals tested. These values were in keeping with the frequency of positive reactors expected with an antibody against the antigen allelic to Zw[a] or Pl[A1]. Thus the Zw or Pl[A] blood group system is firmly established.

Although the gene-dosage of erythrocyte antigens can be detected in some groups, such as MNSs, by agglutination technics, the effect usually is indistinct[43] and even with elaborate technics, it is not possible to determine quantitative differences in a clear-cut manner.[44] In contrast, the heterozygous and homozygous antigenic content of cells appears to be readily ascertainable in some platelet antigen systems (but not in all). The ability to translate phenotypes directly into genotypes can be most helpful in identifying allelic antigens, particularly if there is marked disparity in the frequencies of the allelic genes. For instance, if the frequency of a gene, p, were .97, the frequency of its allele, q, would be .03 and 99.9% $(.97^2 + 2 \times .97 \times .03)$ of the population would

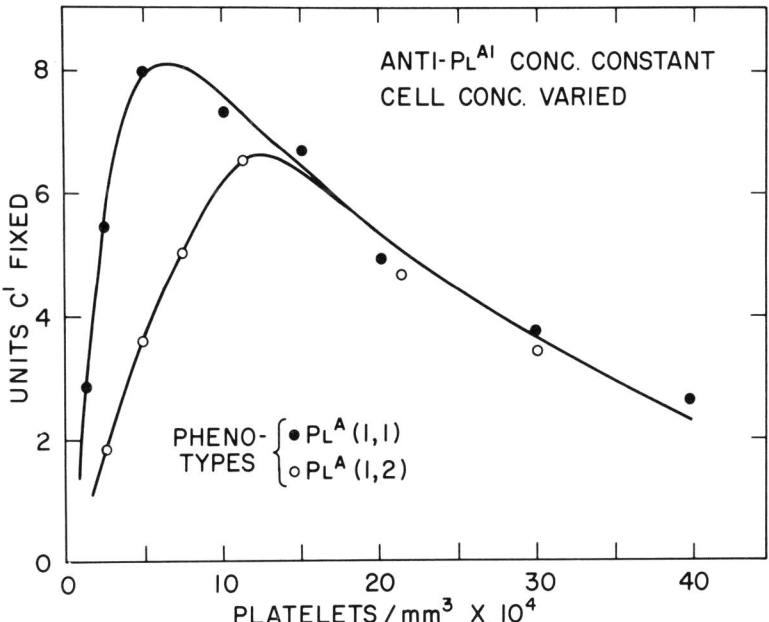

Fig. 5—Complement fixation with various concentrations of homozygous PlA(1,1), or heterozygous PlA(1,2) platelets and a fixed concentration of anti-PlA1. The serum used was the same as that in figure 4. The serum concentration was kept constant at 0.015 ml/0.4 ml. of reaction mixture.

react with an antibody against the antigen controlled by the gene, p. It would be much easier to identify the product of the allelic gene, q, by detecting it in the 5.9 per cent $(2 \times .97 \times .03)$ of heterozygous reactors than in the 0.1% $(.03^2)$ of homozygous non-reactive individuals. This type of analysis did in fact, permit identifying alleles in the PlE system described below.

Reactions other than C' fixation

In its ability to inhibit clot retraction,[32] anti-PlA1 resembled an antibody reported by Zucker et al.[45] A simple test of qualitative inhibition of clot retraction, in which antibody was added to 1 or 2 ml. of whole blood and the presence or absence of retraction noted after two hours (see Appendix), could be used as a rapid and simple phenotyping procedure. This was possible because anti-PlA1 caused complete inhibition of retraction in the blood of all reactive individuals. Unfortunately, the inhibition of clot retraction test has not been as reliable with isoantibodies against other platelet antigens.

The C'-fixing form of anti-PlA1 also agglutinated platelets and although relatively insensitive,[32] this test could be used reliably for phenotyping. Since van Loghem et al.[27] used the agglutination technic exclusively with their example of anti-PlA1 (anti-Zwa), it is not known whether it fixed C' or inhibited clot retraction.

The anti-gamma globulin consumption technic has been used by a number of investigators in attempts to detect[24, 25, 46] or measure[9] platelet and leukocyte

TABLE 1.—*Anti-Globulin Consumption by Anti-Pl^{A1}*

1 Anti-globulin final dilution	2 Preliminary titration	3 Pl^A(2,2) platelets + normal serum	4 Pl^A(2,2) platelets + anti-Pl^{A1}	5 Pl^A(1,1) platelets + normal serum	6 Pl^A(1,1) platelets + anti-Pl^{A1}
1/40	4+	4+	4+	4+	2+
1/80	4+	3+	4+	3+	2+
1/160	3+	3+	3+	2+	1+
1/320	3+	3+	2+	2+	0
1/640	2+	1+	1+	1+	0
1/1280	1+	0	0	0	0

General technic described in Ref. 46. The initial adsorption mixtures consisted of 10^9 platelets suspended either in patient's serum containing sufficient anti-Pl^{A1} to saturate this number of platelets, or in normal serum from an individual with type AB erythrocytes. After incubation for 30 minutes at 37°C. and 5 washes, 10^8 platelets from each mixture were suspended in 0.2 ml. of anti-globulin serum at 1/20, 1/40, 1/80, 1/160, 1/320, and 1/640 dilutions. Supernatant anti-globulin serum from these mixtures was then added to an equal volume of a suspension of sensitized erythrocytes to give the final dilutions listed in column 1. The preliminary titration of plain anti-globulin serum against erythrocytes sensitized with anti-D is shown in column 2. In columns 3, 4, 5 and 6, the adsorption mixtures used and the degree of agglutination obtained with the indicator erythrocytes are listed. Columns 3, 4, and 5 are controls for column 6. Similar results were obtained in 4 separate experiments with platelets from different donors each time.

isoantibodies. We have obtained reproducible but weakly positive results in the anti-gamma globulin consumption test with anti-Pl^{A1}, as shown in table 1. Although this test was consistently positive with the C′-fixing form of anti-Pl^{A1}, in our experience it has been negative with most other platelet and leukocyte isoantibodies.

Van de Wiel and co-workers[25] have described numerous pitfalls of the anti-gamma globulin consumption technic when it is applied to blood cells other than erythrocytes. An anti-non-gamma globulin or anti-C′ globulin consumption test that involves the use of C′-coated indicator cells[39] did not give positive results with C′-fixing anti-Pl^{A1} or other platelet and leukocyte isoantibodies. The amounts of certain C′ components fixed by isoantibodies apparently were much less than amounts adsorbed nonspecifically by platelets and leukocytes.[39]

Differences evident in the C′ fixation reaction with homozygous and heterozygous cells were not detectable by agglutination, inhibition of clot retraction or anti-globulin consumption technics.

It is noteworthy that the three examples of post-transfusion anti-Pl^{A1} reacted in all serologic tests (table 5) but the one example of an antibody against the allelic antigen Pl^{A2} (Zw^b), was an agglutinin only. It did not fix complement, inhibit clot retraction or give a positive anti-globulin consumption test.

The Incomplete or Blocking Form of Anti-Pl^{A1}

Application of complement fixation technics to the problem of detecting the elusive maternal isoantibodies responsible for neonatal purpura was rewarding in that several C′-fixing antibodies were found to account for the disorder.[33, 34, 35, 47] However, in most instances, sera of mothers strongly suspected of being isoimmunized (see section on neonatal purpura) did not fix with C′, or agglutinate platelets of their husbands or infants. When platelets from these mothers were phenotyped with anti-Pl^{A1}, 13 of 37 tested lacked the Pl^{A1} antigen, whereas platelets of their husbands and infants contained the antigen. In view of the infrequency of Pl^{A1}-negative individuals (3 per cent), identification of maternal fetal incompatibility for Pl^{A1} in the first few families studied[33] provided overwhelming evidence that some form of anti-Pl^{A1} was the cause of neonatal purpura. Attempts were therefore made to detect a non-C'-fixing, non-agglutinating antibody that might interfere with activity of the known C'-fixing form of anti-Pl^{A1}, in a manner analogous to that of incomplete or blocking antibodies interfering with erythrocyte isoagglutinins. Typical results with a single concentration of serum from a Pl^A(2,2) mother sensitized by fetal platelets Pl^A(1,2) are shown in table 2, and results of varying the amount of maternal serum in mixtures with the C'-fixing form of anti-Pl^{A1} are shown in figure 6. Of a total of 72 mothers in whom isoimmunization against fetal platelets was suspected, 17 had a blocking form of anti-Pl^{A1} measurable in this way. To test for a blocking antibody, as shown in table 2, a C'-fixing antibody of corresponding specificity had to be available. Examples of maternal and post-transfusion blocking antibodies against isoantigens other than Pl^{A1} are described below.

Since normal serum at $\frac{1}{4}$ dilution or less may inhibit one or two units of C' fixation, a positive blocking antibody should inhibit more than 3 units of C' fixation at $\frac{1}{4}$ dilution, and preferably at $\frac{1}{8}$ dilution. The *quantitative* C' fixation technic, described in the Appendix, in which excess C' is used, proved to be most suitable for detecting blocking antibodies. *Qualitative* C' fixation tests did not detect blocking antibodies as readily, for when blocking antibodies competitively displaced C'-fixing antibodies usually sufficient C'-fixing sites remained (see fig. 6) to fix the minimum amounts of C' employed in qualitative procedures. Examples of the blocking form of anti-Pl^{A1} identified so far inhibited only C' fixation and did not inhibit the agglutination reaction of the complete form of anti-Pl^{A1}. Of 10 incomplete anti-Pl^{A1} antibodies, clearly measurable at dilutions

TABLE 2.—*Inhibition of the C'-Fixing Activity of Anti-Pl^{A1} by Serum from a Mother Whose Child Had Neonatal Purpura*

Tube	Mixture	Units C' Fixed
1	Anti-Pl^{A1} + platelets	9.5
2	Anti-Pl^{A1} + platelets + normal serum	9.0
3	Anti-Pl^{A1} + platelets + maternal serum	1.2
4	Mother's serum + platelets	0
5	Anti-Pl^{E1} + platelets	9.0
6	Anti-Pl^{E1} + maternal serum	8.8

The amount of anti-Pl^A used in the mixture with 50,000 type Pl^{A1}(1,1) platelets/mm^3 was slightly suboptimal (see fig. 1). The maternal serum used in tubes 3, 4 and 6 was from a mother whose platelets were type Pl^A(2,2) and whose thrombocytopenic infant had type Pl^A(1,2) platelets. Maternal serum was used at $\frac{1}{4}$ final dilution in the reaction mixtures. C'-fixing anti-Pl^{A1} was the same as that used in figures 4 and 5. It was used at a concentration of 0.015 ml./0.4 ml. reaction mixture. C'-fixing anti-Pl^{E1} (described below) is an example of isoantibody of different specificity that was not inhibited by the blocking form of anti-Pl^{A1}.

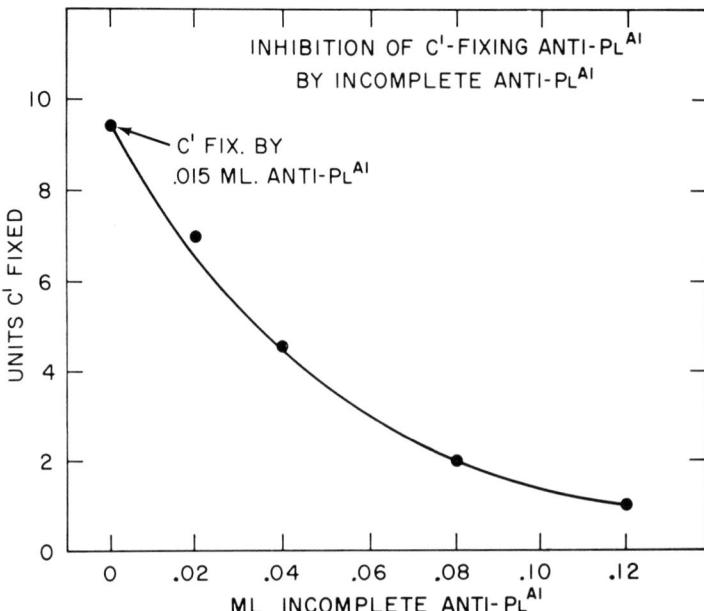

FIG. 6—Effects of various concentrations of the incomplete form of anti-Pl[A1] on complement fixation by the complete form. Conditions of this experiment were the same as those in table 2, with platelet concentration constant at 50,000/mm.[3] and concentration of serum containing C'-fixing anti-Pl[A1] constant at 0.015 ml/0.4 ml. of reaction mixture.

of $\frac{1}{8}$ or more by their ability to inhibit C' fixation, 3 gave a weakly positive and 7 gave a negative reaction in the anti-globulin consumption test performed as in table 1.

Mixtures of the C'-fixing and blocking forms of anti-Pl[A1] gave reaction patterns different from plain C'-fixing anti-Pl[A1] with respect to the amount of C' fixed as the concentration of cells or antibody was varied. The graph on the left of figure 7 shows the effects of increasing cell concentrations as in figure 5, but with sufficient blocking antibody (.045 ml.) in mixture with C'-fixing antibody (.015 ml.) to cause approximately 50 per cent inhibition. Blocking antibody not only decreased the maximum amount of C' fixed, but also changed relationships in the region of antigen excess, such that increasing cell concentrations did not produce the expected decreases in C' fixation. For comparison, the upper curve of the graph on the left of figure 7 is a duplication of the curve in figure 5 obtained with plain C'-fixing antibody. The same mixture of blocking and C'-fixing antibody as that in the graph on the left of figure 7 was used in the graph on the right. The maximum amount of C' fixed by increasing concentrations of the antibody mixture was less than that fixed by plain C'-fixing antibody (see figure 4) and the mixture produced decreases in C' fixation rather than an asymptotic value in the region of antibody excess. The upper curve in the graph on the right shows results obtained with a plain C'-fixing antibody.

The curves in figure 7 with mixtures of blocking and C'-fixing antibodies are similar to curves that were obtained with 6 of 30 C'-fixing antisera we have studied. Quantitative relationships of the type shown in figure 7, rather than

REACTIONS OF ARTIFICIAL MIXTURE OF BLOCKING
AND C'-FIXING FORMS OF ANTI-PL^AI

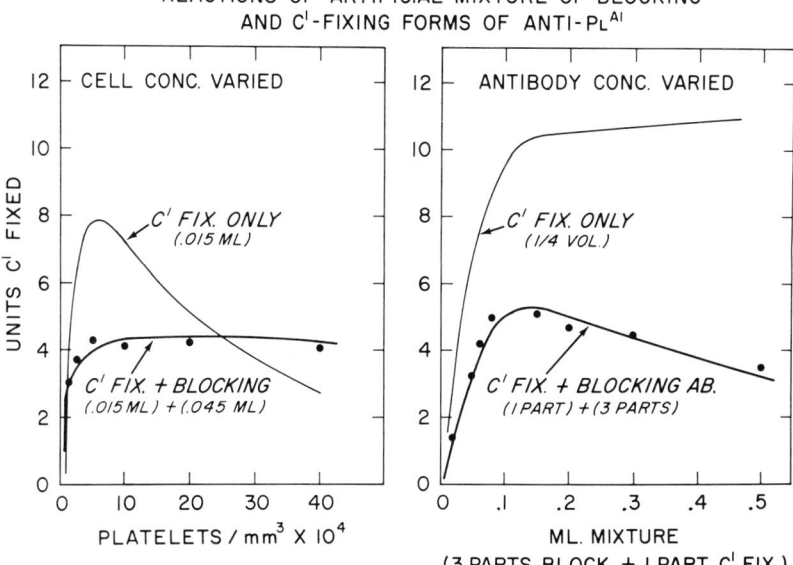

Fig. 7—Comparison of C' fixation by plain anti-Pl^A1 and mixtures of the blocking and C'-fixing forms. The experimental conditions are described in the text. The upper curves in the graphs on the left and right have been reproduced from figures 5 and 4, respectively. Table 2 and figure 6 contain additional information on effects of incomplete antibody. The amount of blocking anti-Pl^A1 in mixture with the C'-fixing form was selected to give approximately 50 per cent inhibition. The *ratio* of blocking antiserum to C'-fixing antiserum was constant at 3:1 in all tubes as the total amount of mixture was varied in the graph on the right.

those shown in figures 4 and 5, indicated that an antiserum contained a mixture of C'-fixing and blocking antibodies. Sometimes the two types of antibody could be separated by adsorption and elution technics, as described below. We have observed one patient in whom a predominantly C'-fixing form of post-transfusion anti-Pl^A1 changed to a predominantly blocking form over a period of two weeks. The reverse occurrence has not been observed.

The PlGrLy^B1 Antigen

Reactions of platelets and leukocytes.—Because the initial two examples of anti-PlGrLy^B1 were found in mothers of infants with neonatal purpura, the antigen was at first considered to be present only on platelets.[33] Shortly thereafter, by the use of pure granulocyte and lymphocyte suspensions and by cross-adsorption experiments, the antigen was found to be on granulocytes and lymphocytes as well.[34, 35] Killmann,[48] van Rood and co-workers,[8] and Dausset and co-workers[49] had suggested that isoantibodies might be directed against antigens shared by platelets and leukocytes.

C' fixation was found to be the only serologic procedure that could be used to measure the 13 different examples of anti-PlGrLy^B1 we have seen. Figure 8 shows the relationship between C' fixation and cell concentration when antibody concentration was kept constant. The optimum platelet concentration nec-

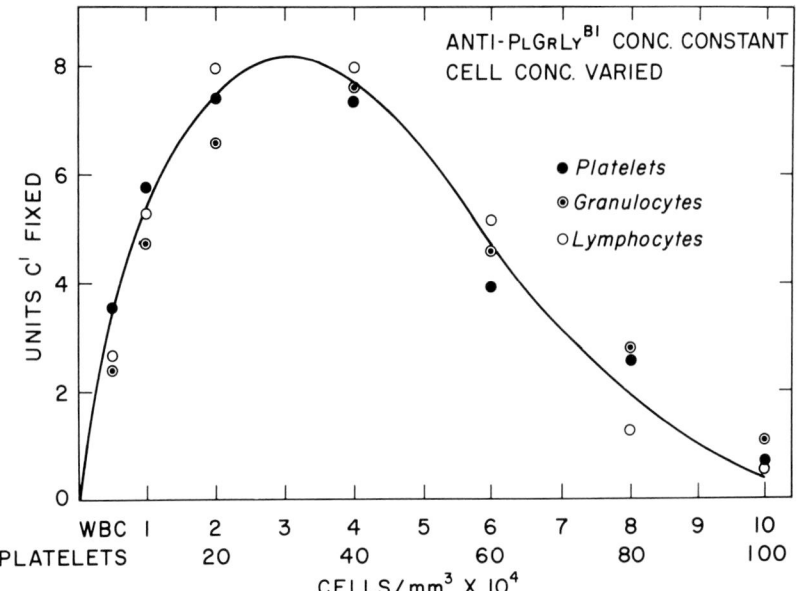

FIG. 8—Complement fixation with various concentrations of platelets, granulocytes, or lymphocytes and a fixed concentration of anti-PlGrLy[B1]. Experimental conditions were the same as in figure 5, but with different antiserum. Twelve examples of C′-fixing anti-PlGrLy[B1] have shown similar quantitative reactions with the same cells.

essary to fix eight units of C′ with the different samples of this antibody was approximately 300,000/mm.³ compared to 60,000/mm.³ required for the same amount of C′ fixation with anti-Pl[A1] (fig. 5). Granulocytes or lymphocytes could be substituted at approximately 1/10 the concentration of platelets to produce identical curves of C′ fixation. Standard curves for titering antibody could be prepared with platelets, granulocytes or lymphocytes, as shown in figure 9. The cells used in figures 8 and 9 were from a patient with chronic granulocytic leukemia. Platelets and granulocytes were obtained from peripheral blood and lymphocytes from a lymph node of the same patient.

There was no problem in comparing the reactions of platelets with a mixture of granulocytes and lymphocytes from normal blood, for the usual platelet preparations were practically free of leukocytes, there being only one per 1,000 to 5,000 platelets, and the usual leukocyte preparations contained an approximately equal mixture of granulocytes and lymphocytes with only one or two platelets per ten leukocytes (see Appendix). In view of the low reactivity of platelets compared to leukocytes, a 10 per cent platelet contamination was relatively insignificant.

Reactions of normal and leukemic leukocytes.—Since the different types of leukocytes could not be readily separated in sufficient quantities from normal blood, special suspensions, such as those in table 3, were used to compare reactions. The panel of leukocytes in table 3 was used in tests with three different antibodies listed on the right. Anti-PlGrLy[B1] and anti-PlGrLy[C1] reacted with granulocytes and lymphocytes, as well as platelets, and anti-Ly[D1] reacted with

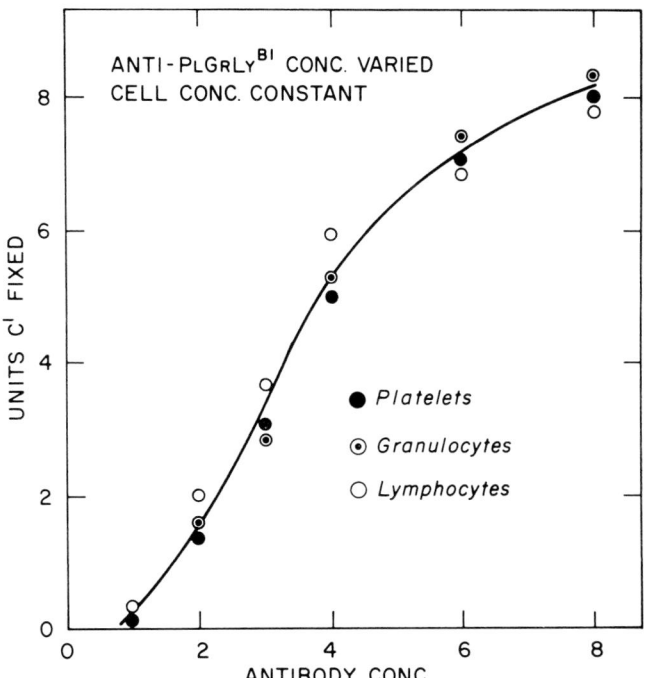

ANTI-PlGrLy^{B1} CONC. VARIED
CELL CONC. CONSTANT

● *Platelets*
◉ *Granulocytes*
○ *Lymphocytes*

Fig. 9—Complement fixation with various concentrations of anti-PlGrLy[B1], and fixed concentrations of platelets, granulocytes or lymphocytes. Experimental conditions were the same as in figure 4, but with different antiserum and different cells. Platelet concentration was constant at 300,000/mm.³; granulocyte or lymphocyte concentration was constant at 30,000/mm.³ Antibody concentration is expressed simply as a number to indicate activity of relative amounts of antibody. The absolute amounts of different sera (ml/0.4 ml. reaction mixture) that gave similar curves varied with the titers of antibody.

lymphocytes only. The PlGrLy[C1] and Ly[D1] antigens are described below. Lymphocytes were obtained from the spleen or thymus of patients who had undergone surgery for removal of these organs, from one or two Gm. of lymphoid tissue obtained during diverse operations, and from peripheral blood of patients with chronic or acute lymphocytic leukemia. Pure suspensions of granulocytes were obtained from patients with chronic or acute myelogenous leukemia. It was possible to obtain a pure platelet preparation from 107 of the 109 individuals from whom pure leukocyte suspensions were obtained. The reactions of leukocytes and platelets with anti-PlGrLy[B1] and anti-PlGrLy[C1] were concordant in every instance. Anti-Ly[D1] did not react with granulocytes or platelets. The apparent antigenic content of cells in the different leukocyte preparations listed in table 3 was similar in that variations of quantitative reactions, as in figures 8 and 9, were no greater with the different leukemic cell preparations than with normal cell preparations. The frequency of positive reactors with the different preparations was also similar.

To establish a more precise frequency of reactors, further phenotyping was performed with platelets, using the qualitative C′ fixation procedure described in the Appendix. Of a total of 888 individuals tested, 46 per cent were

TABLE 3.—*Panel of Leukocytes*

Type of Cell	Number of Donors	Number of Positive Reactors with Anti-		
		PlGrLy^{B1}	PlGrLy^{C1}	Ly^{D1}
1. Mixture of granulocytes and lymphocytes from normal blood	50	22	15	17
2. Normal lymph node lymphocytes	10	4	4	5
3. Normal thymus lymphocytes	3	2	0	1
4. Normal spleen lymphocytes	4	1	2	1
5. Chronic lymphatic leukemic blood lymphocytes	12	5	3	7
6. Acute lymphatic leukemic blood lymphocytes	4	2	1	2
				33/83 = 40%
7. Chronic myelogenous leukemic blood granulocytes	22	8	7	0
8. Acute myelogenous leukemic blood leukocytes	3	1	1	0
9. Acute undifferentiated leukemic blood leukocytes	1	1	0	0
	109	46/109 = 42%	33/109 = 30%	

positive reactors. The PlGrLy^{B1} antigen is inherited as a dominant character and no genetic inconsistencies with this type of inheritance were observed in 102 children of 28 families. The gene frequency and calculated genotype frequencies, assuming 2 alleles, are listed in table 6.

Lack of a gene dosage effect.—In the initial description of the PlGrLy^{B1} antigen,[33] it was found that platelets from some individuals had higher C′-fixing activity than others. In view of experience with the Pl^{A1} antigen, it was considered that high-activity platelets might be from individuals homozygous for the antigen, and low-activity platelets from heterozygous individuals. However, subsequent quantitative determinations of the antigenic content of platelets from 27 individuals (fig. 10) showed a continuum of values over an approximate two-fold range. Since one would expect only 7 per cent, or 2 of 27 individuals to be homozygous for this antigen, it is apparent that there is no clear relationship between gene dose and the amount of C′ fixed per cell with anti-PlGrLy^{B1}, as there is with anti-Pl^{A1}.

The blocking form of anti-PlGrLy^{B1}.—The blocking form of anti-PlGrLy^{B1}, when detected, usually was present in mixture with the C′-fixing form. Two such mixtures were seen in post-transfusion sera and one in a maternal serum. One example of blocking antibody alone was found in another maternal serum. The lower curve of figure 11 shows the activity of a serum containing a mixture of the blocking and C′-fixing forms of anti-PlGrLy^{B1}, and the upper curve of figure 11 shows the activity of an eluate made from the same serum. The platelet concentration is the same and constant in both curves. Note the resemblance in shape of the lower curve in figure 11 to the curve obtained with an artificial mixture

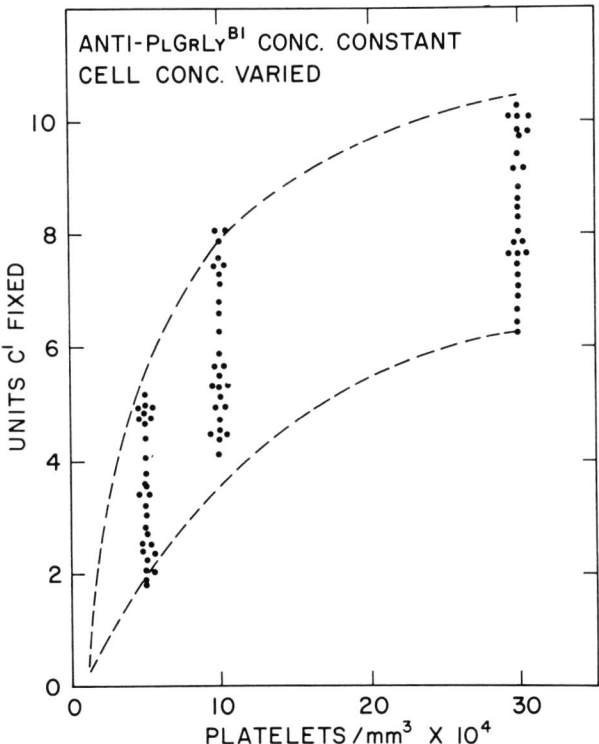

Fig. 10—Quantitative reactions of platelets from random donors with anti-PlGrLy[B1]. The three final platelet concentrations used were 50,000, 100,000, and 300,000 per mm.[3] in reaction mixtures containing excess antibody. Variation in reactions of leukocytes from 12 individuals at 30,000/mm.[3] was similar to that of platelets at 300,000/mm.[3]

of the C′-fixing and blocking forms of anti-Pl[A1] in the graph on the right of figure 7. By contrast, the eluate in figure 11 has the properties of a plain C′-fixing antibody. The eluate was made in a straightforward manner by incubating reactive platelets or leukocytes in the serum, and then acidifying the rinsed button of cells to detach antibody (see Appendix). It is important to realize that differences in the curves in figure 11 are not due to changes in antibody concentration, for in each instance an excess of antibody was added to a constant concentration of cells. The absolute increase of C′-fixing activity in the eluate could be attributed to selective separation of C′-fixing and blocking antibodies that were present in the original serum. This was possible to accomplish by an adsorption and elution procedure probably because the different forms of antibody had different affinity for antigen under the conditions that were used. Acidification of serum alone did not produce this change. In each of 6 sera (3 with anti-PlGrLy[B1] specificity) in which evidence for mixtures of C′-fixing and blocking antibodies was obtained by curves of the type shown in figure 7, eluates of the sera contained antibodies of higher C′-fixing activity. The elution procedure sometimes could be used to prepare an excellent C′-fixing antibody from an antiserum otherwise too weak to use for phenotyping.

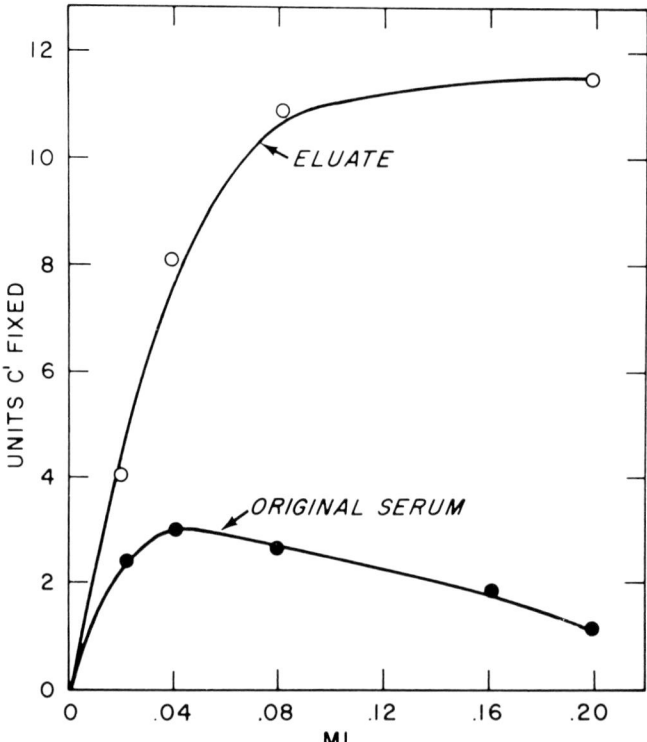

Fig. 11—Demonstration of a naturally-occurring mixture of blocking and C'-fixing isoantibodies. Antibody activity was measured using a fixed concentration of platelets with various amounts of the original serum or its eluate. Final platelet concentration was 300,000/mm.³ in all tubes, as in figure 9.

Reactions other than C'-fixation.—None of 13 different examples of anti-PlGrLy^{B1} reacted reliably in serologic tests other than C' fixation. Direct agglutination tests with platelets were consistently negative and with leukocytes were typically equivocal as shown in table 4.

Anti-globulin consumption tests were never positive. The low-affinity anti-PlGrLy^{B1} was readily detached from cells by the washing procedure necessary before the cells were exposed to anti-globulin serum (fig. 12). This is in contrast to the high-affinity anti-Pl^{A1} that remained on cells and gave a positive reaction in the anti-globulin test.

Inhibition of clot retraction tests were weakly positive with some, and negative with other cells known to contain the antigen. Since inhibition of clot retraction was variable and never complete as with anti-Pl^{A1}, this technic could not be used for phenotyping with anti-PlGrLy^{B1}. Although we have observed inhibition of clot retraction only with C'-fixing isoantibodies, it is evident that C' fixation alone is not the only factor that determines the outcome of this phenomenon. Affinity of antibody for antigen may also be involved.

The PlGrLy^{C1} Antigen

The first antibody identifying this antigen was found in the serum of a mother whose child had neonatal purpura, and the second was separated by adsorption

TABLE 4.—*Leukocyte Agglutination*

Panel of PlGrLy[B1]-Positive Cells	Agglutination Reaction with Anti-PlGrLy[B1]			Panel of PlGrLy[B1]-Negative Cells	Agglutination Reaction with Anti-PlGrLy[B1]		
	Serum A	Serum B	Serum C		Serum A	Serum B	Serum C
1	0	1+	1+	11	0	0	1+
2	0	0	1+	12	1+	±	1+
3	0	1+	3+	13	0	0	1+
4	0	±	0	14	0	0	1+
5	±	0	2+	15	1+	0	1+
6	0	0	0	16	0	0	0
7	±	1+	1+	17	0	0	0
8	±	1+	2+	18	0	0	0
9	0	0	2+	19	±	0	0
10	0	1+	0	20	0	0	0

Each of the sera, A, B and C, reacted to fix 10 units of C′ at $\frac{1}{8}$ or greater dilution in reaction mixtures containing leukocyte preparations 1 to 10 at 30,000/mm.³ final concentration as in figure 9. Leukocyte preparations 11 to 20 did not fix C′.

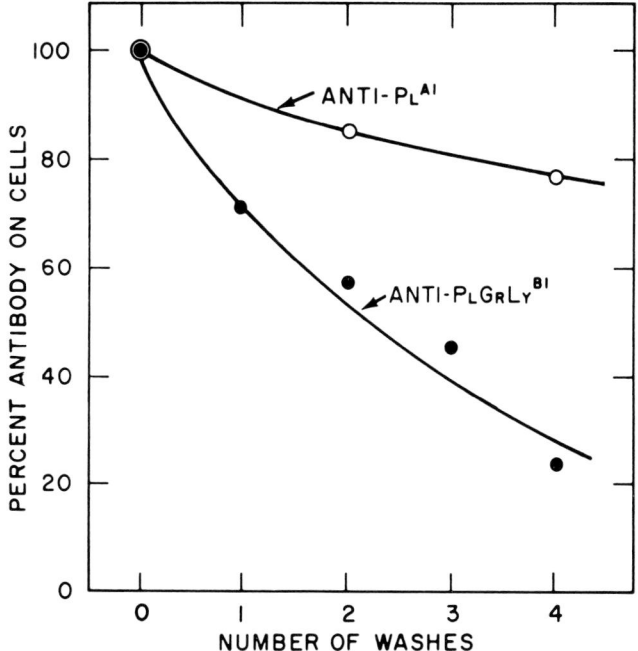

FIG. 12—Effect of repeated washing on the amount of antibody remaining attached to cells sensitized with anti-Pl[A1] or anti-PlGrLy[B1]. Platelets were sensitized with either anti-Pl[A1] or anti-PlGrLy[B1] by incubation in the presence of excess antibody for one hour at 37°C., following which platelets were sedimented at 3000 g and resuspended in 0.147 M NaCl at a concentration of 10⁶/mm.³ An aliquot of the resuspended platelets was saved and the remaining suspension was brought to 3 ml. with 0.147 M NaCl, incubated for 10 minutes and centrifuged again. The washing procedure was repeated 4 times and after each wash an aliquot of the platelet suspension containing 1.2×10^8 platelets sensitized by anti-PlGrLy[B1] or 2×10^7 platelets sensitized by anti-Pl[A1] were mixed immediately with C′ in a final volume of 0.4 ml. The amount of C′ fixed was measured as usual; and the amount of antibody remaining on cells was determined from standard curves as in figures 4 and 9.

and elution technics from a mixture of antibodies in the serum of a patient who had received over 200 transfusions.[34, 35] As indicated by the symbols of the locus, the antibody reacted with platelets, granulocytes and lymphocytes. When the 109 leukocyte preparations that were tested with anti-PlGrLy[B1] (table 3) were tested with anti-PlGrLy[C1], 30 per cent of the panel reacted; platelet preparations from 107 of the same donors reacted concordantly. Further phenotyping was performed only with platelets and 30 per cent of a total of 252 individuals tested were positive reactors. The frequency of reactions of anti-PlGrLy[C1], anti-PlGrLy[B1] and anti-Pl[A2] with the same cells was that expected for antibodies against unrelated antigens. The PlGrLy[C1] antigen was inherited as a dominant character with no inconsistencies in 78 children of 21 families. The gene frequency of PlGrLy[C1] is 0.17, which is identical with that of Pl^{A2}, but from the specificity of reactions of the respective antibodies with different cell types and different panel members, the two genes were clearly different.

C' fixation curves with anti-PlGrLy[C1] and platelets, granulocytes or lymphocytes were similar in all respects to those obtained with anti-PlGrLy[B1] in figures 8 and 9. Quantitative assays of the antigenic content of 10 platelet preparations with anti-PlGrLy[C1] gave a wide spread of values without segregation, similar to that in figure 10. Adsorption studies performed as in figure 2 with high- and low-activity platelets showed that C'-fixing activity was indeed related to the antigen content per cell.

A blocking form of anti-PlGrLy[C1] was present in mixture with the C'-fixing form in the maternal serum that contained this antibody. Antibody obtained from the maternal serum by adsorption and elution gave much higher activity than the initial serum, in the manner shown in figure 11. Approximately 15 per cent of the cell preparations that gave little or no C' fixation with the maternal serum reacted in a clear-cut manner with the eluate. The presence of a blocking antibody in this particular serum appeared to cause relatively more inhibition of C' fixation with low-activity cells than with high-activity cells. The difference in reaction of cells with different antigenic content may account for a similar phenomenon of "adsorption-positive, reaction-negative" cells found by van Rood[31] when phenotyping in the 4[a], 4[b] antigen system he described.

Agglutination tests with anti-PlGrLy[C1] and platelets or leukocytes were negative, as were anti-globulin consumption tests.

The Ly[D1] Antigen

Anti-Ly[D1] was at first thought to be a very weak and variable antiplatelet antibody at a time when we were not yet routinely employing leukocytes, as well as platelets, in screening sera. It was found that unusually high platelet concentrations, on the order of $10^6/\text{mm.}^3$ and above, gave increasing amounts of C' fixation with serum from a repeatedly transfused patient. Since platelet concentrations this high had never been required previously for C' fixation, a reactive contaminant was sought and found to be lymphocytes. Although platelet suspensions prepared in the suggested manner (see Appendix) contain only one lymphocyte per 1000 to 5000 platelets, suspensions prepared using a slower rate of sedimentation to obtain platelet-rich plasma (300 g for 10 minutes, rather than 1100 g for 4 minutes) contained approximately 10 to 20 lymphocytes per 1000 platelets. This degree of lymphocyte contamination accounted for the positive reactions obtained with some platelet preparations. Lymphocyte-free preparations made from the same donors did not react. Tests with a panel of leukocytes showed lymphocytic specificity (table 3). None of the 26 granulocyte preparations reacted, whereas 40 per cent of the suspensions containing either pure lymphocytes, or lymphocytes mixed with granulocytes, did react. Further proof of lymphocytic specificity was indicated by positive reaction with lymph node lymphocytes obtained from two patients with myelogenous leukemia whose granulocytes and platelets did not react or adsorb antibody. Moreover, quantitative aspects of the reaction between anti-Ly^{D1} and lymphocytes (shown in fig. 13) were not changed by the presence of high concentrations of platelets or granulocytes from the same donor. Therefore, for convenience, lymphocyte-rich platelet preparations could be utilized for additional phenotyping, the final concentration of cells in reaction mixtures being based solely on the lymphocyte count. Of a total of 113 individuals tested, 36 per cent were positive reactors.

Three examples of antibodies with the same specificity have been found, two in repeatedly transfused patients, one in the serum of a multiparous woman who had received no transfusions and whose children were normal. No genetic family studies have been performed as yet.

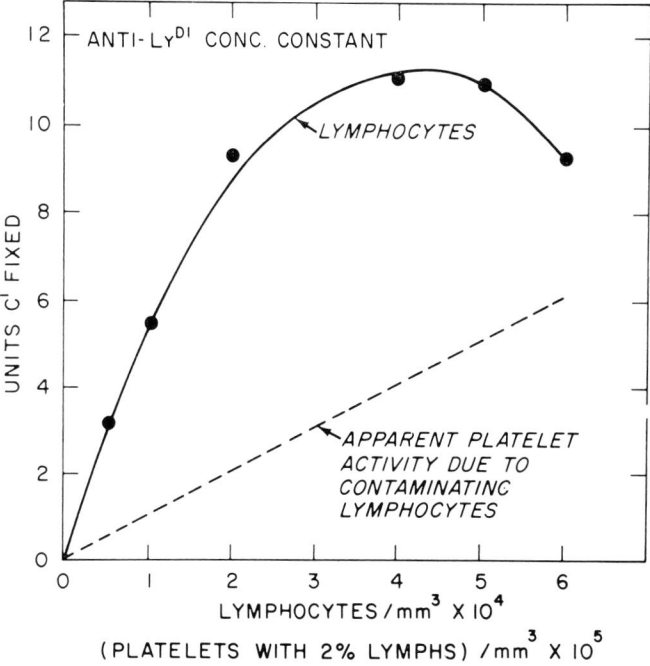

FIG. 13—Complement fixation by anti-Ly^{D1} with plain lymphocytes and lymphocytes contaminating a platelet suspension. Experimental conditions were similar in all respects to those used with lymphocytes in figure 8. Note that the quantitative activity of lymphocytes contaminating the platelet suspension was the same as that of lymphocytes alone; e.g., 500,000 platelets/mm.³ containing 10,000 lymphocytes/mm.³ fixed 5 units of C'.

The Pl^E System

The antibody that recognized the Pl[E1] antigen was one of two high titered complement-fixing antibodies in the serum of a patient who had received over 200 transfusions, and the antibody that recognized the Pl[E2] antigen was from the mother of a thrombocytopenic infant.[34, 47] Anti-Pl[E1] has reacted with all of 945 platelet preparations tested, but not with platelets of the patient that developed the antibody, and anti-Pl[E2] has reacted with 5 per cent of 147 preparations. Both antibodies react only with platelets. The manner in which the Pl[E] system was established demonstrates the utility of quantitative phenotyping in detecting alleles.

The likelihood that anti-Pl[E1] recognized only a single antigen despite the high frequency of its reactions, was established by finding that each of 25 platelet preparations from different individuals completely adsorbed out antibody for all others, that the eluate from each of these preparations reacted with all others, and that quantitative reactions of the antibody with platelets from 16 random donors were alike (fig. 14, solid symbols). In view of the almost universal presence of Pl[E1], it was evident that the allelic antigen would be found infrequently. We had on hand three maternal isoantibodies responsible for neonatal purpura

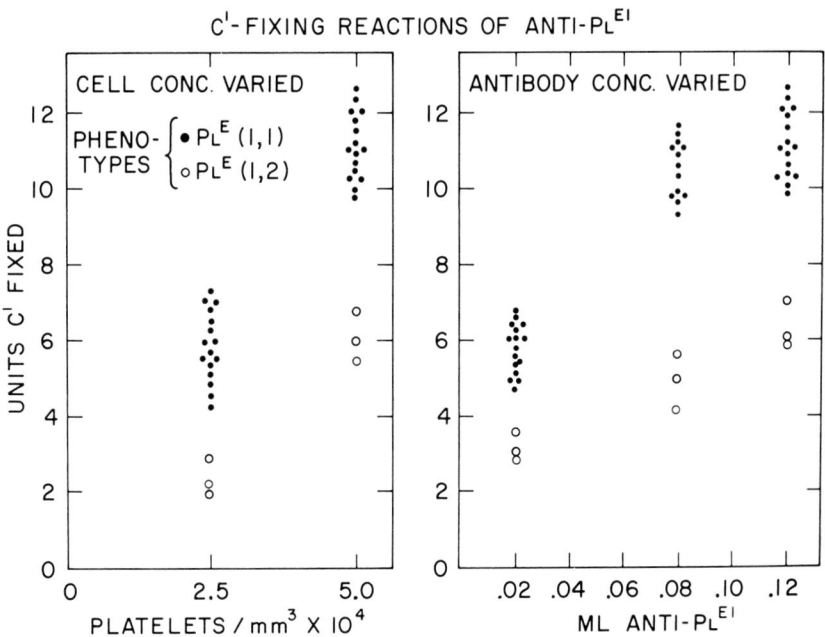

Fig. 14—Quantitative activity with anti-Pl[E1] of platelets from random donors and from 3 individuals who reacted with a maternal antiserum subsequently called anti-Pl[E2]. Experimental conditions were the same as those in figures 1 and 4, but with a different antibody. In the graph on the left, anti-Pl[E1] was present in excess (0.14 ml/0.4 ml. reaction mixture) and the two final platelet concentrations used were 25,000/mm.³ and 50,000/mm.³ In the graph on the right, platelet concentration was constant at 50,000/mm.³ in all tubes. Amounts of serum used are shown on the abscissa. The solid symbols are random donors; the open symbols, individuals who reacted with the maternal antisera.

that reacted with platelets of approximately 5 per cent of donors. Each conceivably could have identified the antigen allelic to Pl^{E1} on the basis of the frequency expected for the heterozygous state of a gene that is present in approximately 99.9 per cent of the population. The manner of performing such calculations was described in discussion of the Pl^A system. One of these maternal antibodies did react with the platelets of the Pl^{E1}-negative patient who had developed anti-Pl^{E1}. Platelets from members of the family of that patient were tested with anti-Pl^{E1} and with the maternal isoantibody subsequently considered to be anti-Pl^{E2}. The phenotypes are shown at the top of figure 16. The bottom of figure 16 shows the phenotypes of the family of the sensitized mother whose antibody was subsequently considered to be anti-Pl^{E2}.

Because random platelet samples reacted with anti-Pl^{E1} in quantitative assays to give a narrow range of high activity (fig. 14) similar to that seen with platelets homozygous for Pl^{A1} (fig. 1), it was reasonable to perform quantitative tests on platelets suspected of being heterozygous for the Pl^{E1} antigen. The three possible heterozygous individuals whose fresh platelets could be obtained for quantitative tests were the brother and son of the patient who had developed anti-Pl^{E1} (fig. 16) and a random platelet donor whose platelets reacted with both anti-Pl^{E1} and the maternal isoantibody. Results of the quantitative studies are shown in figures 14 and 15. Platelets that reacted with the maternal isoantibody (open symbols) fixed half as much C′ per platelet with anti-Pl^{E1} and ad-

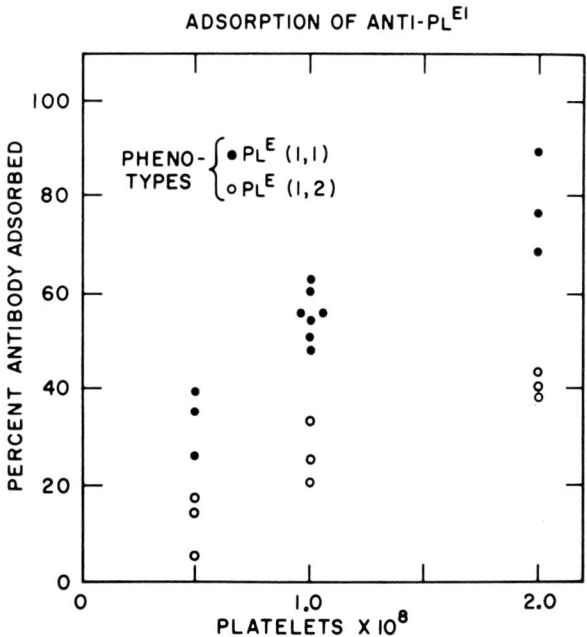

Fig. 15—Adsorption of anti-Pl^{E1} by high-activity and low-activity platelets. The adsorption experiments were performed as in figure 3, using anti-Pl^{E1} with platelets from 7 random donors (solid symbols) that showed high-activity in figure 14 and with 3 examples of low-activity platelets that reacted with a maternal antiserum that was subsequently called anti-Pl^{E2}.

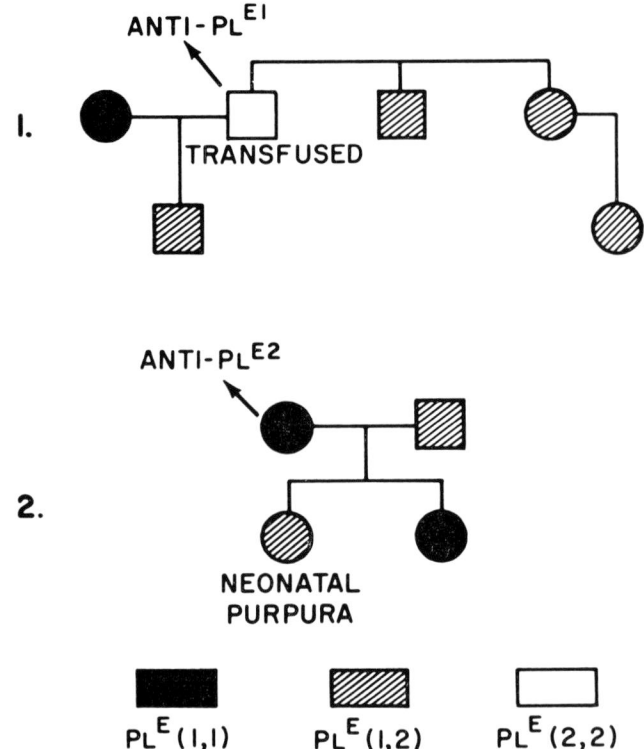

FIG. 16—Quantitative activity of platelets from family groups with anti-Pl[E1]. Platelets were phenotyped at a concentration of 50,000/mm.[3] in the presence of excess anti-Pl[E1] as in the graph on the left of figure 14. Individuals whose platelets fixed less than 8 units of C′ under the conditions are represented by hatched symbols. All of these individuals reacted with the maternal antiserum subsequently called anti-Pl[E2]. The solid symbols are individuals whose platelets reacted with anti-Pl[E1], but not with the maternal antiserum (anti-Pl[E2]). The one open symbol represents the patient who developed anti-Pl[E1] and whose platelets did not react with that antibody, but did react with the maternal serum that was considered to contain anti-Pl[E2]. Platelets from the patient who developed anti-Pl[E1] could not be used to obtain meaningful quantitative data with anti-Pl[E2] because the patient had Glanzmann's disease associated with large bizarrely shaped platelets that reacted more like leukocytes. Association of the rare phenotype Pl[E](2,2) and the rare disease suggested possible linkage, but the large misshapen platelets of another patient with Glanzmann's disease had the usual phenotype Pl[E](1,1).

sorbed half as much anti-Pl[E1] per platelet as did platelets that did not react with maternal isoantibody. The quantitative differences were clear-cut and in all respects similar to quantitative assays of platelets proven to be homozygous and heterozygous for the Pl[A1] antigen (see figs. 1, 2, 3, 4). It was therefore concluded that the maternal serum recognized the antigen allelic to Pl[E1] and this antigen was called Pl[E2]. Further proof will await finding that other nonreactors with anti-Pl[E1] (besides the patient who developed the antibody) react with the maternal isoantibody. Family studies involving 130 children of 40 matings were not helpful, as might be expected, for platelets from every one reacted with anti-Pl[E1]. In three families in which one parent was Pl[E2]-positive, four of the total of seven children were Pl[E2]-positive.

Anti-Pl[E1] did not agglutinate platelets, reacted weakly in the antiglobulin consumption test, and only partially inhibited clot retraction. Since partial inhibition of clot retraction could not be read accurately, this test was not used in phenotyping; however the qualitative C' fixation procedure described in the Appendix was precise and convenient to use for phenotyping large numbers of donors. Anti-Pl[E2] gave negative reactions in all serologic tests other than C' fixation.

The Ko[a] Antigen

In 1961 van der Weerdt and co-workers[29] described a platelet agglutinin that reacted with 21.3 per cent of the Dutch population and subsequently found three other examples of agglutinins with the same specificity.[28] These examples of anti-Ko[a] were the result of testing the serum of 204 individuals who had received three or more transfusions. Dausset and Berg[30] reported a fourth example of an agglutinin that recognized the antigen Ko[a]. Additional studies by these investigators have shown that the Ko[a] antigen is present on closer to 17 per cent of platelets, is not present on leukocytes and is inherited in the dominant manner characteristic of most other blood cell antigens.

All four examples of anti-Ko[a] did not react in the anti-globulin test and did not fix C'. It was interesting that the anti-Ko[a] reaction was not interfered with by high titered C'-fixing antibodies of different specificity in the same serum sample.

The 4 System

In 1963 van Rood and van Leeuwen[31] reported a leukocyte antigen system defined by leukoagglutinins. The antibodies used were obtained from a panel of 66 maternal sera containing a variety of isoagglutinins that had been detected on the basis of screening over 400 mothers.[8, 50] The 66 sera were each reacted with a panel of 100 cell suspensions, and reactions of each serum were compared with all other sera by computer analysis to select those that were either similar in their specificity or were likely to be recognizing products of allelic genes. There was a problem with reproducibility of results and failure of some cells to agglutinate although they contained the antigen as shown by adsorption studies. Nevertheless it was possible to obtain 5 good antisera identifying the antigen called 4[a] and 7 good antisera identifying the allelic antigen 4[b]. Anti-4[a] was found to react with 63 per cent of a panel of 347 individuals and anti-4[b] was found to react with 87 per cent of the same panel. The antigen was inherited as a dominant character and there were no inconsistencies with this type of inheritance in 140 children of 33 families. By adsorption experiments it was found that placental tissue, kidney tissue, lymphocytes, and platelets removed anti-4[a] and anti-4[b].

Other Antigens

Dausset[10] found a pattern of similar reactions of 20 leukocyte suspensions with 7 antisera and named an antigen that was present on 12 of these leukocytes, MAC. Moulinier[9] used the anti-globulin consumption test and papain-treated platelets in an attempt to determine the frequency of a platelet antigen in the general population, with serum of a normal mother who had given birth to a thrombocytopenic infant. He had difficulty with false-positive reactions, but concluded that approximately 22 per cent of platelets were positive for the antigen that he called DUZO. Payne and Hackel[51] in a report on the inheritance of leukocyte antigens, did not establish a clear-cut antigen group, but estimated that the gene frequency of some leukocyte antigens would be in the range of 0.2 to 0.8, based on frequencies of reactions with antisera containing mixtures of antibodies.

Summary of Serology of Specific Antibodies

Table 5 summarizes the serological characteristics of antibodies that are directed against a single antigen. The source of the monospecific antibodies, the frequency of reactors in the general population, and calculations of gene and genotype frequencies are listed in table 6.

By comparing reactions of specific antibodies in different laboratories through an exchange of sera, it was found that PlGrLy^{B1} and PlGrLy^{C1} differ from Ko^a, 4^a and 4^b, and that the 4^a and 4^b antigens differ from MAC. Zw^a and Pl^{A1} are identical. Characteristics of the Ly^{D1}, Pl^{E1} and Pl^{E2} antigens clearly distinguish them from other known antigens.

Five technics have been used to characterize platelet and leukocyte isoantigens: platelet agglutination, leukocyte agglutination, anti-globulin consumption, inhibition of clot retraction and C′ fixation. Each has its own advantages and disadvantages and there is no single test that is reliable for measuring all antibodies. The advantages of the platelet agglutination test of Dausset and Malin-

TABLE 5.—*Serologic Characteristics of Monospecific Antibodies Against Platelet and Leukocyte Antigens*

Anti-	Aggl.	Anti-glob. Consumption γ	C′	C′ Fix.	Inhib. Cl. Retr.	Inhib. C′ Fix.	Cell Specificity
1. Pl^{A1} or Zw^a	+	+	0	+	+		Platelets
Incomplete form	0	±	0	0	0	+	
2. Pl^{A2} or Zw^b	+	0	0	0	0		Platelets
3. PlGrLy^{B1}	0	0	0	+	0		⎧ Platelets
Incomplete form	0	0	0	0	±	+	⎨ Granulocytes
							⎩ Lymphocytes
4. PlGrLy^{C1}	0	0	0	+	0		⎧ Platelets
Incomplete form	0	0	0	0	0	+	⎨ Granulocytes
							⎩ Lymphocytes
5. Ly^{D1}	0	0	0	+			Lymphocytes
6. Pl^{E1}	0	±	0	+	±		Platelets
7. Pl^{E2} (Probable)	0	0	0	+	0		Platelets
8. Ko^a	+	0	0	0	0		Platelets
9. 4^a	+				0		⎧ Granulocytes
10. 4^b	+				0		⎨ Platelets*
							⎩ Lymphocytes*
11. DUZO		+					Platelets
12. MAC	+						Leukocytes

* By adsorption only. Reactions of these cells not tested.

TABLE 6.—*Source of Antibodies, Percent Reactors, and Genotype Frequencies*

Anti-	Source		Panel		Approx. Gene Frequency	Approximate Genotype Frequency	
	Post-Trans-fusion	Ma-ternal	Total	% Positive		Homo-zygous	Hetero-zygous
1. Pl^{A1}(Zw^a)	4	17	452	97	.83	.69	.28
			*287	97.6			
2. Pl^{A2}(Zw^b)	1		435	26	.17	.03	.28
			† 75	27			
3. PlGrLy^{B1}	5	8	888	46	.26	.07	.39
4. PlGrLy^{C1}	1	2	252	30	.17	.03	.28
5. Ly^{D1}	2	1	113	36	.20	.04	.32
6. Pl^{E1}	1		945	>99.9	.975	.95	.049
7. Pl^{E2}		1	147	5	.025	.0006	.049
8. Ko^a	4		435	17	.08	.005	.145
			‡ 75	12			
9. 4^a		5	347	63	.38	.15	.47
10. 4^b		7	347	86	.62	.38	.47
11. DUZO		1	82	22	.12	.014	.21
12. MAC	5		20	60	.37	.14	.47

* This panel was tested by van Loghem et al.[27] by agglutination.

† This panel was tested by us with serum sent by van der Weerdt et al.[28]

‡ This panel was tested by us with serum sent by van der Weerdt[29] and by Dausset.[30]

vaud[26] are its simplicity and clarity, but the test is infrequently applicable because of the rarity of strong agglutinins, and it is inconvenient for use with large panels because fresh cells are required. Leukocyte agglutination[31] is a sensitive test with some antibodies but does not detect others, is subject to many technical pitfalls, is particularly difficult to use for selecting antibodies against single antigens and requires fresh cells. The anti-globulin consumption test[46] requires large amounts of antibody and fresh cells, is cumbersome to perform with more than a few cell samples, and is subject to great variation in results with minor changes in procedure.[26, 52] Anti-globulin consumption is, however, the only test available for detecting those incomplete antibodies that are not measurable by inhibition of C' fixation. The very simplest technic, inhibition of clot retraction, may be useful only on rare occasions to identify an isoantibody and phenotype cells. C' fixation, performed as described herein, is a sensitive technic for measuring both platelet and leukocyte isoantibodies, can be used with stored or shipped cells, detects some blocking antibodies, can sometimes be used to determine gene dosage effects, permits quantitative measurements of antigen and antibody, and when used for qualitative measurements, gives clear-cut results and is easily applied to a large panel of cells.

Other technics that have been used in an attempt to detect isoantibodies and heteroantibodies, but have not been applicable in defining antigenic specificity are: agglutination technics involving prolonged incubation at 5°C.,[53, 54] fluorescent antibody methods,[55, 56] the mixed anti-globulin reaction,[57] the tanned erythrocyte hemagglutination test[58] and technics involving labeling of antisera or anti-globulin with I[131].[59] Not all of these tests have been given a thorough trial with each type of antibody, but the indications are that these technics either are useless, or offer no improvement over simpler technics that have been used to define specific antibodies. Other approaches involving various measurements of cytotoxicity effects[60] or mitogenic effects in tissue culture[61] have not yet been explored with human isoantibodies.

Chemical Characteristics of Antigens and Antibodies

The Pl^{A1}, PlGrLy^{B1}, PlGrLy^{C1}, Ly^{D1}, Pl^{E1} and Pl^{E2} antigens are all surface antigens associated with the stromal fraction of lysed cells. Cells that were heated at 56°C., incubated at pH 3 or 10 at 20°C. for 30 minutes, frozen or lyophilized, retained full capacity to adsorb antibody but lost much of their C'-fixing activity. Cells heated at 100°C. for 10 to 15 minutes usually lost their ability to adsorb antibody. The Pl^{A1} antigen could not be obtained in soluble form from cells,[32] and by inhibition tests, none of the above antigens were found to be secreted in saliva. In one attempt to purify Pl^{A1}, the ratio of nitrogen to hexose at each step of fractionation remained essentially unchanged. Treatment with high concentrations of trypsin[32] did not inactivate the Pl^{A1} antigen. The chemical nature of the various platelet and leukocyte antigens remains uncertain, but information obtained so far is consistent with the possibility that the antigens are polysaccharides, like erythrocyte isoantigens.

A variety of simple sugars and oligo- or poly-saccharides, some of which competitively inhibit reactions of antibodies against erythrocyte A, B, Le^a and Le^b antigens,[62, 63] did not inhibit the C'-fixing reaction of anti-Pl^{A1}, -PlGrLy^{B1}, -PlGrLy^{C1}, and -Pl^{E1}. The sugars that did not produce inhibition were: L-fucose, d-galactose, N-acetyl-d-galactosamine, d-glucose, d-glucosamine, N-acetyl-d-glucosamine, d-glucuronic acid, d-mannose, d-ribose, d-melibiose, d-raffinose, oligosaccharides from human milk, dextran and glycogen. All sugars were used at a final concentration of 1.5 mg/ml. One sugar, d-galactosamine HCl, at a concentration of 1.5 mg./ml., completely inhibited C' fixation by all four isoantibodies. Whether d-galactosamine is a component of the isoantigens, or interferes with the C' fixation reaction, rather than the primary antigen-antibody reaction, is presently under study.

No correlations have been noted between 19 different erythrocyte antigens and the above platelet and leukocyte antigens,[32, 33, 34] the Ko^a antigen[28] or the Zw^b (Pl^{A2})[28] antigen.

All of 17 isoantibodies against platelet and leukocyte antigens that we have studied were 7S gamma globulin, as determined by ultracentrifugation in a sucrose gradient[32, 34] or more recently by the relatively simple technic of gel filtration with Sephadex G-200.[64] The isoantibodies studied included post-transfusion and maternal C'-fixing antibodies, as well as three examples of the blocking form of anti-Pl^{A1} and one example of the blocking form of anti-PlGrLy^{B1}. These blocking and C'-fixing forms of the same isoantibody could not be separated by physical technics.

Heterologous Reactions

Some isoantibodies against human erythrocytes react with cells of many different non-human primates[65] and of a few different mammalian orders.[66] Table 7 shows the similar property of some human platelet and leukocyte

TABLE 7.—*Heterologous Reactions of Human Platelet and Leukocyte Isoantibodies*

Platelets From	Antigenic Specificity of Human Antibody									
	Pl^{A1}		$PlGrLy^{B1}$		$PlGrLy^{C1}$		Ly^{D1}		Pl^{E1}	
	No. Tested	% Pos.	No. Tested	% Pos.	No. Tested	% Pos.	No. Tested	% Pos.	No. Tested	% Pos.
Man	452	97	888	46	252	30	113	36	945	>99.9
Chimpanzee	54	100	32	0	37	0			56	100
Orangutan	35	100	21	0	22	0			36	100
Baboon	26	100	23	0	23	0			32	100
Rhesus Monkey	12	100	9	0	10	0	12	0	9	100
Gibbon	10	100							10	100
Dog	21	100	20	0	20	0	6	0	12	0
Rabbit	35	100	20	0	20	0	6	0	12	0
Guinea Pig	12	0	10	0	10	0	6	0	6	0
Rat	16	0	10	0	10	0			6	0

isoantibodies. Those isoantigens that were products of genes occurring frequently in the human population (table 6) were found on cells of all other primates tested, whereas antigens that were products of human genes that occur relatively infrequently were absent on cells of other primates. Van der Weerdt et al.[28] reported that Ko^a and Zw^b could not be identified on 20 platelet samples from Macacus Cynomolgus monkeys. No human platelet or leukocyte isoantibody has been found to react with guinea pig or rat platelets, and anti-Pl^{A1} is the only platelet or leukocyte isoantibody that has reacted with cells of dogs and rabbits. This conclusion is based on testing all sera that contained C'-fixing antibodies, whether singly or in undifferentiated mixtures. It is interesting that with animal platelets anti-Pl^{A1} reacted only to fix C' and did not cause agglutination as it did with human platelets. The species specificity of anti-Pl^{A1} reactions is sufficiently distinctive to permit tentative identification of this antibody in other laboratories without an exchange of sera.

All of our attempts to immunize rabbits, guinea pigs, rats and dogs against human platelets and leukocyte isoantigens have been unsuccessful. These animals developed high-titered anti-human platelet and leukocyte antibodies, but the antibodies did not discriminate isoantigens. Any one human platelet or leukocyte preparation adsorbed out heterologous antibodies for all other cell preparations. An attempt made to stimulate anti-Pl^{A1} by immunizing rats that are Pl^{A1}-negative with Pl^{A1}-positive platelets from a more closely related species, rabbit, did not produce antiserum that would react with Pl^{A1}-positive human platelets. Possibilities of developing type-specific antisera against human platelets and leukocyte isoantigens in lower animals have not been fully exploited, but the likelihood of success seems slight.

As Landsteiner,[67] and more recently Wiener and Moor-Jankowski[68] and Moor-Jankowski et al.,[69] have pointed out, not only can blood-grouping reagents prepared for human cells be used to study reactions of different primate species, but also antisera prepared in monkeys and anthropoid apes can be used to differentiate human blood groups. In studies done in association with Dr. Moor-Jankowski, it was found that chimpanzees immunized with human whole blood or buffy coat suspensions developed antibodies that reacted with platelets and/or leukocytes of some, but not all, human beings. The C'-fixing antibodies developed in chimpanzees had all the characteristics of human non-agglutinating isoantibodies that are directed against specific human isoantigens. A detailed report of this work will appear shortly. In addition, cells from non-human primates could sometimes be used as effectively as human cells to dissect mixtures of isoantibodies. Table 8 shows reactions of serum from a repeatedly transfused patient containing a mixture of antibodies that fixed C' with all human and chimpanzee platelets tested and with some baboon, orangutan and gibbon platelets, but not with rhesus monkey platelets. An eluate made from this serum with chimpanzee platelets contained an antibody that reacted with some chimpanzee and human platelets and not with others; and an eluate prepared from the serum with human cells that had reacted with the chimpanzee eluate contained an antibody that reacted concordantly with all of the same cells. The chimpanzee and human eluates therefore appeared to contain the same monospecific antibody. By using cells from a species that has some, but not all, human antigens, the chances of obtaining a monospecific eluate from mixtures of human isoantibodies may be better than with human cells. Baboon cells that had reacted with the whole serum did not react with the chimpanzee or human cell eluates (table 8). Had they been sufficiently available, baboon cells would have been the cells of choice to use for preparing an eluate in an attempt to identify a second monospecific isoantibody. This type of analysis need not be done near the source of nonhuman primates, for C' fixation procedures permit using shipped and stored cells. Opportunities to use human isoantibodies to identify antigens of other primates, and to use cells of various primates to identify human antigens, are numerous, for we have found that 5 of 6 sera with mixtures of human isoantibodies cross-reacted with platelets and/or leukocytes from members of one or more primate species.

EXPERIMENTAL PATHOPHYSIOLOGY

By infusing well defined isoantibodies to produce thrombocytopenia or leukopenia, quantitative aspects of in vivo cellular sensitization have been

TABLE 8.—*Dissection of a Human Antiserum with Cells from Other Primates*

Platelets From	Serum from Patient K. I.					
	Whole		Eluate Chimp.		Eluate Human	
	No. Tested	Pos.	No. Tested	Pos.	No. Tested	Pos.
Man	80	80	46	31	46	31
Chimpanzee	38	38	12	3	12	3
Baboon	28	11	6	0	6	0
Orangutan	20	13				
Gibbon	10	9				
Rhesus Monkey	12	0				

studied and the findings interpreted in terms of quantitative relationships established in vitro.[32, 34, 36, 37, 38] The role of the spleen and liver in immune cellular destruction has been evaluated with respect to the degree of cellular sensitization,[39, 40, 70] and the effects of splenectomy and adrenocorticosteroid hormones on immune thrombocytopenia have been elucidated.[39, 40] Isoantibodies have served as models for establishing the properties of the factor responsible for thrombocytopenia in idiopathic purpura.[36, 37, 39] In addition, comparisons have been made of the in vivo response of leukemic and normal leukocytes to isoantibodies.[34]

Technic of in vivo Infusion

Experimental induction of thrombocytopenia was a symptomless and relatively safe procedure, whereas induction of leukopenia could be uncomfortable and even hazardous. In most instances it was not possible to predict accurately by in vitro tests the degree of thrombocytopenia, leukopenia or systemic reaction that might be produced by an in vivo infusion of a particular plasma containing a platelet or leukocyte isoantibody.[34, 39] However, by using the principle of gradual in vivo titration that had been used to produce symptomless controlled thrombocytopenia with anti-platelet drug antibodies,[71] it was possible to establish a safe dose for platelet isoantibodies. The in vivo potency of some isoantibodies made it advisable to use an initial dose of antibody-containing plasma not exceeding 0.12 ml./Kg. of body weight, infused over a 30-minute period.[39] Doses that did not produce systemic symptoms or more than approximately 20 per cent decrease in cell count could be safely doubled after 24 hours. Although the rate of infusion, as well as the dose, influenced the degree of cellular depression produced by a platelet or leukocyte isoantibody,[34] it was generally best to maintain the infusion period for 30 to 60 minutes and vary the dosage.[39] Granulocytopenia induced by isoantibodies was almost always associated with temperature elevation and sometimes with chills, headache, nausea and vomiting. With the doses of isoantibodies used, however, destruction of leukocytes was not so acute as to cause the more alarming symptoms of shock, cyanosis or convulsions that may occur with buffy coat reactions.[4, 6, 72, 73]

Although untoward symptoms caused by immune reactions can be controlled by appropriate dose-rates of antibody, serum hepatitis remains a possible major hazard of infusing homologous plasma. Plasma from patients who have received multiple transfusions should be given only to volunteers who have had documented serum hepatitis. All recipients of homologous plasma should receive injections of pooled normal human gamma globulin for its possible protective effect against hepatitis. Use of gamma globulin fractions of plasma, rather than whole plasma, as a source of isoantibody, is feasible[39] and minimizes the risk of transferring hepatitis.

In vivo Effects of Various Isoantibodies

In figure 17 the thrombocytopenic effects of isoantibodies, drug antibodies, and plasma from patients with idiopathic thrombocytopenic purpura (ITP) are compared. Doses of the different isoantibody-containing plasmas varied from

THROMBOCYTOPENIA INDUCED BY ISOANTIBODIES, DRUG-ANTIBODIES
AND ITP PLASMA

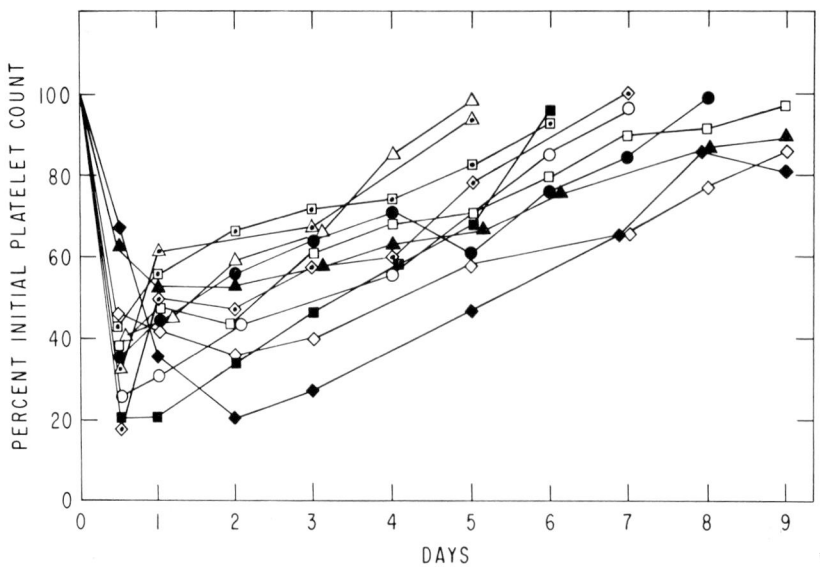

Fig. 17—Thrombocytopenia induced by isoantibodies, drug antibodies and ITP plasma. The squares with a dot show results obtained with a C′-fixing form of anti-Pl^{A1} given to a normal recipient at a dose of 0.4 ml. per Kg; the open triangles show results with a blocking form of anti-Pl^{A1} given at 0.8 ml./Kg; the open square, the same plasma used for the open triangle, given at 1.7 ml./Kg; the open diamond, a blocking form of anti-Pl^{A1} given at 1.3 ml./Kg; the diamond with a dot, a C′-fixing form of anti-Pl^{E1} given at 6.0 ml./Kg; the triangle with a dot, a C′-fixing form of anti-PlGrLy^{B1} that reacts with leukocytes as well as platelets, given at 5.0 ml./Kg; the solid circle, an isoantibody detectable only by failure of transfused platelets to circulate, given at 2.7 ml./Kg; the open circle, effects of giving 15 micromoles of quinidine intravenously to a patient with the antibody of quinidine purpura;[75] solid triangle, plasma from ITP patient P. F., given at 1.25 ml./Kg; solid diamond, plasma from ITP patient H. W. given at 2.0 ml./Kg; and solid square, plasma from ITP patient B. S. given at 0.7 ml./Kg. The 100 per cent value varied for different recipients from approximately 200,000 to 300,000/mm.³ and was based on the average of platelet counts done daily on each recipient for 3 to 7 days before an infusion. This figure is taken from Ref. 39, courtesy of the publisher.

0.4 to 6.0 ml./Kg; but variation in the amounts of the different plasmas required for a particular thrombocytopenic effect were similar whether they contained a C′-fixing or incomplete form of isoantibody. For example, if a C′-fixing and blocking form of anti-Pl^{A1} were infused on separate occasions in amounts proportional to the in vitro mixture that produced 50 per cent inhibition of C′ fixation in blocking tests (table 2 and fig. 6), a similar degree of thrombocytopenia developed (figure 18). None of the antibodies infused in figures 17 or 18 caused a prolonged bleeding time, petechiae, or subjective symptoms, except one, anti-PlGrLy^{B1}. This antibody, directed against an antigen shared by platelets and leukocytes, caused a slight febrile reaction and a transient leukopenia along with the thrombocytopenia. Depression of platelets to the lowest level shown in figure 17 by the other antibodies was not associated with signifi-

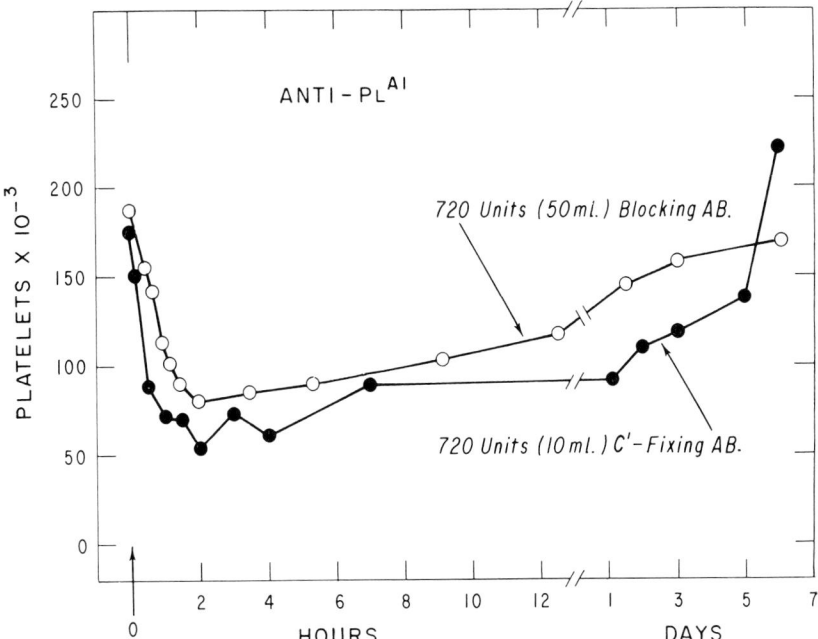

ANTI - PL^AI

720 Units (50 ml.) Blocking AB.

720 Units (10 ml.) C'-Fixing AB.

FIG. 18—In vivo effects of a C'-fixing and blocking antibody against the same antigen. Values plotted with solid circles were obtained by infusing a C'-fixing form of anti-Pl[A1] obtained from a Pl[A1]-negative patient sensitized by transfusion (see section on post-transfusion purpura) and values plotted with open circles were obtained by infusing an incomplete form of anti-Pl[A1] obtained from a Pl[A1]-negative mother sensitized by Pl[A1]-positive fetal platelets. The same volunteer received both antibodies one year apart. The amounts of the different forms of antibody used were chosen on the basis of their apparent effectiveness in competing for equal numbers of platelet antigen sites. A 5:1 mixture of blocking:C'-fixing serum produced 50 per cent inhibition of C' fixation in mixtures, as described in table 2. This figure is taken from Ref. 34, courtesy of the publisher.

cant changes in total or differential leukocyte count or in serum C' levels determined at the same intervals as platelet counts.

Quantitative Aspects of in vivo Responses

Figure 19 shows the relationship between the in vitro and in vivo activity of anti-Pl[A1]. Results are typical of those obtained with anti-PlGrLy[B1], anti-PlGrLy[C1], anti-Pl[E1], and some less well-defined platelet and leukocyte antibodies. Depression of cells was obtained with in vivo isoantibody concentrations, generally 10-fold lower than the minimum concentrations that could be detected by the most sensitive in vitro serologic technics.

The molar concentration of antibody present in vivo when thrombocytopenia occurred was determined by measuring the molar concentration of antibody*

* Concentration of isoantibody was measured in purified acid eluates (see Appendix) by Kjeldahl nitrogen or ultraviolet absorption methods. Values were converted to molar concentrations assuming a molecular weight of 160,000 and 16 per cent nitrogen content or an $E_{1\,cm.}^{1\,per\,cent}$ of 13 at 280 mμ for 7S antibody protein.[36] Nonspecific protein in the eluates was accounted for by the difference in values before and after adsorption with stroma of

in the infused plasma and accounting for its dilution in the recipient's plasma. The average number of antibody molecules attached per cell when thrombocytopenia occurred could then be estimated, providing the association constant,* or avidity, of the antigen-antibody reaction was determined. As shown in figure 19, infusion of 10 ml. of 10^{-7} M antibody into a 60 Kg. individual with Pl^A (1,1) platelets caused an immediate and sustained thrombocytopenia. The in vivo concentration of antibody after dilution in the recipient's plasma was approximately 4×10^{-10} M. With an association constant of 2×10^9 for the reaction, almost all of the antibody was complexed with antigen, and essentially 4×10^{-10} antibody was distributed over the circulating platelets. Therefore the number of antibody molecules per cell was equal to the molar concentration of antibody (Ab) multiplied by Avogadro's number and divided by the number of platelets per liter of plasma:

$$\frac{[4 \times 10^{-10} \text{ M Ab}][6 \times 10^{23}]}{3.2 \times 10^{11} \text{ platelets/L}} = 750 \text{ antibody molecules/cell}$$

Although 500 to 1000 antibody molecules were sufficient to sensitize a cell for destruction in vivo, they represented a small fraction of the number of antibodies that could be adsorbed per cell. The concentration of antigen sites on 3.2×10^{11} platelets/L was 6.4×10^{-8} M (see footnote). Hence, cells were $4 \times 10^{-10}/6.4 \times 10^{-8}$ or approximately 1 per cent saturated with antibody when thrombocytopenia occurred. In view of the requirement of nearest neighbor pairs of antibodies for C' fixation[75] and higher concentrations of antibody for agglutination,[32, 75] it is apparent that these reactions did not occur when cells were destroyed in vivo. Moreover, incomplete antibodies that neither agglutinated cells nor fixed C' were as effective as C'-fixing antibodies in causing cellular destruction (figs. 17, 18). Therefore the critical concentration of antibody that caused in vivo cellular destruction did not agglutinate or lyse cells directly but only

---

cells containing the specific antigen. The C'-fixing activity of the antibody in the eluate was then related to a molar concentration of antibody. The effective molar concentration of cell sites for combination with antibody was determined by the amount of antibody adsorbed on cells under conditions that saturated cells with antibody. For example, Pl^A(1,1) platelets at a concentration of 50,000/mm.^{3} adsorbed approximately 10^{-8} M anti-Pl^{A1}.

* By converting the number of cells per cu. mm. into a molar concentration of cell sites for antibody attachment, association constants for antibody-cell complexes were calculated from equilibrium concentrations of free cell sites and free antibody in mixtures such as those shown in figure 20. In this figure, the initial concentration of antibody was constant at 10^{-8} and the amount of antibody adsorbed by various platelet concentrations was measured (open triangles). When the initial concentration of both reactants was 10^{-8} M (at 50,000 platelets/mm.^{3}), 0.8×10^{-8} M antibody was adsorbed. The association constant of the reaction therefore was:

$$K_a = \frac{[\text{AbPl}^{A1}]}{[\text{Ab}][\text{Pl}^{A1}]} = \frac{[0.8 \times 10^{-8}]}{[0.2 \times 10^{-8}][0.2 \times 10^{-8}]} = 2 \times 10^9 \text{ liters per mole}$$

This association constant is the highest obtained for isoantibodies studied so far, but is similar to values that have been obtained for other human antibodies, e.g., anti-insulin.[74] The K_a of anti-Pl^{E1} was approximately 10^8, and a rough estimate of the K_a for anti-PlGrLy^{B1} was less than 10^7. Values obtained with anti-PlGrLy^{B1} were relatively inaccurate because cells used for eluates could not be washed extensively to remove nonspecific protein without losing antibody as well (fig. 12). Different antibodies with the same antigenic specificity will no doubt be found to have different degrees of avidity for antigen.

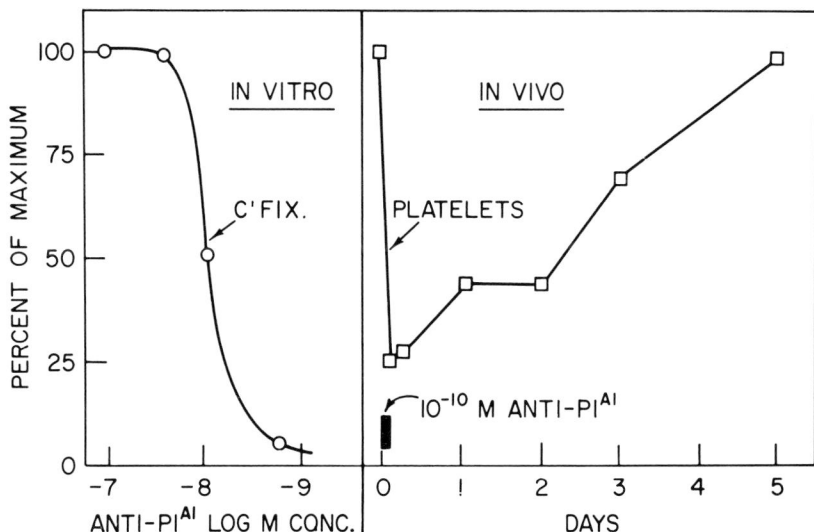

F𝜄ɢ. 19—Comparison of the in vitro and in vivo sensitivity of reactions of an anti-platelet isoantibody. The left graph shows the amount of complement fixed in a standard in vitro system as anti-Pl[A1] concentration was varied in a mixture with platelets. The right graph shows thrombocytopenia produced in vivo by infusing anti-Pl[A1] into a Pl[A1]-positive normal individual at concentrations too low to measure in vitro. The recipient's initial platelet count was 195,000/mm.[3] and his hematocrit was 40 per cent. The platelet concentration in plasma therefore was 320,000/mm.[3] This figure was taken from Ref. 37, courtesy of the publisher.

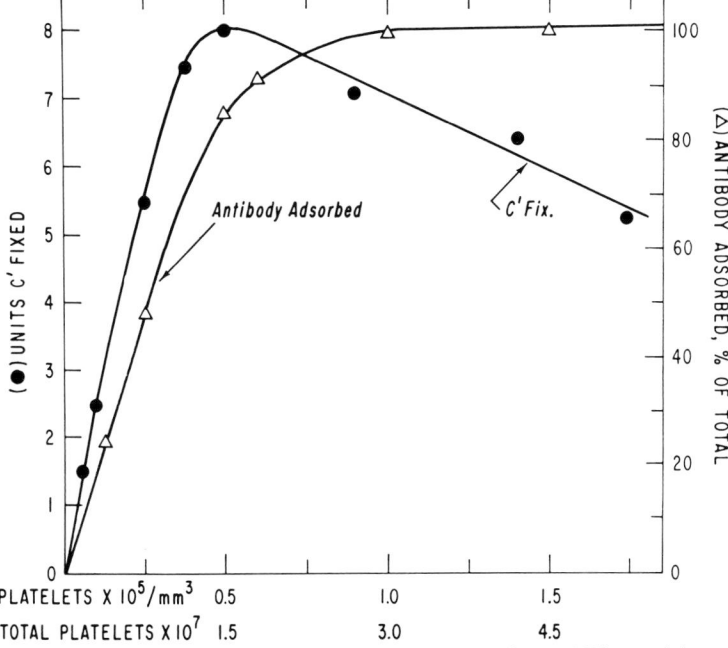

F𝜄ɢ. 20—Adsorption of anti-Pl[A1] by different concentrations of Pl[A1]-positive platelets. Initial anti-Pl[A1] concentration was constant at 10^{-8} M and the amount of antibody adsorbed (open triangles) by different concentration of platelets was determined as in figure 3. At the lower cell concentration, cells were essentially saturated with antibody and the concentration of antigen sites was found to be approximately 10^{-8} M for 50,000 platelets/mm.[3] When this concentration of platelets was present in mixture with 10^{-8} M antibody, 80 per cent of the antibody was adsorbed. This figure is taken from Ref. 36, courtesy of the publisher.

sensitized them for sequestration.[32, 71] Similar quantitative considerations appear to pertain to leukocytes since the amounts of antibody required to produce leukopenia and thrombocytopenia were alike (e.g., fig. 26).

Destruction of platelets by infusion of isoantibodies appeared to be an all-or-none phenomenon.[39] Cells that remained after induction of thrombocytopenia survived normally thereafter, even if half of the initial platelets present were destroyed within an hour (fig. 21). Information presented in figure 21 is relevant to the problems of platelet reserve, production and survival, as well as to immune thrombocytopenia. The stippled area shows the mean and one standard deviation of values for survival of Cr51-labeled platelets in normal persons. In measuring platelet survival, the number of platelets in buttons separated from blood for radioactive measurement were counted and radioactivity was expressed as counts per minute per platelet, or specific activity. The large black symbols

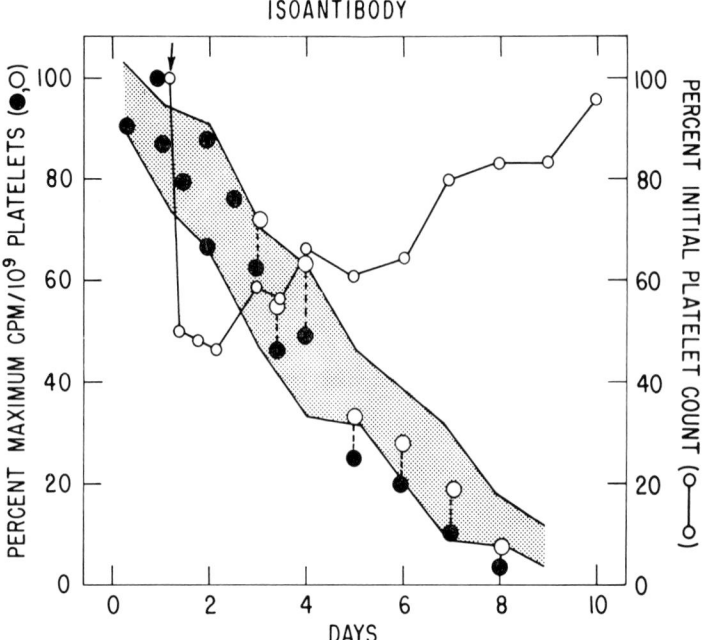

Fig. 21—Thrombocytopenia produced in a normal individual by an isoantibody. Autologous platelets were tagged with Cr151 24 hours before anti-PlA1 was infused. The solid circles are cpm/10⁹ platelets (specific activity) expressed as percent of the maximum, and the stippled area is the range of results obtained in 7 normal individuals over a 9 day period. The large open circles connected to the solid circles are corrections for apparent dilution of tagged platelets by newly formed platelets that entered the circulation in sufficient numbers to increase the count. The platelet count is shown by the small open circles, the arrow indicating the infusion of anti-PlA1. When platelet count increased, for example from the minimum of approximately 50 per cent on day 1 to 80 per cent on day 7, the observed value for cpm/10⁹ platelets (a solid circle) was multiplied by 8/5 to obtain the value shown by the open circle above it.

The initial platelet count was 220,000/mm.³ Drop in platelets to approximately 50 per cent of initial value occurred within 1 hour after start of the infusion. This figure is taken from Ref. 39, courtesy of the publisher.

represent individual measurements of specific activity one day before, during, and for 7 days after infusion of isoantibody. Experiments of this type with both the blocking and C'-fixing forms of several different isoantibodies, have given uniform results.[39] Platelet specific activity did not change during the induction of thrombocytopenia, indicating the absence of any reserve to counteract the thrombocytopenic effects of infused antibodies. After induction of thrombocytopenia, specific activity remained in the normal range, providing corrections were made for return of unlabeled platelets to the circulation (large white symbols above the solid symbols). Thus platelets that initially were insufficiently sensitized for immediate sequestration survived normally, and there was no evidence of return of platelets that were sequestered. In all respects, the effects of isoantibodies on platelets were found to be the same as those of simple mechanical removal of platelets by plasmapheresis.[39, 76]

Similarities between Isoantibodies and ITP Factor

Evidence indicates that the humoral factor responsible for thrombocytopenia in idiopathic purpura is an antibody,[1, 53] namely: the occurrence of thrombocytopenia in infants of mothers with ITP; the ability of ITP plasma to cause thrombocytopenia in normal individuals; and similarities between the clinical picture of ITP and thrombocytopenia caused by heterologous antibodies in animals or drug antibodies in man. Although ITP sera frequently have been found to be non-reactive in immunologic tests in vitro,[39, 77, 78, 79] the platelet-depressing factor in plasma of patients with typical ITP recently has been shown to be present in the 7S gamma globulin fraction of plasma, to be adsorbed by platelets, to affect autologous as well as homologous platelets, and to be species specific.[39, 40] It has been suggested that the inability to measure the ITP factor by serologic technics may simply reflect its low concentration in plasma, for it has been shown that isoantibodies produce thrombocytopenia at concentrations too low to be detected in vitro.[32, 37] However, quantitative aspects of the adsorption of ITP factor by platelets in vitro were similar to those of known platelet isoantibodies, and amounts of plasma from ITP patients that were effective in producing thrombocytopenia by passive transfer were comparable to amounts of plasma from isosensitized individuals.[39, 40] Therefore failure of the ITP factor to react in immunologic tests did not appear to be due to its low concentration, but was explicable on the basis of its serologic similarity to the incomplete forms of platelet isoantibodies. These incomplete or blocking antibodies were identified only fortuitously because a C'-fixing form of antibody with the same specificity was available (see Pl^{A1} and $PlGrLy^{B1}$ antigens), but they proved to be as effective as complete antibodies in causing thrombocytopenia (figs. 17, 18).

*Role of the Spleen and Liver in Thrombocytopenia Induced by Isoantibodies and
    ITP Factor*

The thrombocytopenic response to a given dose of isoantibody was rather uniform for different normal individuals and for the same individual on different occasions. The stippled area of figure 22 shows variations in platelet counts of 4 normal Pl^{A1}-positive individuals given 1.6 ml./Kg. of plasma containing a

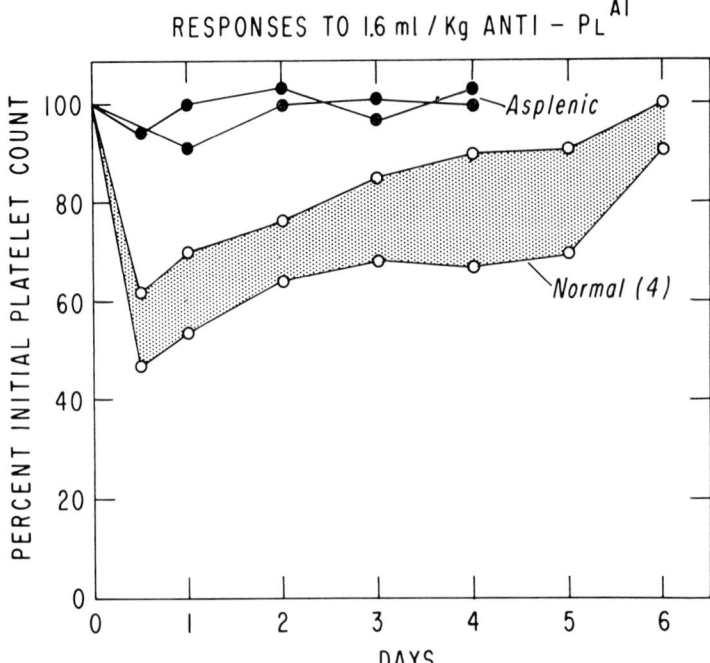

Fig. 22—Responses to one dose of a single isoantibody. The blocking form of anti-Pl[A1] that was used was in the plasma of a mother sensitized by fetal platelets. The dose given was 1.6 ml./Kg. This figure is from Ref. 40, courtesy of the publisher.

blocking form of anti-Pl[A1] from a mother sensitized by fetal platelets. At the top of figure 22 are shown data on two splenectomized individuals who did not respond to the dose that produced sustained thrombocytopenia in normal individuals. However, doses of isoantibodies 5- to 7-fold higher than that used in figure 22 did cause thrombocytopenia in splenectomized individuals. Similar observations have been made on the resistance of splenectomized animals to the thrombocytopenic effect of heterologous anti-platelet serum[80, 81] and on the resistance of splenectomized individuals to the thrombocytopenic effect of ITP plasma.[1, 39] Since it has been found that splenectomy *per se* does not prolong survival[39, 79] of normal platelets or appear to cause increased platelet production,[39] the protection afforded by splenectomy against the thrombocytopenic effect of low doses of isoantibody, heteroantibody or ITP factor can be attributed to removal of a major site for sequestration of lightly sensitized platelets. The fact that splenectomy did not protect against high doses of platelet-depressing agents, indicated that highly sensitized platelets were removed by organs other than the spleen. Intravascular agglutination or C' fixation were not prerequisites for sequestration by the spleen or other organs, for incomplete antibodies were as effective as C'-fixing or agglutinating antibodies in causing sequestration.

Conclusions concerning the patterns of sequestration based on differences in the response of splenectomized and normal individuals were strengthened by studies of organ localization of Cr[51]-labeled platelets sensitized by different concentrations of isoantibodies.[39, 70] Figure 23 shows the accumulation of radioactivity that occurred only in the splenic area when a dose of anti-Pl^{A1} similar to that used in figure 22 was given to an individual whose platelets had been labeled with Cr^{51} prior to infusion of antibody. This dose of anti-Pl^{A1} produced thrombocytopenia in normal, but not in splenectomized individuals. Increases in radioactivity confined to the splenic area occurred also with doses of ITP plasma that produced thrombocytopenia in normal, but not in splenectomized individuals (fig. 23). On the other hand, when isosensitized patients, whose

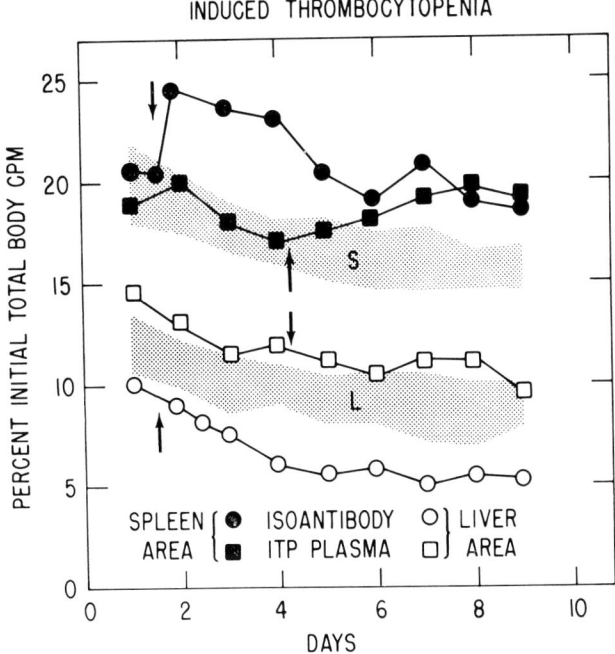

FIG. 23—Localization of radioactivity in normal individuals made thrombocytopenic with isoantibody and ITP plasma. Radioactivity in organ areas is expressed as percent of total body cpm. All counts are corrected for physical decay from the day of infusion. The total body count was obtained with the 18 detectors in a whole-body counter and the spleen or liver count with the one detector nearest each organ. The total count after one day was proportional to the amount of Cr^{51} attached to infused platelets; hence the ratio on the ordinate makes the data from different individuals comparable, even though they were given platelets containing different amounts of Cr^{51}.

The upper shaded area marked S covers one standard deviation from the mean of values for splenic localization of radioactivity in 9 normal individuals and the lower shaded area marked L shows the values for liver localization. The normal S/L ratio of approximately 1.7/1.0, on calibration with a phantom, indicated approximately equal distribution of radioactivity in the two organs; hence about equal participation of spleen and liver in platelet sequestration normally.

The isoantibody experiment (arrows, day 1) is the same as that used to obtain data for figure 21 and the ITP plasma experiment (arrows, day 5) is similar to one shown in figure 17. The decrease in platelets to approximtely 50 per cent after infusion of isoantibody caused an abrupt rise in splenic radioactivity while hepatic radioactivity continued to fall. The amount of radioactivity accumulated in the spleen accounted for almost all of the radioactivity in platelets that were sequestered. The ITP plasma infusion produced a more gradual fall in platelets and a more gradual increase in splenic radioactivity. This figure is from Ref. 39, courtesy of the publisher.

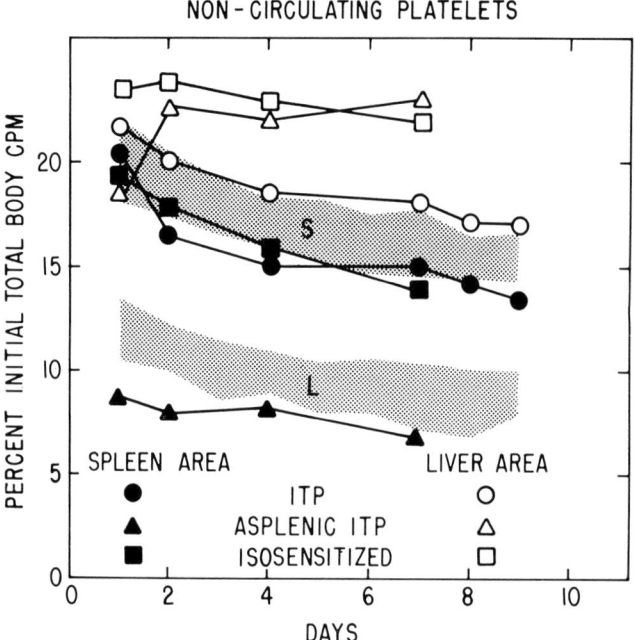

FIG. 24—Localization of radioactivity in patients in whom transfused platelets did not circulate. The isosensitized individual had received a total of 12 transfusions at intervals over a 2-year period for surgical procedures. Autologous Cr[51]-labeled platelets survived normally but the homologous Cr[51]-labeled platelets used did not circulate. Although isoantibody could not be measured in this individual's serum by in vitro tests, her plasma produced thrombocytopenia on passive transfer (fig. 17, solid circles). The patients with ITP had mild symptoms at the time labeled platelets were infused; one ITP patient had been splenectomized. Radioactivity in organ areas was measured as in figure 22 and the shaded areas marked S for spleen activity and L for liver activity of normal individuals are the same as those in figure 23. Note that the open symbols referring to *liver* activity are above normal *splenic* values. These values were consistent with sequestration of approximately 75 per cent of platelets by the liver. The solid circles and squares representing splenic activity were in the normal range when rapid platelet elimination occurred, for the spleen took part in sequestration. The very low splenic level near background activity shown by the solid triangles was obtained on the splenectomized patient. This figure is from Ref. 39.

plasma contained excess antibody, or ITP patients with high levels of ITP factor, were given Cr[51]-labeled homologous platelets that did not circulate, an accumulation of radioactivity appeared predominantly in the hepatic area (fig. 24). Details of the radioactive experiments are given in the legends of figures 23 and 24 and fuller explanation of the methods of measuring organ localization is in Ref. 39.

The findings that platelets lightly sensitized by antibodies are removed mainly in the spleen, whereas highly sensitized platelets are removed primarily in the liver, parallel the findings of Jandl et al.[82] and Cutbush and Mollison[83] on sequestration of red cells altered by isoantibodies. Although the minimum number of antibody molecules required to effect sequestration of erythrocytes has not been determined, comparison of the work of Masouredis[44] with that of Jandl et al. and Cutbush and Mollison, suggests that a similar concentration of antibody on the cell surface of platelets and erythrocytes predisposes to sequestration by the spleen. Masouredis found that D-positive erythrocytes contained 6,400 to 10,300, and C-positive cells, 4,600 to 7,400 antigen sites per cell. Jandl et al. and Cutbush and Mollison found that cells coated with anti-D or anti-C were sequestered primarily in the spleen. In view of the methods used for sensitizing erythrocytes in vitro with anti-D or anti-C, the number of antibodies present on the sequestered erythrocytes were no doubt similar to the values obtained for antigen sites by Masouredis. Since platelets contained 500 to 1000 antibody molecules per cell when sequestered in the spleen by anti-Pl[A1] (see above), and since the surface area of platelets is approximately 1/10 that of erythrocytes, the surface concentration of antibody on both types of cells appears to be similar when splenic sequestration occurs. Erythrocytes approaching saturation with anti-D or anti-C reacted like platelets minimally (1 per cent) saturated with anti-Pl[A1].* Platelets sensitized with 5- to 7-fold, the minimum concentration of anti-Pl[A1], were sequestered primarily by the liver. Some degree of hepatic sequestration was obtained by injecting D-positive or C-positive erythrocytes into patients with high titers of anti-D and anti-C,[82] but erythrocytes more highly sensitized by antibodies other than anti-D or anti-C were sequestered almost completely by the liver.[82, 83]

Effect of Adrenocorticosteroid Hormones

Beneficial effects of adrenocorticosteroid hormone therapy in apparent immune blood cell deficiency states have been ascribed to a variety of possible actions: interference with antigen-antibody union,[84] increased production of cells,[85] decrease in antibody synthesis,[86] direct inhibition of the sequestering function of the reticuloendothelial system,[87] or indirect effects on hepatic sequestration through hemodynamic changes.[88] The effects of prednisone on the thrombocytopenic response to a dose of isoantibody that produced only splenic sequestration is shown in figure 25. Two control infusions, one before and one after steroid therapy, produced the same degree of thrombocytopenia, whereas the infusion given during steroid administration produced almost no response, as though the recipient had been splenectomized. Similar protection was afforded by prednisone against the thrombocytopenic effect of infusions of ITP plasma that produced primarily splenic sequestration.[39] Adrenocorticosteroids therefore appeared to act by inhibiting splenic sequestration of lightly sensitized platelets. Other possible explanations, such as an increase in platelet production, nonspecific prolongation of platelet survival, or interference with antibody attachment, were untenable, for it was found that steroid hormones did not alter platelet survival or increase platelet production in normal individuals and did

* Quantitative aspects of this comparison were corroborated by anti-globulin consumption tests performed as in table 1, with erythrocytes sensitized by anti-D and platelets sensitized by anti-Pl[A1]. It was found that 8×10^8 red cells saturated with anti-D and 10^8 platelets saturated with anti-Pl[A1] bound approximately the same amount of anti-globulin (the value for platelets having been corrected for nonspecific binding). In view of the 10-fold larger erythrocyte surface area, the concentration of antibody on cell surfaces of platelets 1 per cent saturated with anti-Pl[A1] and erythrocytes saturated with anti-D appear to be similar. Antibody distributed this sparsely on cellular surfaces cannot fix measurable amounts of C'.[36, 75]

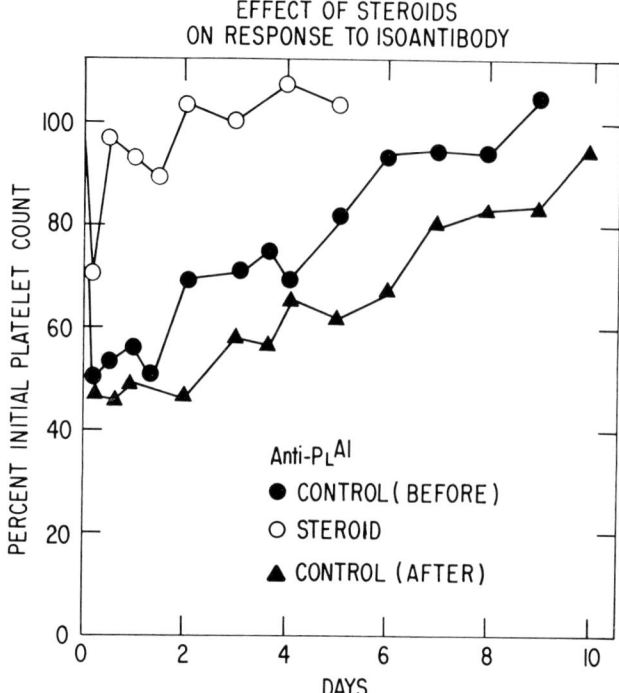

FIG. 25—Effect of prednisone on the response to an isoantibody. Five weeks after receiving 2.0 ml./Kg. of a plasma sample containing a blocking form of anti-Pl^{A1} from a sensitized mother (solid circles), the same recipient received the identical isoantibody infusion, while on 60 mg. prednisone/day for a total period of 8 days beginning 3 days before the second infusion (open circles). The 100 per cent platelet count was 220,000/mm.^{3} for the first control curve and 222,000/mm.^{3} for the curve with steroids. One week after steroids were stopped, when the platelet count was 217,000/mm.^{3}, the same dose of anti-Pl^{A1} produced results shown by the solid triangles. This figure is from Ref. 39, courtesy of the publisher.

not change in vitro reactions of platelets with isoantibodies.[39] Previous observations on failure of adrenocorticosteroids to protect against induction of thrombocytopenia by heterologous anti-platelet serum,[89] barring species difference, may have been due to use of excessive antibody, for the protective effect of adrenocorticosteroids, just like that of splenectomy, could be overcome by increased doses of isoantibody or high concentrations of ITP factor.[39] Beneficial effects of steroid therapy and splenectomy in ITP therefore have the same implications. If the ITP factor is relatively low in titer, and platelets lightly sensitized, splenectomy or steroid inhibition of splenic, and to a lesser extent hepatic, sequestration prevents thrombocytopenia, whereas splenectomy and steroid therapy are not as effective against titers of ITP factor that heavily sensitize platelets and cause primarily hepatic sequestration. These observations also explain the beneficial effects of adrenocorticosteroids in isoimmune neonatal thrombocytopenia.[35]

Experimental Isoimmune Leukopenia in Normal Individuals

Initial investigations of the in vivo effects of isoantibodies that react with leukocytes were prompted by the observation that several different maternal isoantibodies directed against antigens shared by platelets and leukocytes caused only neonatal thrombocytopenia and not concomitant leukopenia[34, 35] (see section on neonatal purpura). The reason for this apparent paradox was evident when maternal antibodies were infused into adult volunteers (fig. 26). During the infusion, initially both platelets and leukocytes fell, as expected, but with continued infusion of antibody, platelets remained low, whereas the leukocyte count increased. If the effects had been measured only after three hours, a deceptive picture of a specific effect on platelets would have been obtained. It could therefore be postulated that maternal isoantibodies cause neonatal thrombocytopenia more often than leukopenia because compensatory mechanisms for maintaining cell levels are much more effective for leukocytes than for platelets. There is essentially no platelet reserve (fig. 21)[39, 76] but the capacity of the marrow to replace granulocytes through reserve pools and regeneration has been calculated to be from 20- to 70-fold that of the circulating cells.[90, 91] This no doubt accounts for the rarity of isoimmune neonatal leukopenia[92] compared to neonatal thrombocytopenia.[35]

The well characterized isoantibodies described above (table 5) were specific for antigens limited to platelets or lymphocytes, or were shared by platelets, granulocytes and lymphocytes. However, in addition to these antibodies, other less well characterized isoantibodies have been found that react with granulocytes and lymphocytes but not platelets (fig. 27), and it can be expected that

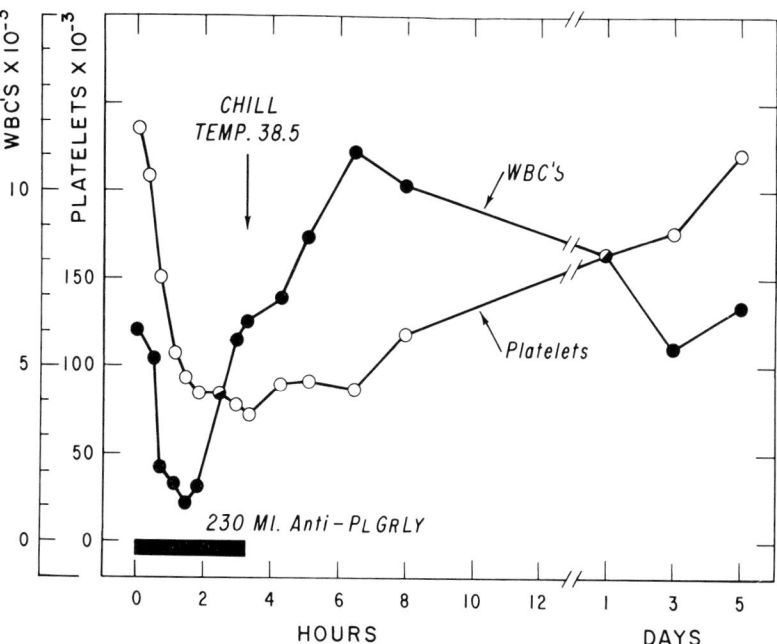

FIG. 26—Transient leukopenia and persistent thrombocytopenia caused by an antibody against an antigen shared by platelets, granulocytes and lymphocytes. The differential leukocyte count remained approximately the same with respect to the proportion of granulocytes and lymphocytes during induction of leukopenia. A marked preponderance of immature granulocytes was present during recovery from leukopenia. This figure is from Ref. 34, courtesy of the publisher.

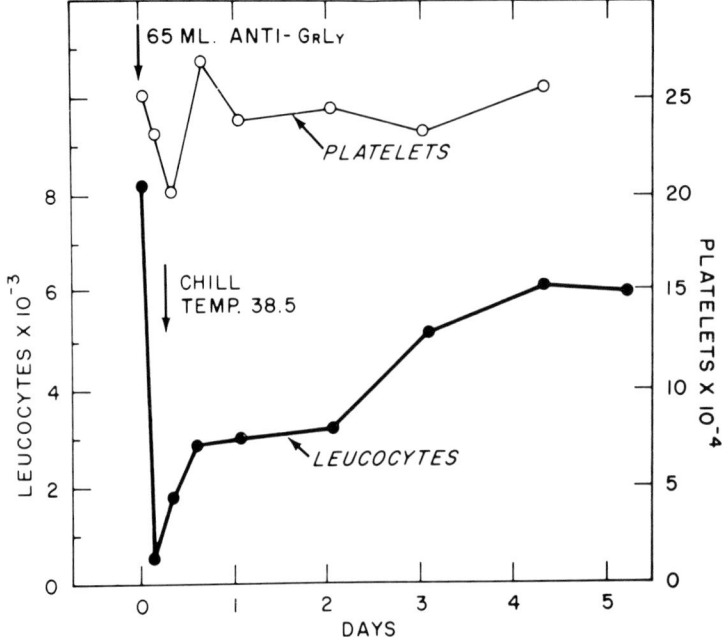

FIG. 27—Persistent leukopenia produced by an antibody against an antigen present on granulocytes and lymphocytes only. An infusion of half this dose in the same individual several months previously had caused less sustained leukopenia and no systemic symptoms except for slight temperature elevation. The differential leukocyte count with respect to the proportion of lymphocytes and granulocytes remained approximately the same during induction of and recovery from leukopenia. There was a marked shift to the left of the granulocytic series during recovery.

antibodies will be found that react with granulocytes only.[93] Although several isoantibodies directed against antigens shared only by granulocytes and lymphocytes have been detected by C′ fixation, the particular antibody used in figure 27 was an incomplete one that could not be studied in vitro because it was detectable only by passive transfer. The marked degree of leukopenia produced by the incomplete isoantibody was associated with only a slight chill and a maximum temperature elevation to 38.5°C. Similar depression of leukocytes with C′-fixing isoantibodies has been associated with more severe symptoms, such as nausea, vomiting, shaking chills and temperature elevation to as high as 40°C. However, too little information is available to know whether C′-fixing leukocyte isoantibodies predispose to more severe reactions than the incomplete forms. Antibodies that react only with leukocytes, as in figure 27, may be suitable for assessing granulocyte reserve in the same manner that endotoxin[94] and typhoid vaccine[95] have been used.

In vivo Effects of Isoantibodies on Leukemic Leukocytes

An example of the in vivo response of chronic lymphatic leukemic cells to a C′-fixing isoantibody is shown in figure 28, and of chronic granulocytic leukemic cells, in figure 29. The amounts of isoantibodies used were selected on the basis of the degree of leukopenia produced in normal individuals by prior infusions of the same antibody. In both instances, many more leukemic cells left the circulation than expected, even though leukemic leukocytes fixed C′ quantitatively like normal leukocytes in vitro (table 3). The same amount of antiserum that caused a depression of 80,000 lymphocytes/mm.³ in the patient with chronic lymphatic leukemia (fig. 28) caused a fall of 5000 leukocytes/mm.³ in a normal individual, and a similar apparent increase in susceptibility to isoantibody was noted in the patient with chronic granulocytic leukemia (fig. 29). Considering the relatively high initial amount of antigen present in leukemic blood by virtue of the elevated white count, and that the amounts of antibody used had caused only moderate leukopenia in normal individuals, it is evident that leukemic cells were highly unsaturated with antibody when sequestered. If the observation reported by Perry et al.[95] that normal leukocytes, once having left the vasculature are unable to re-enter in any significant numbers, applies in the case of leukemic cells under conditions of the experiments shown in figures 28 and 29, then one may conclude that circulating leukemic cells are unusually susceptible to destruction by isoantibodies.

Exploration of the possibilities that isoantibodies may be used as therapeutic agents, either alone or in conjunction with other forms of therapy, in an attempt

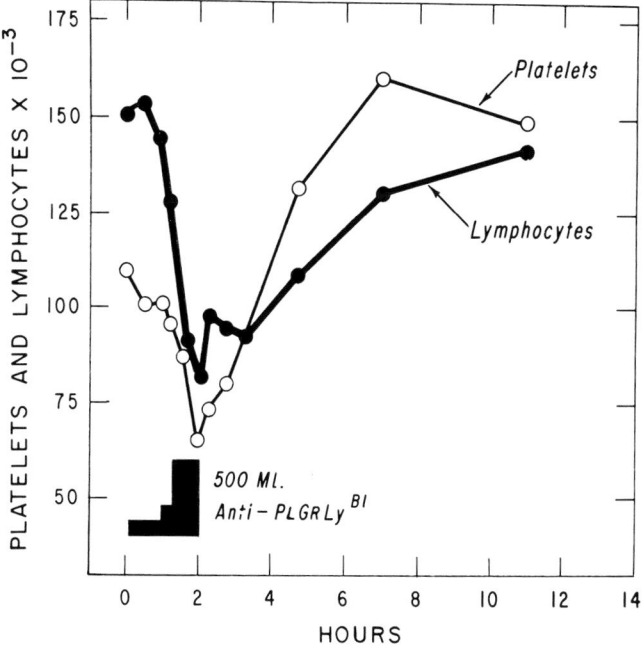

FIG. 28—Marked decrease in a patient with lymphocytes of chronic lymphocytic leukemia caused by isoantibody against shared antigens. The fall in lymphocytes did not cause any subjective symptoms. Five hours later a temperature elevation to 37.8°C. without chills was noted. The unusual increase in platelets within a matter of hours has not been seen in any normal individual in whom thrombocytopenia was produced by isoantibodies. This may represent an instance of temporary sequestration of platelets by a readily reversible antibody that conceivably transferred to lymphocytes. The peculiar platelet response may have been related to the marked splenomegaly that this patient had. This figure is from Ref. 34, courtesy of the publisher.

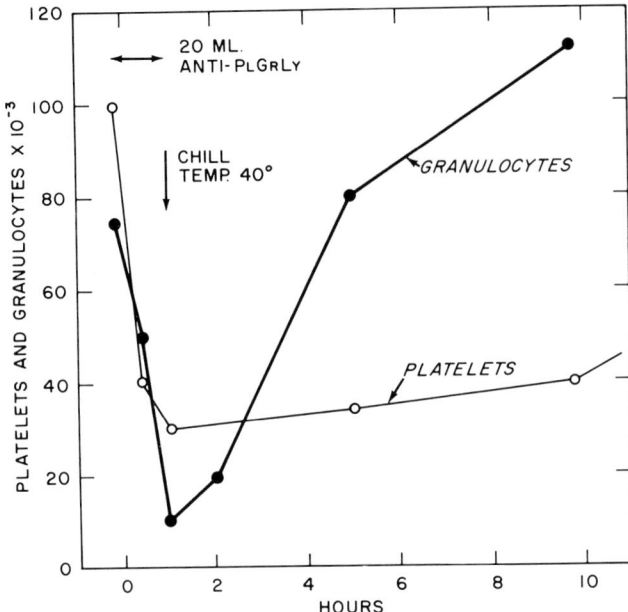

FIG. 29—Marked decrease in granulocytes of chronic myelogenous leukemia caused by an isoantibody against shared antigens. This same antibody had been infused in a normal individual at a dose of 4.6 ml./Kg. to produce the cellular changes shown in figure 26. The dose used in this instance was 1.8 ml./Kg. and the effect was more marked than expected. The temperature elevation was accompanied by shaking chills, cyanosis and transient hypotension.

to produce remissions in leukemia, seems warranted. Under some circumstances, it appears that isoantibodies may be able to affect bone marrow cells in addition to circulating cells, for amegakaryocytosis sometimes accompanies isoimmune neonatal purpura[33, 35] and reduced granulopoiesis has been seen in apparent isoimmune neonatal neutropenia.[93] Although tested in only a few instances (table 3), very immature leukocytes were found to contain the usual concentration of some isoantigens in much the same way that normoblasts at all stages of development contain the blood group antigens, A, B, and H.[96] It is reasonable to expect that antibodies against leukocyte isoantigens may be able to affect bone marrow precursors of malignant cells. The usual isoantibodies found in transfused patients appear to be as suitable for potential therapeutic use as "anti-leukemic leukocyte serum" that might be made by injecting leukemic cells into normal individuals.[97] Caution is indicated in exploring the therapeutic use of isoantibodies in leukemia, not only because of possible serious toxic side effects due to systemic reactions or destruction of normal cells, but also because isoantibodies have been known to enhance tumor growth, albeit not leukemia, in some animal experiments.[98, 99]

Other Applications for Leukocyte and Platelet Isoantibodies

Quantitative C' fixation procedures are uniquely suited for measuring iso-antigenic differences of leukocytes or platelets in mixtures of cells from different individuals, as well as in mixtures of different types of cells from the same individual (figure 13). For example, leukocytes or platelets of distinct antigenic specificity present as a 1 or 2 per cent minority can be easily differentiated by an appropriate isoantibody with which they react if the other 98 or 99 per cent of cells does not contain the same antigen.

By quantitative C′ fixation procedures we have detected antigenically dissimilar platelets and have followed their survival in recipients of usual transfusions; and in one instance, detected an apparent platelet graft in an acute leukemic transfused with chronic myelogenous leukemic blood. Hematopoietic grafts have been reported in some patients with acute leukemia who have been given white cell transfusions obtained from donors with chronic myelogenous leukemia,[100, 101] and occasionally after excessive radiation.[102] The chronic myelogenous leukemic blood grafts are usually detected by the Ph[1] chromosome characteristic of these cells,[100] but a graft detected by a change in erythrocyte blood group from type O to AB has been reported by Bronson et al.[101] It appears possible with C′ fixation procedures not only to detect leukocyte and platelet grafts by changes in blood groups, but also to quantify the proportion of circulating autologous and grafted cells.

In view of the reports of the loss of erythrocyte antigens or blood group modification in association with leukemia or other malignancies,[43] it will be interesting to see what quantitative or qualitative changes may occur in the isoantigens of malignant cells themselves or in normal cells in tissue culture. Mononuclear cells cultured from peripheral blood by the general methods of Hungerford et al.[103] react with isoantibodies against antigens present on lymphocytes (unpublished observations made in association with Dr. William McFarland). These isoantibodies may be useful in distinguishing or selectively destroying mononuclear cells of a particular antigenic type and may even prove useful in identifying precursors of particular cell lines, either in culture or in instances of acute undifferentiated leukemia.

As yet well defined animal platelet and leukocyte isoantibodies comparable to those of human isoantibody systems are not available for physiologic studies. However, the finding by Borel et al.[104] that repeated blood transfusions in rabbits produced isoimmunity detectable by shortened platelet survival and occasionally by formation of platelet agglutinins, suggests that it may be possible to produce type-specific isoantibodies in this species. It is evident that antibodies against the surface isoantigens of leukocytes form in various common laboratory animals, as shown by the frequent development of leukocyte agglutinins in association with transplantation immunity[105] or tumor homograft enhancement.[98, 99] The serologic characteristics and specificity of these isoantibodies are not yet well defined. Physiologic studies in some animals may not be applicable to man in view of the marked quantitative differences in responses of dog and man to a cross-reacting human isoantibody.[32] However, the finding that human isoantibodies frequently react with platelets and leukocytes from a variety of nonhuman primates (tables 7 and 8) promises to permit animal studies that are relevant to human physiology.

Some of the platelet and leukocyte isoantibodies appear to be uniquely suited for studying certain fundamental aspects of antibody function. For instance,

C′-fixing and incomplete antibodies with identical immunologic specificity may afford an opportunity to determine the physical-chemical or structural basis for differences in serological activity; and the C′-fixing monospecific isoantibodies may be used for studying immune damage to platelet and leukocyte membranes in systems analogous to those developed by Green et al.[106, 107] and applied by Sears et al.[108] in characterizing the membrane defects produced by erythrocyte isoantibodies.

CLINICAL CONSIDERATIONS

Clinical consequences of sensitization to platelet and leukocyte isoantigens include (1) refractoriness to therapeutically transfused platelets or leuko-cytes[1, 2, 39, 79, 109] and febrile "buffy coat" reactions common in patients who have received multiple transfusions over protracted periods,[4, 6, 49, 52, 110, 111, 112, 113] (2) neonatal thrombocytopenia and possibly leukopenia due to trans-placental transfer of maternal isoantibodies,[1, 9, 35, 92, 93, 114, 115, 116] and (3) a unique form of purpura resulting from sensitization to transfused Pl^{A1} anti-gen.[32, 36, 38] Information on the frequency of isosensitization with respect to degree of exposure, antigenicity of particular antigens, and anomalous or obscure in vivo reactions of isoantibodies, is pertinent not only to the clinical problems mentioned, but also to prospective problems in the rapidly progressing fields of homo- and hetero-transplantation and immunologic tumor therapy.

Isosensitization by Transfusion

Frequency.—There is general agreement that the frequency with which platelet and leukocyte isoantibodies are detected in the serum of transfused patients increases with increasing numbers of transfusions. After 10 or 11 transfusions, the frequency of detectable antibodies was 5 to 10 per cent, after 11 to 50 trans-fusions, 20 to 35 per cent, and after more than 50 transfusions, 25 to 50 per cent, whether agglutination,[6, 25, 49, 52, 110, 111, 112, 113] anti-globulin consumption,[25, 52, 117] or C′ fixation[25] technics were used. Platelet isoantibodies were found about as frequently as leukocyte isoantibodies. Since none of the various serologic tests is capable of detecting all isoantibodies[25, 52, 117] (table 5), the frequency with which antibodies were found by utilizing one technic and either platelets or leukocytes, was much less than it would have been if all techniques and both types of cells had been used. Moreover, it is apparent that isoimmunization may occur with production of incomplete antibodies that cannot be detected by usual serologic technics, as in the case of blocking antibodies (see Serology) and anti-bodies detectable only by passive transfer of plasma (e.g. figs. 17 and 27) or by shortened survival of transfused cells[79, 109] (e.g. fig. 24). Therefore the true frequency of isosensitization by transfusion may be as high as double the reported values.

The patients that we tested for isoantibodies are listed in table 9. This series is somewhat selected, for a number of patients came to our attention because of febrile transfusion reactions or refractoriness to platelet transfusion. Most of the sera in which antibodies were detected could not be utilized for blood grouping studies because the antibodies either were too weak to be efficiently concentrated or were in mixtures that were difficult to separate. The highest

TABLE 9.—*Relationship between Number of Transfusions and Frequency of Developing C'-Fixing Isoantibodies*

Number of Transfusions	Number of Patients Tested	Number with C'-Fixing Platelet or Leukocyte Isoantibodies	Antigenic Specificity of Sera		
			Multiple	Single	Uncertain
1–10	97*	7*	2	4*	1
11–50	44	7	4	1	2
>50	69	14	10	0	4
>50 + reactions	18	8	8	0	0

* Including 3 patients with post-transfusion purpura whose serum contained anti-Pl^A1.

Most of the patients who were repeatedly transfused received small amounts of blood at intervals over a period of several weeks to several years. Patients exposed to large doses of antigen all at once, as in cardiac surgery with extracorporeal circulation, were not included in this series. The type of transfusion reactions referred to is described in the section on "buffy coat" reactions.

titered C'-fixing isoantibodies were usually found in those patients who had received more than 50 transfusions and had frequent febrile, "buffy coat" reactions. Antibodies were detected in approximately 50 per cent of this group, and although their sera contained mixtures of isoantibodies (table 9), individual antibodies were usually present in sufficiently high titer to permit efficient separation by adsorption and elution techniques.

The frequency with which C'-fixing platelet isoantibodies were detected in individuals refractory to platelet transfusions, or in whom homologous Cr^51-labeled platelets did not circulate, is shown in table 10. All patients were presumed to be isosensitized by virtue of having received previous transfusions. Most of the patients with aplastic anemia, chronic leukemia or lymphoma had received more transfusions over longer periods of time than the other patients

TABLE 10.—*Detection of C'-Fixing Isoantibodies in Patients in Whom Homologous Platelets Did Not Circulate*

Diagnosis	Number	Number Having C'-Fixing Antibody
Aplastic anemia	14	9
Chronic leukemia	6	3
Lymphoma	3	2
Acute leukemia	11	2
Surgery	2	0
Total	36	16

Patients with aplastic anemia, chronic leukemia and lymphoma had been treated for four months to several years with from 8 to over 50 transfusions. Many of these patients had typical "buffy coat" reactions with some transfusions. The patients with acute leukemia had been treated for a period of several weeks to several months with 6 to 20 blood and platelet transfusions. The patients treated for surgical hemorrhage had received a total of 8 and 12 transfusions, respectively, two or three at a time, over a period of approximately one year for different procedures.

and many had febrile transfusion reactions. The patients with acute leukemia generally had received fewer transfusions over much shorter periods of time. About half the patients with decreased platelet survival had isoantibodies in their sera detectable by C' fixation and none had platelet agglutinins. Results of anti-globulin consumption tests performed with eight of the sera containing C'-fixing antibodies were negative in seven instances and weakly positive in one.

Shortened platelet survival without detectable platelet isoantibodies may reflect either early low-titered isoimmunization, as suggested by the work of Borel et al. in rabbits[104] and observations of Baldini et al. in man,[109] or simply formation of a type of antibody that will not give positive results with immunologic tests currently available. The latter was found to be the case in two patients listed in table 10 whose plasma was non-reactive in vitro but contained high-titered incomplete platelet and leukocyte isoantibodies when assayed by passive transfer (e.g., fig. 17). Erythrocyte isoantibodies on occasion also may be undetectable by serologic tests, yet cause cellular destruction in vivo.[118, 119]

Experimental immunization.—Few systematic studies of isosensitization have been carried out. In 1958 Marchal et al.[120] immunized six individuals with 75 ml. of whole blood from single donors each week for 12 to 19 weeks. Leuko-agglutinins appeared in 4 of the recipients by the 7th transfusion, but only a single very weak platelet agglutinin appeared after the 18th transfusion in one recipient. The leukoagglutinins, although stimulated by blood from single donors, reacted as though they were mixtures of antibodies with a broad pattern of activity similar to sera from patients who had received multiple transfusions. Brittingham and Chaplin,[121] on immunizing a normal individual with leukemic leukocytes, obtained a leukoagglutinin that reacted with almost all normal leukocytes. The leukoagglutinin appeared after 10 intravenous infusions of leukemic leukocytes from one donor over a period of 20 weeks, but in vivo survival of the infused leukocytes was shortened after only five infusions. A very weak platelet agglutinin developed in association with the strong leukoagglutinins. Baldini et al.[109] infused 10 normal individuals with platelet concentrates from 500 ml. of blood at weekly intervals and found that after 2 to 8 weeks all had developed isoimmunity as demonstrated by reduced survival of Cr51-labeled homologous platelets although no isoantibodies were detected by serologic technics.

In contrast to the frequent immunization observed in these studies, Freireich et al.[122] found that 28 children with acute leukemia who were treated with multiple platelet transfusions from one or two donors over periods up to 18 weeks did not develop resistance to platelet transfusions. Salmon and Schwartz[110] also noted that isoimmunization after multiple transfusions was relatively rare in acute leukemia. Failure to become sensitized could not be attributed entirely to the immunosuppressive effect of anti-leukemic therapy, for the antibody response of a similar group of acute leukemics to other antigens was found to be nearly normal.[123] Since the donors studied by Freireich et al. were usually one or both of the patient's parents, the likelihood of transfusing antigens was no doubt less than if random donors had been used. Moreover, there may have been a degree of immune tolerance against dissimilar antigens on maternal platelets and leukocytes that are known to cross the placenta.[124] The patients studied by Freireich et al. therefore are a very special group, not necessarily comparable with patients with acute leukemia treated with transfusions from random donors (table 10) and certainly not comparable with patients who receive multiple transfusions for other disorders.

"Buffy coat" reactions.—Recipients of many transfusions[6, 49, 52, 110, 111, 112] and multiparous women[4, 8, 34, 52] show an increased frequency of isoimmunization against not only leukocyte and platelet antigens, but also against minor erythrocyte blood group antigens[110, 111, 112] and plasma components.[125] Any of these isoantibodies may be responsible for transfusion reactions. However, isoantibodies against minor erythrocyte antigens usually are detected in the major cross-match by appropriate serologic tests[126] and the antigens are not transfused; isosensitization against protein constituents very rarely has been implicated in transfusion reactions,[127, 128] and there is general agreement that isoimmune destruction of platelets is usually a relatively asymptomatic occurrence.[6, 10, 16, 25, 34, 49, 73] By exclusion and also by appropriate tests with leukocyte-rich and leukocyte-poor fractions of whole blood,[6, 10, 52] immune destruction of leukocytes has been found to be the most frequent cause of significant febrile transfusion reactions characterized[6] by (1) immediate flush and tachycardia with transient leukopenia and subsequent leukocytosis, (2) an asymptomatic latent period of 15 to 60 minutes after beginning of the transfusion, and (3) delayed onset of frank rigor and rapid rise in temperature associated with diastolic hypertension, headache and prostration.

The frequency of detecting leukocyte agglutinins in patients who had "buffy coat" reactions varied from approximately 12 per cent to 67 per cent in different series.[52, 110, 111, 112] Generally leukoagglutinins were found more frequently and in higher titer in the patients with more severe reactions. However, some patients had severe reactions in the absence of leukoagglutinins and other patients did not have febrile reactions when leukoagglutinins were present in relatively high titer.[52, 110, 112, 113] We have confirmed these various findings. Patients who had febrile transfusion reactions had the highest incidence of C'-fixing isoantibodies (table 9); serologically undetectable isoantibodies could cause febrile reactions on passive transfer; and an occasional patient whose serum contained high-titered C'-fixing isoantibodies gave inconstant systemic responses to infusions of incompatible leukocytes from different donors. The latter occurrence could be attributed to the varied antigenic make-up of incompatible cells that were infused and mixtures of isoantibodies in the plasma of the recipients that produced a variety of antigen-antibody combinations, some of which caused systemic reactions more readily than others. It is possible that avidity of leukocyte isoantibodies as well as their titer determines the severity of systemic reactions, for the occasional platelet isoantibodies that have caused transfusion reactions[27, 32] have had the highest affinity for antigen (see Footnote, page 254).

Severity of reactions is influenced not only by the nature of the antibody, but also by the amount of antigen and the rate at which it is infused. "Buffy coat" reactions can be greatly diminished by transfusing washed or dextran-sedimented[52, 129] erythrocytes that contain 20 per cent or less of the leukocytes in whole blood, or sometimes by simply decreasing the rate at which blood is given. When these measures are not effective, it should not be forgotten that prophylactic administration of antipyretics and/or adrenocorticosteroids are most helpful in ameliorating or preventing febrile transfusion reactions.

Isoimmune Neonatal Purpura

Isoimmune neonatal thrombocytopenic purpura occurs only about once or twice per 10,000 births and is frequently benign and self-limited.[35, 114, 130, 131] However, serious complications and death may occur in the more severely affected infants.[35, 130, 131] In our own series, and in a review of reported cases,[35] the mortality without treatment was approximately 13 per cent. Recently C' fixation technics have been found to be most useful in detecting and characterizing the isoantibodies responsible for neonatal purpura[33, 34, 55] and in distinguishing the isoimmune form from that due to metabolic or anatomic disorders, infections, or trans-placental transfer of maternal ITP factor. If the physician is alerted to the possibility of neonatal thrombocytopenia by its previous occurrence in a family, the likelihood of recurrence frequently can be predicted by serologic tests during subsequent pregnancies;[35] and on the basis of these findings and the condition of the infant shortly after birth, appropriate effective therapy can be instituted.

Serologic aspects.—Table 11 shows the frequency of detecting isoantibodies in sera of 72 normal mothers whose infants had neonatal purpura. Agglutination tests, C' fixation tests and tests for blocking antibodies were performed with these sera. Agglutinins alone were detected in approximately 5 per cent of these sera, but were not sufficiently strong to give the clear-cut results necessary for establishing blood group antigen specificity. Approximately 17 per cent of the maternal sera contained C'-fixing isoantibodies and an additional 29 per cent had detectable blocking antibodies. The remaining 49 per cent had no detectable antibodies by the three serologic tests used. Sera containing C'-fixing or blocking antibodies did not agglutinate platelets. All maternal sera that were positive in the C' fixation test, and 7 sera containing the blocking form of anti-Pl^{A1}, gave negative anti-globulin consumption tests; 3 sera containing blocking anti-Pl^{A1} gave weakly positive anti-globulin consumption tests. A sporadic additional antibody may have been detected had the anti-globulin consumption test been used with all negative sera.[9] Since half the detected antibodies were the blocking type, it appears that more instances of maternal isoimmunization will be recognized by blocking tests (see table 2) when additional monospecific C'-fixing isoantibodies are defined.

TABLE 11.—*Serology of Normal Mothers whose Infants Had Neonatal Purpura*

Mothers Tested	Types of Antibodies Found						No Detectable Antibody	
	Agglutin-ating		C'-Fixing		Blocking			
Number	Number	%	Number	%	Number	%	Number	%
72	4	5	12	17	21	29	35	49

Eight of the mothers were reported previously.[33, 34, 35] Tests for blocking antibodies were performed as in table 2, using C'-fixing forms of anti-Pl^{A1}, -PlGrLy^{B1}, -PlGrLy^{C1}, -Pl^{E1} and -Pl^{E2} in mixtures with maternal sera. Agglutination tests were performed with a panel of platelets from 10 donors by the method of Dausset and Malinvaud.[26] Maternal sera were obtained in all instances within a month after birth of the purpuric infant.

Isoantibodies found in maternal serum generally were not detectable in serum from cord blood. Only one of eight cord sera gave positive results and this was in an unusually severe case in which the newborn infant's platelet count was 8000/mm.[3] and megakaryocytes were absent. The responsible antibody was a low-affinity C'-fixing form of anti-PlGrLy[B1] that was barely detectable at 1/10 the titer in maternal serum. High affinity anti-Pl[A1] antibodies have not been detected in cord blood no doubt because they are completely adsorbed by the infant's platelets.

Platelets from the mother, father and infant were phenotyped in 15 of 21 instances in which maternal blocking antibodies were detected and in all 12 instances in which C'-fixing antibodies were measured (table 12). Specificity of all antibodies was consistent with the phenotypic maternal-fetal incompatibility. In 4 instances in which platelets from family members were available for phenotyping, but no maternal antibody was detected, incompatibility in the Pl[A1] system was found. This was rather conclusive evidence for isoimmunization as the cause of neonatal purpura, for Pl[A1] incompatibility occurs rarely in the general population, yet is the most frequent basis for maternal sensitization (table 12). The many families studied were brought to our attention by physicians throughout the country. It was feasible to phenotype these families because 20 ml. of whole blood or 10 ml. of platelet-rich plasma, shipped over periods as long as 3 days with no special precautions (see Appendix) provided sufficient platelets for use in C' fixation tests with 6 to 10 antisera.

Potency of specific antigens.—Specificities of maternal isoantibodies that were detected are shown in table 12. Of 33 maternal sera containing C'-fixing or blocking antibodies, 28 were definitely monospecific and the other 5, although not fully characterized, appeared to be monospecific as well. Anti-Pl[A1], the most frequent cause of neonatal purpura, was always in the blocking form. Although incompatibility of Pl[A1] occurs in less than 3 per cent of pregnancies, anti-Pl[A1] accounted for 46 per cent of detected antibodies and 29 per cent of the 72 suspected cases of isoimmune neonatal purpura. It is evident that Pl[A1] is a relatively potent antigen. The next most potent antigen appeared to be PlGrLy[B1] which is incompatible in 15 per cent of pregnancies and accounted for 20 per cent of

TABLE 12.—*Antigenic Specificity of Maternal Isoantibodies*

Specificity	C'-Fixing Antibodies	Blocking Antibodies
Pl[A1]	0	17
PlGrLy[B1]	5	3
PlGrLy[C1]	1	1
Pl[E2]	1	0
Not established	5	
Total	12	21

Although sera of 10 mothers had antibodies directed against antigens shared by platelets and leukocytes, only neonatal thrombocytopenia occurred. None of the thrombocytopenic infants had significant abnormalities of total or differential leukocyte count. High granulocyte reserve[34, 90, 91] (fig. 26) and essentially no platelet reserve[34, 39, 76] (fig. 21) appears to account for this paradox.

detected antibodies and 11 per cent of suspected cases of neonatal purpura. Too little information was available on other antigens to draw conclusions about their relative potency. In any case, it is not yet clear whether frequency of detecting a specific antibody is related so much to potency of the antigen as to fortuitous characteristics that determine the ease with which an antibody is revealed by serologic tests.

The ability of antigens to sensitize mothers during the first pregnancy may be an index of their potency. Table 13 shows the parity and serology of 51 normal mothers whose children were suspected of having isoimmune neonatal purpura. Of all suspected cases, 49 per cent were in the first, 20 per cent in the second, 14 per cent in the third, and 18 per cent in the fourth or later born children. Limiting the analysis to those mothers in whom serologic evidence of immunization was obtained, including mothers phenotypically incompatible with Pl^{A1}, 41 per cent were immunized during the first pregnancy, 26 per cent during the second, 18 per cent during the third, and 19 per cent during the fourth or subsequent pregnancies. The highest incidence of immunization occurred during the first pregnancy, not only against the Pl^{A1} antigen, but also against other platelet antigens, including those shared with leukocytes. Platelet and leukocyte isoantigens appear to act like A and B erythrocyte antigens that stimulate "immune" antibodies as often in the first as in subsequent pregnancies,[126] in contrast to the Rh antigens that very rarely immunize during the first pregnancy.

Physiologic aspects.—Bone marrow aspirates taken from purpuric infants within two days of birth have shown two general patterns of megakaryocyte activity.[35] Normal to increased numbers of megakaryocytes were seen in six cases and amegakaryocytosis in two cases. The two cases with amegakaryocytosis had severe thrombocytopenia, but equally severe thrombocytopenia was seen in some cases with normal or increased megakaryocytes. The two instances of amegakaryocytosis were associated with C'-fixing isoantibodies (anti-$PlGrLy^{B1}$ and anti-$PlGrLy^{C1}$) whereas the bone marrow of five infants affected by the blocking form of anti-Pl^{A1} and one infant affected by C'-fixing anti-$PlGrLy^{B1}$ contained plentiful megakaryocytes. Megakaryocytes may contain the $PlGrLy^{B1}$ and $PlGrLy^{C1}$ isoantigens as do immature leukocytes (see table 3), and may be

TABLE 13.—*Serology and Parity of Normal Mothers Whose Infants Had Neonatal Purpura*

Para	Number	Specificity of Maternal Antibody					Mother $Pl^A(2,2)$ Infant $Pl^A(1,2)$	No Serologic Evidence
		Pl^{A1}	$PlGrLy^{B1}$	$PlGrLy^{C1}$	Pl^{E2}	Other		
1	25	6	1	1	1	1	1	14
2	10	4	1				2	3
3	7	3				1	1	2
4 or >	9	1	3					5
Total	51	14	5	1	1	2	4	24

Detailed histories and cells for phenotyping were available on these 51 families. Phenotypic incompatibility in the Pl^A system (next to last column) was strong evidence for isoimmunization being the cause of neonatal purpura (see text). Only the first instance of neonatal purpura in each family is included.

unusually susceptible to the cytotoxic action of isoantibodies, compared to the granulocytic precursors that were not affected. However, additional observations are needed to determine whether the effect on megakaryocytes is due primarily to the C′-fixing property of certain isoantibodies, the presence of only certain isoantigens on megakaryocytes, or to factors not related to direct cytotoxic effects. That obscure, indirect factors may be involved is suggested by the occasional association of hypomegakaryocytosis with non-isoimmune forms of neonatal purpura, for instance, due to septicemia or Fanconi syndrome.[35, 130, 131, 132]

The maternal platelet and leukocyte isoantibodies studied so far have all been 7S gamma globulin (see section on Serology) and would be expected to pass freely across the placenta.[133, 134] Titers of maternal isoantibodies have varied from the more usual low levels that most likely would sensitize fetal platelets for sequestration only by the spleen (see figs. 18, 22, 23) to occasional high levels that could sensitize fetal platelets for hepatic sequestration (e.g., fig. 24). Most infants who develop neonatal purpura are not born severely thrombocytopenic or purpuric, but become so within several minutes to several hours after birth. This suggests that sensitized platelets are not sequestered as readily in the fetus as they are in the newborn infant. That the fetal reticuloendothelial system, particularly that of the spleen, may not be fully functioning is suggested by observations on fetal lambs that thorotrast is not removed by the spleen until after cessation of placental blood flow.[135] Therefore, it appears that fetal platelets are protected from relatively low doses of maternal isoantibody by a circumstance equivalent to splenectomy (see fig. 22). Therapeutic agents, such as adrenocorticosteroids, that interfere with sequestration of minimally sensitized platelets (see fig. 25), given ante partum may traverse the placenta in sufficient amounts to exert a protective effect on the infant during the stresses of birth. If relatively high levels of maternal isoantibody enter the fetal circulation, sensitization of platelets may be sufficient to produce a degree of hepatic sequestration that cannot be overcome by steroid therapy (see section on Pathophysiology). This form of sequestration no doubt has occurred when severe thrombocytopenia and extensive hemorrhage is present at birth. Under these circumstances, exchange transfusion is the only effective therapy.

Therapeutic aspects.—Because the severity of neonatal purpura varies markedly, it has been difficult to compare therapeutic requirements in different small series of cases. However, it seems clear that the major cause of death is intracranial hemorrhage. The following findings, premonitory of this serious complication, therefore should be considered indications for exchange transfusion:[35] thrombocytopenia below 30,000/mm.³ at birth and below 10,000/mm.³ several hours thereafter, high reticulocytosis or normoblastemia, amegakaryocytosis, early jaundice, and melena or hematuria in addition to extensive petechiae, ecchymoses and hematomas. Exchange transfusion has been immediately and completely effective in stopping hemorrhagic manifestations of severely affected infants.[35] On occasion exchange transfusion has been necessary to prevent kernicterus (e.g. fig. 31) when extensive tissue hemorrhage resulted in formation of excessive bilirubin that was not excreted because of the physiologic deficiency of hepatic glucuronyl transferase in the neonatal period.[35]

When platelet levels were 50,000/mm.³ or above at birth and did not fall precipitously, and hemorrhagic manifestations were not extensive, evaluation of effectiveness of therapy was difficult because of the tendency for spontaneous improvement. By comparing results of different forms of therapy in sequential pregnancies (figs. 30, 31), taking into account antibody titers, it appeared that prophylactic ante partum steroid therapy may have benefitted infants in those instances in which neonatal thrombocytopenia could be anticipated on the basis of serologic tests.[35] Steroid therapy to the infant also appeared to shorten the duration of thrombocytopenia.

An attempt was made to predict the occurrence of neonatal purpura by performing serial tests for antibody on eight mothers whose previous infants had had isoimmune neonatal purpura. Three of the mothers who had been sensitized to Pl^{A1} developed anti-Pl^{A1} again during the 6th to 9th month of pregnancy and their infants had neonatal purpura, as predicted. One infant was so severely affected that immediate exchange transfusion was necessary. Four of the mothers, one previously sensitized to Pl^{A1}, two to PlGrLy^{B1}, and one to PlGrLy^{C1}, did not develop detectable antibodies during subsequent pregnancies and their infants were unaffected. In one instance neonatal thrombocytopenia was predicted on the basis of finding an increased titer of a pre-existing anti-PlGrLy^{C1} during the 7th to 9th month of pregnancy, but the infant was not thrombocytopenic although his cells contained the antigen. This circumstance also occurs in ABO hemolytic disease of the newborn, for the chances that an incompatible infant will show hemolysis are about 1 in 3 if the mother's serum contains an

Platelet Types of Family H Determined With Anti-Pl^{A1}

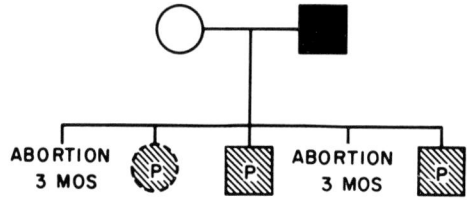

Fig. 30—Pedigree of a family in which three children had neonatal purpura due to anti-Pl^{A1}. Symbols are the same as in figure 2. The first and fourth pregnancies ended in abortion. The full term infant resulting from the second pregnancy was covered with petechiae at birth, had a large cephalohematoma and remained severely thrombocytopenic for at least one week (see fig. 31). This child died at 18 months of extreme hydrocephalus, possibly related to neonatal intracranial hemorrhage. Maternal serum was not available during the second pregnancy. During the third pregnancy, antibody could not be detected in the mother's serum. During the 5th pregnancy, maternal antibody was not detected from the fourth to the sixth month, but during the seventh month a blocking form of anti-Pl^{A1} appeared at ¼ titer and persisted at the same titer until term. The ability of this isoantibody to cause thrombocytopenia was tested by giving 275 ml. of maternal plasma, obtained two days postpartum, to a 55 Kg. Pl^{A1}-positive normal individual. Platelets in the recipient fell from 290,000/mm.³ to 120,000/mm.³ within 60 minutes and remained depressed for three days. The dilution of maternal plasma in the recipient when thrombocytopenia occurred was ⅑, a dilution too high to give positive in vitro tests for blocking antibody. This family and 5 other families in which isoimmune neonatal purpura occurred are presented in detail in reference 35, courtesy of the publisher.

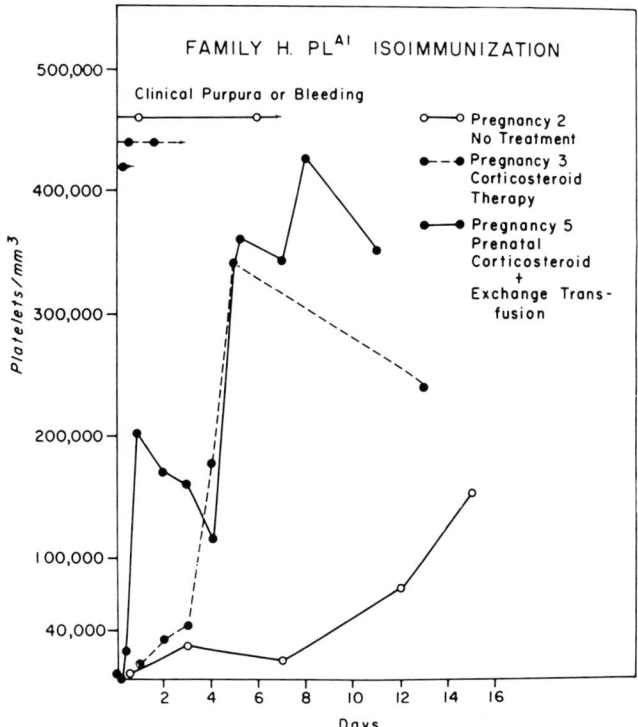

FIG. 31—Platelet counts and clinical courses of three infants with neonatal purpura in the family of figure 30. No specific therapy was given to the first full term infant (pregnancy 2). The second infant (pregnancy 3) was treated with 40 mg. of cortisone/day for 4 days. Neonatal thrombocytopenia was anticipated in the fifth pregnancy on the basis of serologic findings. Since steroids pass the placenta, the mother was given 60 mg. of prednisone/day at term in an attempt to produce a therapeutic steroid level in the infant for its possible beneficial effects during birth. Labor was induced by amniotomy after two days of steroid therapy and four hours later the infant was born. Generalized petechiae appeared within two minutes after delivery and progressed over the next two hours. The platelet count on cord blood was 4000/mm.^{3} and the count on the infant's blood, 1000/mm.^{3} four hours after birth. Megakaryocytes were normal. Exchange transfusion, performed at four hours with fresh Pl^{A1}-positive blood, caused no symptoms; six hours following the exchange, platelet count was 22,500/mm.^{3} and twelve hours later, 210,000/mm.^{3} Bilirubin rose over the next four days to 24.2 mg. per cent and another exchange transfusion was performed at this time to prevent kernicterus. This figure is from reference 35, courtesy of the publisher.

immune form of anti-A or anti-B.[136] When serologic tests are performed on multiparous women, it should be realized that, although most maternal isoantibodies decay to undetectable levels within several months to a year, some may persist at relatively high titers for many years.[33] Therefore, finding a platelet isoantibody in a pregnant multiparous woman does not necessarily mean that the fetus under gestation stimulated it. Moreover approximately 3 per cent of multiparous women have C'-fixing platelet isoantibodies with no history of an affected infant.[34]

In the event that exchange transfusion may be necessary, fresh blood containing non-reactive platelets probably would be optimal. Donors can be typed for this purpose within a matter of hours, but some types, such as Pl^{A1}-negative platelets, are rarely available. However, antigenic platelets can be infused in the face of high-titered C'-fixing or blocking forms of platelet isoantibodies usually without causing systemic reactions, particularly if the infusion is carried out slowly. Moreover, combination of antibody with infused antigenic platelets results in sequestration of the complex, hence more effective removal of antibody than by mechanical exchange alone (see fig. 33). If the antibody happens to be against antigens shared by leukocytes and platelets, transfusions may produce serious reactions for immune destruction of leukocytes is not as innocuous as that of platelets (see section on "buffy coat" reactions).

Neonatal Isoimmune Leukopenia

Neonatal leukopenia caused by transplacental transfer of maternal isoantibodies must be extremely rare, for there are only a few reports of its occurrence.[93, 116, 137, 138, 139] Differentiation of suspected isoimmune neonatal neutropenia from that caused by sepsis has been difficult because most reported cases have had infections when the cellular deficiency was first discovered (see discussion in Ref. 92). The usual maternal agglutinating and C'-fixing isoantibodies against fetal leukocytes do not cause neonatal leukopenia, for in large surveys these antibodies have been detected in up to 20 per cent of multiparous mothers of normal infants.[8, 34, 50, 111] Most maternal leukocyte isoantibodies no doubt cross the placenta, for all those tested so far have been 7S gamma globulin (see Serology). The apparent refractoriness of the fetus to these antibodies can be explained by compensatory leukocyte production sufficient to overcome the effects of the usual relatively low-titered maternal isoantibodies (see fig. 26). However, compensatory mechanisms can be inadequate against relatively high-titered antibody, as shown in figure 27. Neonatal neutropenia may be limited to those instances in which the titer of maternal isoantibody is unusually high, perhaps because of an exceptional exposure to antigen. This appeared to be the case in a family report by Braun et al.[93] The mother had received a blood transfusion from her husband prior to the birth of the first of 3 affected children. The high-titered isoantibody that was measured in her serum at the birth of the third affected child apparently destroyed the infant's granulopoietic cells in the bone marrow as well as circulating granulocytes.

Post-Transfusion Purpura

Destruction of autologous cells usually is not considered among the possible consequences of isoimmunity. However, we have described a syndrome[35,36] in which sensitization to a transfused platelet isoantigen causes destruction of platelets and purpura in the sensitized individual. This syndrome of post-transfusion purpura closely resembles drug purpura in its initiation by a foreign antigen, its acute onset, and its fulminant but self-limited course. Both drug purpura and post-transfusion purpura were differentiated from acute ITP only by demonstrating that a foreign antigen caused sensitization. The mechanism by which sensitization to foreign antigens can destroy autologous blood cells has implications in the pathogenesis of idiopathic blood cell deficiency states and other suspected autoimmune disorders.

Clinical observations.—Table 14 and figure 32 summarize the course of post-transfusion purpura in 3 patients we observed,[32, 36] and in 2 cases from the litera-

TABLE 14.—*Summary of the Clinical Course of Five Cases of Post-Transfusion Purpura*

Case	Sex/Age	Initial Trans-fusion Units	Post-transfusion Thrombocytopenic State							Treatment
			Purpura Onset Days	Mega-karyocytes	Antibody			Duration		
					Anti-	Maxi-mum* Titer	Pre-sent† Days	Pur-pura Days	Low Plates Days	
1	F 40	2	7	Normal	Pl[A1]	100	20	3	6	Exchange Transfusion
2	F 42	1	6	Normal	Pl[A1]	15	18	20	30	ACTH + Prednisone
3	F 41	6‡	3 to 7‡	Normal	Pl[A1]	12	24	3	24	ACTH + Prednisone
4	F 56§	1	5	Normal	?	~100	>15	20	25	ACTH + Prednisone
5	F 51‖	1	7	Increased	Pl[A1](Zw)	~100	>60	8	25	None

* Titer in patient of Zucker and associates[45]§ and patient of van Loghem, Dorfmeijer, and van der Hart[27]‖ (last 2 patients) estimated from reported agglutinin titer. Specificity of antibody in Zucker's case not known; that of van Loghem's case same as Pl[A1] by exchange of serum.

† At level unequivocably detectable in vitro.

‡ Patient transfused on 4 successive days.

§ A case reported by Zucker and associates[45] that appears to fit the picture.

‖ A case reported by van Loghem, Dorfmeijer, and van der Hart[27] that seems to fit the picture. This table is taken from reference 36.

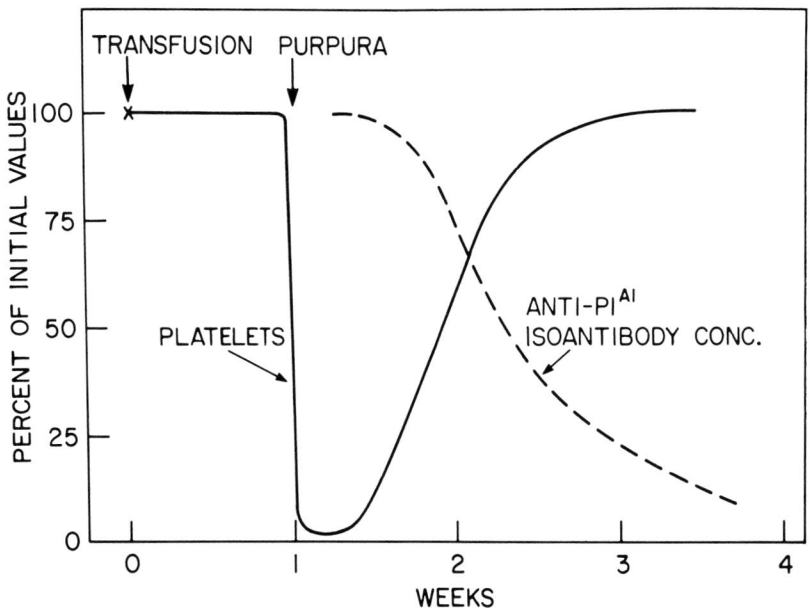

FIG. 32—Salient points of post-transfusion purpura: transfusion, 1-week's delay, precipitous onset of thrombocytopenia associated with isoantibody against foreign platelet antigen, spontaneous recovery, sometimes when antibody is still present (see table 14). This graph is taken from reference 37, courtesy of the publisher.

ture that appeared similar.[27, 45] A transfusion of one or more units of blood was given, usually at operation. The patients recuperated normally for about a week, then developed fulminant purpura with practically no circulating platelets. At this time, the patients' sera contained an antibody against an antigen that was present on donor platelets but absent on the patients' own platelets that were tested after purpura cleared. In the four instances in which the specificity of the antibody was established, it proved to be anti-Pl[A1]. Patients with post-transfusion purpura so far have been the only source of C'-fixing anti-Pl[A1] in contrast to the relatively numerous examples of the blocking form of anti-Pl[A1] found in normal mothers sensitized by fetal platelets (see above). Development of an isoantibody against a foreign antigen in post-transfusion purpura was understandable, but destruction of the recipient's own platelets was paradoxical.

Observations on one patient (Case 1, table 14) who was treated by exchange transfusion (fig. 33) helped clarify the problem. This form of treatment was used because it was felt that the unusually severe purpura and the rather unique

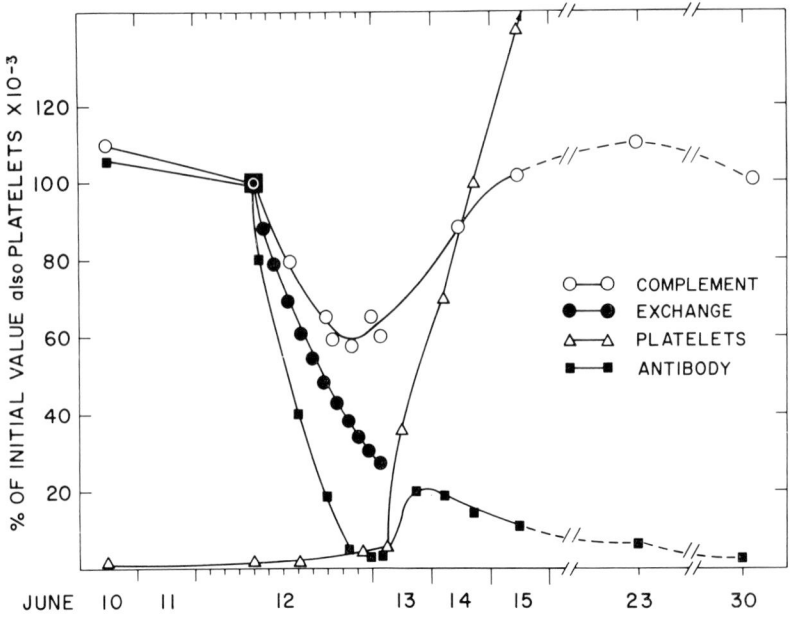

Fig. 33—Effects of exchange transfusion in a patient with post-transfusion purpura. This figure is reproduced from reference 32 and corresponds to Case 1 in table 14. The first serum sample (June 10) was obtained 12 hours after onset of purpura and contained anti-Pl[A1] in high titer. No platelets were present and hemorrhage was profuse and life-threatening. By necessity, the 13 units of fresh blood used in the exchange transfusion contained antigenic platelets, for less than 3 per cent of the population lack the Pl[A1] antigen. Although the patient had a variable febrile reaction to several blood transfusions given rapidly one day prior to the exchange, no reaction occurred during administration of the 13 units of blood given at a slow rate of infusion. It is noteworthy that antigenic platelets caused a significant fall in C' level and were apparently saturated with antibody when sequestered.[32] Antigenic platelets given under these circumstances effected a decrease in antibody rather than perpetuation of the disease. Antibody level on June 13 and 14 was equivalent to a titer of 22 in table 14.

platelet isoantibody were associated in some way. Thirteen 500 ml. units of fresh blood were used in the exchange which was 75 per cent effective as measured by dilution of Cr[51]-labeled red cells, but the antibody level fell much more precipitously due to sequestration of antibody along with transfused antigenic platelets [Type Pl[A](1,1) or Pl[A](1,2)]. During the exchange, hemorrhagic manifestations ceased and at the end of the exchange, although the bleeding time was 6 minutes, the platelet level was less than 5000/mm.[3] That same day, and on subsequent days, rapid return of the patient's own platelets [Type Pl[A](2,2)] occurred. The platelets rose in the face of antibody levels higher than the highest levels present in other patients during severest purpura (table 14). It was apparent that antibody was not the only factor involved in causing thrombocytopenia and that beneficial effects of the exchange transfusion were not due simply to decrease in antibody. The abrupt cure appeared to be caused by removal of an additional factor that must have been present to make the patient's genetically nonantigenic platelets susceptible to antibody during the period of thrombocytopenia. The observed phenomenon could be explained if Pl[A1] antigen in transfused blood not only stimulated antibody, but also persisted in vivo in a form capable of effecting attachment of antibody to non-antigenic platelets. The disorder would then be analogous to drug purpura in which antibodies stimulated by drugs do not attach to platelets in vivo or in vitro unless drug is present.[75, 140] The possible mechanism by which an isoantigen could effect attachment of antibody to cells may be inferred from information obtained on reactions involving drug antibodies, drugs, and cells, discussed in the following section.

Pathophysiology.—In drug purpura, it is generally assumed that drug combines with some cell constituent to form a complete antigen,[140, 141] as shown on the left in Step 1, figure 34, and that in the second step of the reaction, antibody combines with the complete antigen which depends on both the drug and a cellular moiety for its specificity. However, recent evidence obtained from studying the antibodies of quinidine and quinine purpura and of stibophen hemolytic anemia,[36, 38, 75] indicates that the complete antigen consists of a stable complex of drug with some noncellular macromolecule. As shown in Step 1 on the right of figure 34, antibodies elicited by the complete antigen are capable of combining directly with drug alone in accord with classical haptene chemistry, and attachment of antibody-drug complexes onto cells in Step 2 appears to be a relatively nonspecific adsorption step that does not involve cellular antigenicity. The following quantitative considerations support the possibility that adsorption of antigen-antibody complexes is the basis for post-transfusion purpura.

It was found that platelet destruction occurred in vivo when 500 to 1000 anti-Pl[A1] molecules were attached per cell (see *Quantitative Aspects of In vivo Responses* in section on Experimental Pathophysiology). Therefore, in the post-transfusion purpura syndrome, if sufficient transfused antigen survived to permit attachment of roughly 1000 Pl[A1]-anti-Pl[A1] complexes per cell, thrombocytopenia could be expected to occur. This requirement would be met if the antigen from only 5 to 10 per cent of the platelets in the usual 500 ml. unit of blood survived the period of antibody induction.[38] The only additional requisite would be that the nonspecific second step, in which antigen-antibody complexes are adsorbed on platelets, have avidity similar to that for adsorption of antibody-drug complexes onto platelets.[38]

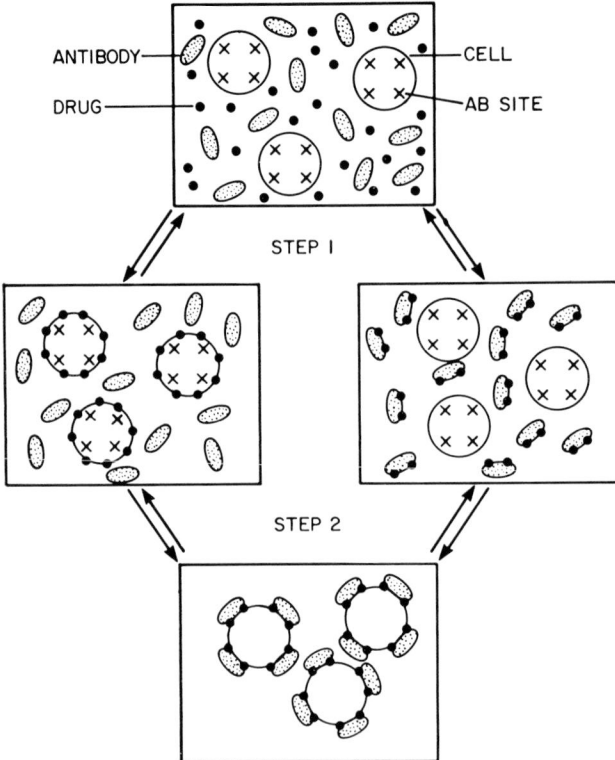

FIG. 34—Two possible mechanisms for the first step of the reaction leading to attachment of drug antibodies to cells. This figure is taken from reference 37, courtesy of the
publisher.

The rapid onset and prolonged course of post-transfusion purpura is consistent
with the proposed immune mechanism. Following adsorption of minimum dam-
aging amounts of antigen-antibody complex, the initial decrease in platelets
would result in relatively more unadsorbed complex available per cell; hence
progressive rapid development of thrombocytopenia in a manner resembling an
autocatalytic reaction. Since the capacity for regenerating platelets is limited, a
thrombocytopenic state could be perpetuated with amounts of complex one or
two orders of magnitude lower than the concentration required to initiate thrombocytopenia. The relatively few newly formed platelets would tend to be more
saturated with remaining complexes, and their sequestration resistant to effects
of adrenocorticosteroid therapy (see Experimental Pathophysiology). Thus a
prolonged thrombocytopenic state could occur despite survival of very small
amounts of antigen. The effectiveness of therapeutic exchange transfusion and
the natural regression of the disease could be interpreted as the result of removal
or gradual intravascular decay, not of antibody, but of the more important
thrombocytopenic agent, circulating antigen-antibody complex.

The missing link in the experimental analysis of this syndrome is identification of a soluble or finely colloidal form of Pl^{A1} antigen that would have to survive
in the transfused individual to combine with antibody. Attempts to produce

such an antigen in vitro so far have not been successful, but it has been possible to make a coarsely colloidal form.[32] Although other antigens could be involved in post-transfusion purpura, only Pl[A1] has been implicated so far. The basis for post-transfusion purpura appears to be the following combination of circumstances: the ability of the Pl[A1] antigen to circulate in free form under some circumstances; the unusual avidity of anti-Pl[A1] that results in complex formation at low concentrations of antigen; and the special properties of the Pl[A1]-anti-Pl[A1] complex that leads to its adsorption by platelets.

Implications in autoimmunity.—That cells can participate as adsorbents for substances involved in immune reactions has been recognized for many years.[142, 143] Most observations made on immune adsorption phenomena involve blood cells, perhaps because their surfaces favor this type of reaction teleologically to rid the circulation of foreign antigens or complexes of foreign antigens with antibodies, or perhaps because these are the most readily available cells to study. In most experimental instances of immune adsorption, the first step is fixation of antigen on cells followed by attachment of antibodies directed only against the adsorbed foreign antigen; for example, adsorption of many bacterial polysaccharides on untreated erythrocytes that leads to agglutination or lysis of the cell by anti-bacterial antibody. The same sequence of events takes place in the more familiar exquisitely sensitive tanned erythrocyte agglutination test for antibodies against a variety of protein antigens. Another adsorption phenomenon called "immune adherence" involves the attachment of certain antigens to primate erythrocytes and guinea pig or rabbit platelets only in the presence of both specific antibody and C'.[1-4] There are also good experimental models for nonspecific cellular adsorption of antigen-antibody complexes in the absence of C'; for instance, adsorption of tuberculoprotein-anti-tuberculoprotein complexes on sheep red cells,[145] or albumin-anti-albumin complexes on rabbit platelets.[146] Although immunologically nonspecific, it is evident that these various adsorption reactions can have predilection for cells of only certain species or for a particular type cell of a given species, and in the latter case even isoantigenic differences in cells can influence the nonspecific reaction.[147] Only recently, however, has experimental evidence been obtained with human antibodies, indicating that nonspecific adsorption phenomena can play a role in disease.[36, 38, 75]

Antibodies elicited by various foreign antigens, in addition to drugs, are well known to cause some self-destructive reactions involving blood cells or other tissues; for example, serum sickness, Arthus's phenomenon, and endotoxin, anaphylactic or Shwartzman reactions.* The basis of these various reactions

---

* Endotoxin, anaphylactic and Shwartzman reactions characteristically are associated with marked transient leukopenia and a variety of systemic symptoms, many of which appear to be secondary to destruction of leukocytes.[148] If nonspecific immune adsorption phenomena play a role in these reactions, the primary target cell is most likely leukocytes, for thrombocytopenia does not occur unless the reactions are unusually severe.[149, 150, 151, 152] Under these circumstances, slight to moderate thrombocytopenia results from intravascular activation of blood coagulation[149, 153] by thromboplastic substances possibly released from disintegrated leukocytes. Platelets are apparently trapped in fibrinous deposits as they are after intravenous injections of thrombin or tissue extracts[149, 153] (thromboplastin) or after severe hemolytic transfusion reactions that release thromboplastic material from erythrocytes.[154]

may be nonspecific cellular adsorption, either of antigen followed by antibody, or of antigen-antibody complexes.[38, 142, 143, 155, 156, 157] Since manifestations of cellular injury by antibodies that combine only with foreign antigens can be so varied, it is evident that diseases caused by sensitization to foreign antigens and those caused by apparent sensitization to autogenous body components or combinations of auto- and hetero-antigens, may be difficult to differentiate. This difficulty is emphasized by comparing for example, "autoimmune" ITP with drug purpura and post-transfusion purpura. In view of current knowledge, it seems likely that sensitization to foreign antigens will prove to be the basis for at least some types of thrombocytopenia that are now idiopathic. Although the humoral factor in the plasma of patients with ITP that causes thrombocytopenia when infused into normal individuals has been identified in the gamma globulin fraction of plasma,[39] it is not yet clear whether this represents (1) an antibody against an autologous platelet constituent, (2) an antibody against an antigen that may be adsorbed on human platelets, or (3) an antibody tightly bound with some foreign antigen as a complex that can be adsorbed nonspecifically by human platelets. If the latter is the case, a macromolecular antigen could be involved, for ITP factor activity is resistant to prolonged dialysis and DEAE cellulose chromatography.[39] Demonstration in post-transfusion purpura that sensitization to a macromolecule can produce the picture of ITP, makes this possibility reasonable.

A Note on Histocompatibility

The possible role of blood group isoantigens in homograft immunity and the relative importance of classical serologic reactions and delayed cellular hypersensitivity in graft rejection have been discussed in a number of recent symposia[158, 159, 160, 161, 162] and reviews.[163, 164, 165, 166] It has been concluded that leukocytes and in some species, possibly platelets and erythrocytes, share skin antigens responsible for homograft immunity because (1) sensitization to blood leukocytes by the intradermal, and to a lesser extent by the intravenous route in certain animals,[168] and by the intradermal route in man,[169] results in immune skin graft rejection; (2) skin grafts sometimes induce antibodies against leukocytes and red cells detectable by serologic tests, particularly in mice,[163, 166] or against platelets detectable by shortened platelet survival in rabbits,[170] and (3) sensitization to grafted skin produces delayed cutaneous hypersensitivity that can be evoked by intradermal injections of leukocytes in guinea pigs[171] and man.[172] Although it is evident that leukocytes elicit transplantation immunity against other tissues, it is not yet clear whether the responsible antigens are the same as those that stimulate circulating antibodies or cause cutaneous hypersensitivity, and if so, whether they are typical blood group isoantigens.

It seems likely from various observations that have been made in man, that homograft rejection usually will not be associated with circulating antibodies against tissues or blood cells that are measurable directly by serologic tests available at present. However, relationships between blood group isoantigens and histocompatibility antigens can be evaluated with current serologic technics using monospecific isoantibodies in the following types of analyses.

Graft rejection and phenotypic incompatibility.—On occasions when skin, kidney, bone marrow or other tissues are transplanted in man, determinations of donor and recipient phenotypes with all available monospecific antisera against platelet and leukocyte isoantigens may permit identifying incompatibilities of significance with respect to graft rejection. Isoantigens not shared by blood cells and immunizing tissues, as determined by serologic procedures (see Serology), could be eliminated as transplantation antigens.

Blood cell survival and homograft immunity.—Individuals who have rejected grafts, but have no serologically active isoantibodies against platelets or leukocytes nevertheless may have developed antibodies detectable by their ability to shorten the in vivo survival of platelets[170] or leukocytes. By using cells that are antigenically well defined in survival studies, it may be possible to associate specific isoantigens with homograft immunity.

Cutaneous hypersensitivity and specific isoantigens.—If transplantation antigens are similar to the usual blood group polysaccharide isoantigens, one would not expect them to cause cutaneous hypersensitivity, for polysaccharides in general have not elicited this type of reaction,[173] and leukocyte,[172] platelet,[32] or erythrocyte isoantigens[174] in particular have not caused delayed cutaneous reactions in individuals sensitized by the intravenous route. However, relatively few isoantigens have been tested in this way, and it is conceivable that the very blood group isoantigens that may be responsible for homograft immunity will elicit cutaneous hypersensitivity. Skin tests performed with antigenically well defined leukocytes on individuals known to be sensitized by transfusion or pregnancy, as well as by grafts, should help resolve this problem.

Heterotransplantation and isoantigens.—In those instances in which heterotransplants in man are performed therapeutically (e.g., dog or monkey parathyroid to man[175] and ape kidney to man[176]) evaluation of heterotransplantation antigens on blood cells may be sought not only by the usual serologic and skin tests, but also by passive transfer of plasma from immunized recipients to donor animals, for suppression of circulating blood cells is frequently the most sensitive test for antibody.[39] If certain isoantigens, common to human and non-human primates, (see tables 7 and 8) prove to be significant in histocompatibility, it may be possible to perform transplantation experiments in animals that will have direct bearing on the problem in man.

Physico-chemical properties.—Pure forms of transplantation antigens and leukocyte or platelet blood group isoantigens are difficult to obtain,[32, 177, 178] hence their chemical characteristics are not established. However, stability properties of transplantation antigens[165] and leukocyte isoantigens under different forms of treatment, e.g., pH, temperature, solvents, enzymes, etc. (see Serology), were consistent with their both being polysaccharides. More recently, analyses on refined transplantation antigens have suggested that they are lipoproteins,[177, 178] but materials used in these studies were insufficiently pure to rule out the possibility that they are polysaccharides. As yet it is not possible to draw conclusions concerning similarities or differences between transplantation antigens and isoantigens on the basis of their physico-chemical characteristics.

Maternal-fetal histocompatibility.—Since maternal sensitization to fetal platelets and leukocytes most often results in formation of monospecific isoantibodies (see Neonatal Purpura) the significance of certain incompatibilities in transplantation immunity may possibly be derived from graft exchanges between immunized mother and offspring in the manner used by Peer *et al.* to evaluate apparent maternally induced tolerance in children.[179] The effect of specific iso-immunization on maternal acceptance of her offspring's skin would be difficult to predict on the basis of observations made in animals, for the ability to reject grafts was found to be weakened by prior intravenous injection of homologous leukocytes or epidermal cells in rabbits,[180] but strengthened by similar injections in mice or rats.[181, 182]

Approximation of placental trophoblastic tissue to maternal circulation would seem to afford an opportunity for immunization, but homograft reactions between mother and fetus do not occur. This is apparently owing to a deficiency of transplantation antigens in the trophoblast in those species that have been studied.[183, 184] If human trophoblastic tissue proves to lack transplantation antigens also, then leukocyte and platelet isoantigens that are shared by placental tissue may be excluded as transplantation antigens. For example, the 4ᵃ and 4ᵇ leuko-cyte antigens of van Rood could be excluded for they are present in the placenta.[8]

Choriocarcinoma.—This malignancy might be expected to elicit isoantibodies, for it is genetically dissimilar to the host. However, sera of patients with advanced choriocarcinoma studied by Schmidt and Hertz[185] did not contain detectable antibodies against erythrocyte blood group antigens of their husbands, and more recently, using 33 of the same sera we did not find C'-fixing antibodies against platelet and leukocyte isoantigens that could be attributed to sensitization by trophoblastic tissue.* Moreover, trials of treating choriocarcinoma in women by immunizing them with their husband's blood have not been successful.[186, 187] These various observations suggest that trophoblastic tissue is deficient in both histocompatibility antigens and isoantigens. However, if rejection of choriocarcinoma in some instances is associated with development of antibodies against a particular isoantigen, or if particular isoantibodies stimulated by choriocarcinoma do not cause tumor rejection, the information may help establish relationships between various tissue antigens and histocompatibility.

Tumor immunity.—Although isoantigenic differences between malignant cells and normal autologous cells generally would not be expected to occur, there are some well documented observations on changes in concentrations or reactivity of red cell blood group antigens in association with leukemia and other malignancies[43] and some suggestions that tumors may contain antigens peculiar to themselves.[188] The latter observation, however, awaits confirmation. If differences in antigenic composition between tumor and host do indeed exist, their identification would provide clues to principles of tissue rejection, equally applicable to problems of immunologic tumor therapy and homotransplantation. If qualitative differences in antigens of malignant and normal cells are not found, quantitative differences with respect to isoantigenic sites per cell may have bearing on the sensitivity of tissues to cytotoxic antibodies[189] (see section on In vivo Effects of Isoantibodies on Leukemic Leukocytes). Monospecific C'-fixing isoantibodies are well suited for these types of studies (see Serology).

---

* We are grateful to Dr. Paul J. Schmidt and Dr. Roy Hertz for the opportunity to study these sera.

APPENDIX

Materials and Methods

Platelet Suspensions

For quantitative C′ fixation.—Platelet preparations were made in siliconized glassware, using disodium ethylenediamine tetraacetate (EDTA, MW 372) adjusted to pH 7.4 as an anticoagulant. The amount of EDTA added, 0.2 ml. of 0.27 M (10 per cent) EDTA/10 ml. of blood, gave a final EDTA concentration of approximately 7×10^{-3} M in plasma. Platelet-rich plasma was obtained by sedimenting blood at 1100 g for 4 minutes and aspirating the supernatant plasma. Platelet buttons were prepared by sedimenting platelet-rich plasma at 1100 g for 20 minutes. Buttons were washed once in 1 per cent ammonium oxalate and twice in 0.147 M NaCl. The final suspension in 0.147 M NaCl (containing 10^{-2} M sodium azide) was adjusted to give a platelet count of 10^6 or 2×10^6/mm.^{3} Platelet counts were performed by the method of Brecher and Cronkite.[190]

Platelet preparations could be standardized on the basis of their nitrogen content more accurately than by count.[32] One ml. of a suspension of 10^6 platelets/mm.^{3} contained 400 μg. N. A convenient method for determining N was by Kjeldahl digestion of 0.12 ml. and 0.24 ml. of a suspension containing approximately 10^6 platelets/mm.^{3}, followed by Nesslerization of the digest. The standard Nesslerization curve covered the range 20 to 150 μg. N.

The yield of platelets from fresh whole blood was 65 to 80 per cent and was the same from blood that was stored for 1 to 2 days at 5° C. Whole blood mailed in plain glass containers without refrigeration gave yields of 20 to 50 per cent despite the usual interval of 2 or 3 days before delivery to the laboratory. Platelet-rich plasma mailed the same way as whole blood gave higher yields.

Platelet suspensions with sodium azide remained stable for at least 6 months when stored at 5° C. Platelets frozen at −20° C. in saline or in glycerol, as used for erythrocytes,[191, 192] lost much of their original C′-fixing activity, no doubt because of disintegration and clumping of platelets. However, frozen platelets retained their normal capacity to adsorb antibody. Lyophilized platelets, reconstituted in water, reacted like frozen platelets.

The initial wash in ammonium oxalate lysed red cells, and contaminating red cell stroma in platelet suspensions, if present, was never sufficient to produce C′ fixation with anti-erythrocyte antibodies. Platelet suspensions contained one leukocyte per 1000 to 5000 platelets and almost all were lymphocytes.

For qualitative C′ fixation.—When many individuals were phenotyped in qualitative C′ fixation procedures, platelets were prepared as described above, except for the final suspension. Platelet buttons were suspended in a volume of 0.147 M NaCl (containing 10^{-2} M sodium azide), equal to 1/10 the volume of blood used for the preparation. Suspensions prepared in this way contained from 1.4 to 2.6×10^6 platelets/mm.^{3} For routine screening tests, platelet counts were not performed; and with the time-consuming step of platelet counting eliminated, preparations from approximately 100 individuals could be made in one day by two technicians.

For agglutination.—Platelets for use in the Dausset and Malinvaud method of agglutination[26] were made as described above, but EDTA buffer was used instead of other washing and suspending fluids. The buffer consisted of 0.025 M Na_2HPO_4 in 0.12 M NaCl containing 0.027 M EDTA; the pH was adjusted to 7.0. Platelets in the final suspension were adjusted to 300,000/mm.^{3}

The agglutination test consisted of adding 0.05 ml. of test serum, heated at 56° C. for 30 minutes and diluted 1/2 in EDTA, buffer to 0.025 ml. of platelet suspension. The mixture was made in a Kline or Boerner plate which was rotated on a Kline shaker in a moist chamber at 80 rotations per minute for 30 minutes at 5° C. and 30 minutes at 37° C. Agglutination was read with a low power objective.

Leukocyte Suspensions

For C' fixation.—Blood in siliconized glassware with EDTA as an anticoagulant, as for platelets, was mixed 5 parts to 1 part of a solution of 5 per cent dextran ("Dextravan" from Bengor Labs. Ltd., Cheshire, England, MW 200,000) in 0.12 M NaCl. The mixture was allowed to settle at a 45° angle at room temperature for approximately one hour, or until a clear line of separation formed between plasma and red cells. The supernatant plasma was removed by aspiration with a siliconized pipette and sedimented at 100 g for 10 minutes to obtain a leukocyte button. More forceful sedimentation resulted in irreversible clumping. The supernatant plasma of the sedimented leukocytes contained platelets that could be processed as described above for a separate platelet preparation. After platelets were removed, the cell-free plasma was recalcified with 1 M $CaCl_2$, fibrin was wound out as it formed, and the resultant serum was heated at 56° C for 30 minutes to inactivate C'. The white cell button from 50 ml. of normal blood was washed twice in 20 ml. of cell-free heated autologous serum. These washes removed platelets trapped in leukocyte buttons as well as fibrinogen adsorbed on leukocytes. Adsorbed fibrinogen appeared to be a major cause of irreversible leukocyte clumping.

The final leukocyte button from 50 ml. of blood was suspended in approximately 1 ml. of autologous heated serum. Serum prepared the same way from a normal group AB donor could be substituted for autologous serum if necessary. A leukocyte count, platelet count, and differential were performed before the final suspension was adjusted to 8×10^5 leukocytes/mm.^{3} in serum. An equal amount of glycerol was then added to bring the final leukocyte concentration to 4×10^5/mm.^{3} in 50 per cent glycerol-serum. The preparations were immediately stored at $-20°$ C. At this temperature the glycerol-serum mixture did not freeze and the cells could be used directly in C' fixation procedures without removing glycerol. Leukocytes frozen in the mixtures of glycerol used for erythrocyte preservation[191, 192] usually were irreversibly clumped on thawing. Suspensions stored at 5° C. in 0.147 M NaCl also clumped irreversibly within 1 or 2 days, whereas cells in glycerol-serum remained discrete and could be evenly suspended over periods longer than a year. Glycerolized cells at 5° C. sometimes became anticomplementary in a few days unless sodium azide was added. Polyvinylpyrrolidone (PVP) has been used instead of dextran, and dimethylsulfoxide (DMSO) has sometimes been used instead of glycerol, but with no apparent advantages. A vortex mixer (Scientific Industries, Inc., Queens Village, N. Y.) was found to produce even suspensions of leukocytes (or platelets) without fragmenting or disrupting cells.

Leukocyte suspensions from normal blood contained about an equal proportion of granulocytes and lymphocytes and 1 to 2 platelets per 10 leukocytes. Suspensions from leukemic blood were more nearly single cell types depending on the differential count and the degree of leukocytosis. Proportionately larger amounts of heated serum were required for washing large yields of leukemic leukocytes to prevent nonspecific clumping.

Other leukocyte suspensions were made from lymphoid tissue, spleens, or thymus glands obtained from individuals on whom operative procedures were performed. The tissue was washed free of blood with 0.147 M NaCl, the capsule was stripped off with forceps and the cellular material was minced and gently mashed and teased in cold 0.147 M NaCl. The crude suspension was then strained through a thin layer of absorbent cotton to obtain discrete lymphocytes that could be resuspended for storage in a 1:1 serum-glycerol mixture. Sufficient cells could be obtained from 1 Gm of lymphoid tissue for phenotyping with approximately 1C antisera. Lymphocytes from lymphoid tissue and thymus glands were not contaminated significantly by other cells. However, suspensions of splenic cells contained so many erythrocytes that the same procedures used for whole blood, including dextran sedimentation, were necessary to obtain pure lymphocytes.

When leukocytes were incubated in mixtures with C′, they frequently clumped. However, reproducible C′ fixation could be obtained if the clumped cells were agitated and pressed against the side of the tube with a glass rod four or five times during the one hour incubation at 37° C. (see C′ fixation procedures).

For agglutination studies.—Leukocytes used in agglutination tests by the method of van Rood[31] were obtained from blood collected in siliconized tubes with 1 ml. of 0.135 M EDTA in 0.147 M NaCl for 8 ml. of blood. To this was added 2.5 ml. of 5 per cent dextran, MW 200,000, in 0.147 M NaCl, buffered at pH 7 with phosphate buffer. Tubes were incubated at 37° C. for 30 minutes at a 45° angle and the upper 4/5 of the superntant plasma, which contained 3000 to 12,000 leukocytes/mm.³, was used in agglutination mixtures. The higher concentration of EDTA in the leukocyte suspensions compared to that used in platelet preparations was apparently necessary to prevent excessive nonspecific leukoagglutination. Some suspensions prepared by this technic were suitable for agglutination studies after 24 hours.

When leukocytes were collected for agglutination by Payne's procedure,[7] blood was defibrinated in an Erlenmeyer flask by gentle rotation for 10 to 15 minutes with 5 glass beads per 10 to 30 ml. of blood. Red cells were then separated by dextran sedimentation. Leukocytes were used at a concentration of 5,000 to 10,000/mm.³ as soon as possible after preparation.

In van Rood's agglutination test, 2 drops of heated serum (30 minutes at 56° C.) were mixed with 2 to 5 drops of leukocyte suspension in 50 × 7 mm. plain glass round bottomed tubes. Two drops of leukocyte suspension were used if the leukocyte count was 8–12,000/mm.³, 3 drops for counts of 6–8,000/mm.³ and 4 to 5 drops for counts below 6,000/mm.³ Tubes were incubated for 1–1/2 to 2 hours at 37° C. in an incubator, the supernatant plasma was removed, and one drop of 6 per cent acetic acid was added to lyse red cells. Leukocytes were then transferred to a clean glass slide and agglutination read at 50 to 100 × magnification.

In Payne's agglutination test, 0.15 ml. of serum heated at 56° C. for 30 minutes was added to 0.05 ml. of leukocyte suspension in 12 × 75 mm. plain glass test tubes. Tubes were incubated in a water bath for 90 minutes at 37° C. without shaking. Then 0.15 ml. of 3 per cent acetic acid was added to the mixture, and after leukocytes had resettled, a drop from the bottom of the tube, removed with a capillary pipette, was deposited on a clean glass slide and agglutination read at 100 × magnification.

Reagents Used in C′ Fixation

Reagents and methods of C′ fixation vary somewhat in different laboratories, but the principles are the same, and the common denominator of standardization is always the C′ content of pooled fresh guinea pig serum. Adaptations of classical methods to measurement of platelet and leukocyte isoantibodies[32, 33, 34, 35, 39] are outlined as a guide for those interested in using the technic. For theoretical aspects of C′ fixation and much practical information, the chapter by Mayer in *Experimental Immunochemistry*[193] is recommended.

Veronal buffer.—Stock buffer, made at a concentration 5 × isotonic, was stored at 5° C. and diluted 1/5 with water for daily use. Deionized water was used throughout. Specific solutions were: (1) 4.6 Gm 5,5 diethyl barbituric acid (MW 184.2, barbital N. F.) dissolved in 500 ml. hot water; (2) 83.3 Gm. NaCl, 2.25 Gm. sodium bicarbonate and 3.0 Gm. 5,5 diethyl barbiturate (MW 206.18, sodium barbital N. F.) dissolved in 1000 ml. water at room temperature; (3) 20.0 grams magnesium chloride 6 H_2O and 4.0 Gm. calcium chloride 2 H_2O in 100 ml. water. All of solutions (1) and (2) were combined; 5 ml. of solution (3) was then added, and the volume brought to 2000 ml. with water. The pH was adjusted to 7.3 to 7.5 with NaOH or HCl, if necessary.

Hemolysin.—Anti-sheep red cell rabbit serum (hemolysin), purchased from Cappel Laboratories, Westchester, Pennsylvania, was titered as described below.

Sheep red cells.—Sheep blood collected in acid citrate dextrose, USP Formula A, or in Alsever's solution, could be used for 4 to 6 weeks, or until excessive spontaneous hemolysis occurred in 0.147 M NaCl. Red cells from different sheep varied greatly in their sensitivity to rabbit hemolysin, sometimes enough to cause a 2-fold difference in C' assay. This may be related in part to inherited differences in the cellular concentration of receptors for rabbit anti-sheep cell antibodies, but also could be attributed to excessive young red cells, resistant to hemolysis, that were present after too frequent bleeding or sometimes after lambing. Therefore it was important to obtain erythrocytes from known sheep or from a commercial source that standardized cells appropriately. More uniform results were obtained if blood was kept at 5° C. for 2 to 3 days before use.

Complement.—Lyophilized pooled guinea pig serum, purchased from Texas Biological Laboratories, reconstituted with 0.147 M NaCl was found to be as potent as fresh pooled guinea pig serum as a source of C'. The lyophilized preparation could be stored for at least six months without loss of potency. Fresh human serum could also be used, but it contained 1/6 the C' activity of guinea pig serum, and the antibodies studied generally fixed less human C'.

Preparation of Sensitized Sheep Cells

Titration of hemolysin.—With each lot of hemolysin, it was necessary to determine the appropriate dilution to use for sensitizing sheep red cells. Two-fold serial dilutions of hemolysin in veronal buffer were made, beginning at 1/400 (with potent antisera, beginning at 1/1200) and 0.1 ml. of each dilution was added to a series of tubes containing 0.2 ml. of guinea pig serum diluted 1/20 and 0.4 ml. veronal buffer. To each tube, 0.1 ml. of a 5 per cent sheep red cell suspension was added. To make a 5 per cent suspension (10^6 cells/mm.³), cells were washed four times with 0.147 M NaCl, then suspended in veronal buffer and adjusted so that a 1/15 dilution of the suspension with distilled water gave an optical density of 0.750 at 540 mμ. The mixtures were incubated at 37° C. for 30 minutes with occasional shaking, then sedimented at 1100 g for 4 minutes. One unit of hemolysin was the minimum dilution that gave complete lysis of sheep erythrocytes.

Sensitizing sheep red cells with hemolysin.—For sensitizing cells, a hemolysin dilution of 4 units was used. Thus, if 0.1 ml. of hemolysin at 1/2400 dilution was the minimum amount that gave complete lysis in the hemolysin titration, then hemolysin at 1/600 dilution was mixed with an equal volume of a 5 per cent suspension of sheep red cells. The hemolysin was added to the cells slowly with swirling and the mixture was incubated at 37° C. for 30 minutes, mixing every 5 to 10 minutes. The sensitized cells were refrigerated at 5° C. for at least 30 minutes before use. Eight ml. of ACD sheep blood provided approximately 50 ml. of a 5 per cent suspension and 100 ml. of sensitized cells.

Titration of C'—The 50 Per Cent Hemolytic Unit

Various aliquots of diluted guinea pig serum were added to a series of 10 × 75 mm. test tubes, keeping the final volume constant at 3.25 ml. with veronal buffer. The amounts of different dilutions of guinea pig serum used in the test system are shown on the abscissa of figure 35. Then 0.5 ml. of sensitized cells was added quickly and the reagents mixed by inverting tubes on parafilm (American Can Company, Menasha, Wisconsin). Tubes were incubated for 30 minutes at 37° C. and inverted once at 15 minutes. After incubation tubes were centrifuged at 1100 g for 4 minutes, supernatant fluid was decanted into 3 ml. spectrophotometer cuvettes and optical density read at 540 mμ. Curves A, B and C in figure 35, obtained with different dilutions of the same guinea pig serum, are symmetrical with respect to each other, although at a glance they may not appear so. There is a direct

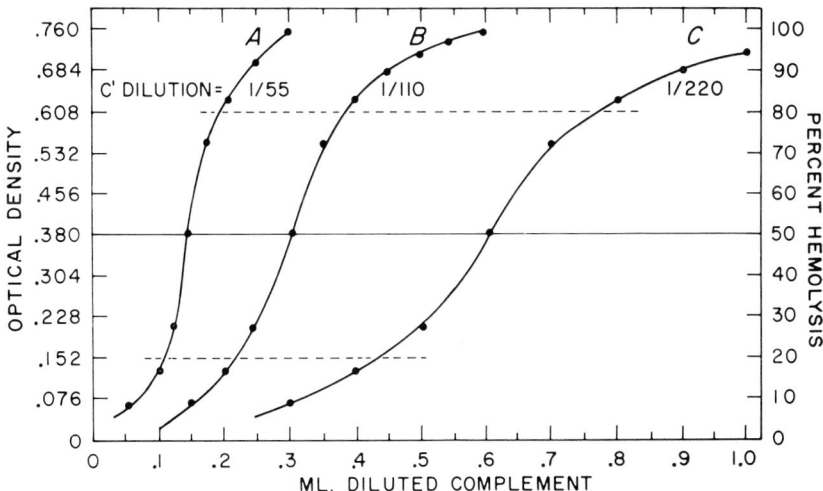

Fig. 35—Standard curves and the 50 per cent hemolytic unit. The points at precisely 50 per cent hemolysis on curves A, B and C are idealized; for in practice, values usually bracket the mid-point that is obtained from the intercept of the line at D = .380 with the line connecting experimental points.

proportionality between the degree of serum dilution and the amount of diluted serum required to lyse a given per cent of cells. Thus, points on the horizontal line marking 50 per cent hemolysis (mid-points) are 0.15, 0.3 and 0.6 ml., respectively, for guinea pig serum at 1/55 dilution, 1/110 dilution and 1/220 dilution. The amount of C' that produces a density of 0.380, i.e., lyses half the cells, is, by definition, a 50 per cent hemolytic unit of C'. Therefore, using any one of the curves for calculating the amount of C' in 1 ml. of undiluted guinea pig serum, the value is the same: (1/0.15 × 55), (1/0.3 × 110), (1/0.6 × 220), or 366 units per ml. If, for example, twelve units of C' were desired for use in an experiment, then 12/366 or 0.0328 ml. of this guinea pig serum would be required. For convenience of pipetting, the guinea pig serum could be diluted 3.28/5.0 and 0.05 ml. of diluted serum used.

The sigmoid curve of C' lysis has been described by an empirical formula, the von Krough equation, that relates units of C' to per cent hemolysis; and a logarithmic transformation of the equation has been used widely for calculating experimental results.[193] However, any curve of C' lysis, such as one of those in figure 35, provides a convenient standard for calculating units of C' with a degree of accuracy equal to that of the von Krough equation. The amount of C' present in an unknown sample is calculated from the optical density (D) produced by an aliquot of the sample through the following simple relationship:

$$\text{Ml. of unknown giving observed D} \times \frac{\text{Ml. on standard curve giving D of 0.380}}{\text{Ml. on standard curve giving same D as unknown}} = \text{Ml. of unknown giving D of 0.380}$$

Calculations are more accurate for degrees of hemolysis within the range 20 to 80 per cent (D = .150 to .610).

The following is an example of calculating the C' content of an unknown solution using curve B in figure 35. Suppose a 0.7 ml. aliquot from 4 ml. of an unknown solution produced an optical density of 0.210. On curve B, 0.25 ml. produced a density of 0.210, and

0.3 ml. produced a density of 0.380. Therefore, $0.7 \times 0.3/0.25$ or 0.84 ml. of the unknown would produce a density of 0.380 and would contain 1 unit of C'. The number of units of C' in the 4 ml. unknown sample would be 4/0.84 or 4.76 units. The same value is obtained using curve A or C for the calculation.

Quantitative C' Fixation

Reaction mixtures.—A reaction volume of 0.4 ml. was suitable for all work described herein. Veronal buffer was used as a diluent to keep the volume constant. The reactants were: (1) antigen as a cell suspension of known concentration, (2) C' in the form of either undiluted or slightly diluted guinea pig serum and (3) antibody either as serum or eluate, added in the order listed. The amount of C' used was determined by the amount expected to be fixed, for not more than 75 per cent of the C' present initially should be fixed to assure completion of the reaction.[75] Twelve or 15 units of C' were used most frequently (see data under Serology). An incubation period of 60 minutes at 37° C. was optimum for all isoantibodies encountered; and tubes were mixed at about 5-minute intervals to keep cells suspended. No benefit was derived from longer periods of incubation at lower temperatures.

Table 15 shows the protocol used for a standard curve that relates amount of C' fixed to concentration of anti-Pl^{A1} (fig. 36, triangles) and table 16 shows a sample protocol used to test sera for platelet and leukocyte isoantibodies. To test for blocking antibodies, unknown sera were added to reaction mixtures containing isoantibodies of known specificity as in table 2 and figure 6.

Calculation of C' fixation.—At the end of the 60-minute incubation period, residual C'

TABLE 15.—*Protocol of Standard Curve of C' Fixation by an Isoantibody*

Tube	a. Cells ml.	b. Buffer ml.	c. C' ml.	c. C' units	d. Serum ml.	e. C' present units	f. C' fixed units
1	.04	.26	.05	12	.05	11.2	.8
2	.04	.21	.05	"	.10	9.0	3.0
3	.04	.16	.05	"	.15	6.1	5.9
4	.04	.11	.05	"	.20	3.8	8.2
5	.04	.31	.05	"	0	11.7	—
6	0	.20	.05	"	.15	11.5	—
7	0	.35	.05	"	0	12.5	—
8	.04	.01	.05	18	.30	4.6	12.7
9	0	.35	.05	"	0	18.3	—

a. Cells were a suspension of Pl^{A1}-positive platelets at a concentration of 2×10^6/mm.^{3}

b. Veronal buffer was used as diluent.

c. Guinea pig serum titered as described above contained 366 units/ml. or 12 units per 0.0328 ml., hence was diluted 3.28/5.00 for tubes 1 to 7 and was diluted 4.92/5.00 to provide 18 units/.05 ml. in tubes 8 and 9. C' was titered before experiments each day by constructing a curve similar to curve B of figure 35. Potency of a given lot of lyophilized guinea pig serum varied no more than ±10 per cent of the mean.

d. Serum containing anti-Pl^{A1} was diluted $\frac{1}{10}$. Usually several more controls for different amounts of serum were included.

e. Titration of residual C' was carried out as described under Calculation of C' Fixation.

f. Controls that did not differ more than 10 per cent were averaged for the final calculation of units of C' fixed.

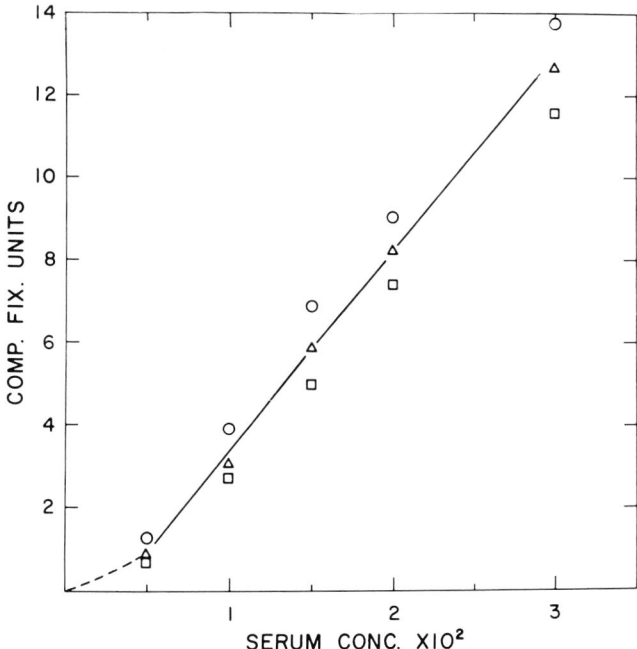

FIG. 36—C'fixation curve from protocol of table 15; values are plotted as triangles. This figure is from ref. 32, courtesy of the publisher.

TABLE 16.—*Protocol of Screening Test for Isoantibodies*

Tube	a. Cells	b. Buffer	c. C' ml.	units	d. Serum
1	.04	.26	.05	12	.05
2	.04	.16	.05	"	.15
3	0	.25	.05	"	.1
4	.04	.31	.05	"	0
5	0	.35	.05	"	0

a. The cells used were platelets at a concentration of 2×10^6/mm.^{3}, or leukocytes at a concentration of 4×10^5/mm.^{3}, containing known antigens. A reasonable screening test involved use of 6 platelet and 3 leukocyte preparations. Mixtures of different cells, each at the concentrations listed were also used. When testing for isoantibodies caused by maternal-fetal incompatibility, the husband's cells were used if possible.

b, c. Buffer and C' dilution as in table 15.

d. Two dilutions of serum were used; for, when blocking antibodies were present in mixture with C'-fixing antibodies, the lower concentration of serum fixed more C' (see figs. 6, 7 and 11). Plasma with Ca^{++}-binding anticoagulants could also be used for testing after recalcification and heating, but heparin plasma was unsuitable because it was anti-complementary. Serum from patients with systemic lupus erythematosus frequently fixed C' with autologous leukocytes (6 of 11 patients); and had to be thoroughly adsorbed with autologous leukocytes before being tested for isoantibodies.

Titration of residual C' was carried out as described in text. If less than 2 units of C' were fixed, the result was not considered positive.

An alternate qualitative procedure for screening sera is described under *A Phenotyping Test*.

See table 2 and figure 6 for protocol of tests for blocking antibodies.

in reaction mixtures was titered as described above. Since known amounts of C' were added to each tube, if none was fixed, the volume of reaction mixture containing 1 unit of C' could be set by diluting appropriately. For convenience and accuracy of measurement, aliquots in the range of those used for curve B in figure 35 were found best. Hence, control tubes containing 12 units of C' were diluted to 3.6 ml. (0.4 ml. reaction mixture + 3.2 veronal buffer) and 0.25, 0.3 and 0.4 ml. of each were used to bracket the mid-point. The one control tube containing 18 units of C' (tube 9, table 15) was diluted to 5.4 ml. and the same aliquots used.

Experimental tubes in which C' was fixed were diluted the same as control tubes according to the initial amount of C' present, but larger aliquots were used for C' titration. For example, if approximately half of the C' was fixed, aliquots in the range of curve C, figure 35, were required to bracket the mid-point. Aliquots of 0.3, 0.4, 0.6 and 0.9 ml. were found to be adequate to cover degrees of C' fixation within the range of accurate measurement. If no C' was fixed in an experimental tube, density values for 0.3 and 0.4 ml. were the same as that of controls, whereas 0.6 and 0.9 ml. aliquots caused complete hemolysis (see curve B, fig. 35). With increasing degrees of C' fixation, values for 0.3 and 0.4 ml. aliquots fell in the inaccurate range of less than 20 per cent hemolysis, while the 0.6 and 0.9 ml. values fell within the 20 to 80 per cent hemolysis range. The volume of diluted reaction mixture containing 1 unit of C' was then calculated as described under Titration of C' − the 50 per cent Hemolytic Unit. Usually two or three aliquots of a given reaction mixture produced hemolysis in the 20 to 80 per cent range and mid-points calculated from these values were averaged. The total volume of diluted reaction mixture (3.6 or 5.4 ml. in the sample experiments) divided by the average mid-point value gave the units of C' in each tube.

Instead of performing a calculation for each density reading using a curve of C' lysis (see above), a table was prepared relating optical density (from .075 to .680 with .005 increments) obtained with a given volume of C' solution (from 0.25 ml. to 1.5 ml. with 0.05 ml. increments) to the volume of solution that would contain one 50 per cent hemolytic unit (the mid-point). This table can be prepared from a C' lysis curve by listing optical density down the left side and ml. of C' solution across the top. By knowing the volume of a C' solution that gave a particular optical density in the titration system, it was possible to read the mid-point directly off the chart. This greatly facilitated calculation and, together with the use of automatic pipettes for adding buffer and sensitized sheep cells, enabled two experienced technicians to run 100 experimental tubes (350 to 400 final titration tubes) and calculate the results in a day's work. One technician could run about 30 experimental tubes conveniently.

Qualitative C' Fixation

Several different qualitative technics have been used for measuring platelet and leukocyte isoantibodies[25, 194] and heteroantibodies.[195] These technics and quantitative methods are about equally sensitive in detecting C'-fixing isoantibodies, but the qualitative C' fixation systems are not suitable for detecting most blocking antibodies (see Serology). Because minimum amounts of C' are employed in qualitative systems, they also have the drawback of being affected by minor anticomplementary activity of some fresh sera and many normal sera or suspensions of cells after storage.

Since the quantitative technic does not involve much additional effort, it appears to be advantageous for use in screening sera for antibodies as well as invaluable for studying their properties. Once the characteristics of an antibody are established, however, the following very simplest qualitative procedure can be used for phenotyping large numbers of individuals.

A phenotyping test.—All reagents were the same as in the quantitative test. Two reaction mixtures were used with each platelet (or leukocyte) preparation to be typed, one with, and one without, antibody. The experimental tubes contained sufficient antibody in .04 ml. to fix approximately 4 units of C′, sufficient cells in .04 ml. for optimum C′ fixation (see Platelet Suspensions, for qualitative C′ fixation) and 2.5 units of C′ in .04 ml. Control tubes contained normal serum instead of antibody. After the mixtures were incubated for 60 minutes at 37° C., 0.5 ml. of sensitized sheep cells were added to each tube, and incubation was continued for 30 minutes at 37° C. Tubes were then sedimented at 1100 g for 4 minutes and observed for hemolysis. Complete hemolysis indicated the absence of antigen in the test cells, and no hemolysis indicated C′ fixation by antigenic cells, providing the control was lysed.

The same procedure can be used to screen sera for antibody by using a panel of platelets and leukocytes (.04 ml. platelets at 600,000/mm.³ or leukocytes at 120,000/mm.³) with .04 ml. of serum both undiluted and diluted $\frac{1}{4}$ to account for possible prozone due to blocking antibodies (see Serology) and .04 ml. of C′.

Adsorption and Elution of Antibody

Cell preparations for use in C′ fixation were suitable for adsorbing antibodies. Stromal fractions of cells could also be used (see Serology). Cell buttons made from suspensions by sedimenting at 1100 g were resuspended in serum containing antibody (heated at 56° C. for 30 minutes). Antibody was completely removed from most sera by two adsorptions, each with 10⁹ platelets/ml. of serum, although an occasional high-titered antibody required four such adsorptions. White cells that shared antigens with platelets were approximately 10 times more effective per cell than platelets in adsorbing antibodies. Adsorption was carried out for one hour at 37° C. and one hour at 5° C., or overnight at 5° C. but most of the antigen-antibody combination took place within the first 15 minutes.

After adsorption, cells and particulate antigen were sedimented at 20,000 g for 15 minutes. Ultracentrifugation prevented trapping of serum in the button and also cleared the supernatant serum of light antigenic particles that interfered with titration of residual antibody. The surfaces of cell buttons and sides of tubes were rinsed with cold 0.147 M NaCl to remove contaminating serum and the cells were then suspended in 0.147 M NaCl for elution. At this stage, antibody titer could be increased above that of unadsorbed serum by appropriate decrease in the volume of suspending fluid.

The saline cell suspension was brought to pH 3.0 by slow addition of 0.1 N HCl using a continuous-reading pH meter and constant stirring, was allowed to stand at room temperature for approximately 10 minutes, and then was sedimented at 1100 g for 10 minutes. Supernatant fluid, containing antibody, was decanted and neutralized immediately with 0.02 N NaOH using the same technique as for acidification. Since pH values above 8.0 were associated with marked losses of antibody activity, it was important to prevent overshooting, and titration was stopped on the acid side of neutrality. Neutralization usually was accomplished with about half as many moles of NaOH as HCl used for acidification. A slight fluffy precipitate that usually formed shortly after the solution was neutralized was removed by centrifugation.

This process of elution consistently has given a 40 to 60 per cent yield of antibody, calculated on the basis of the amount of antibody present on cells that were used for elution. Although other technics that have been recommended for eluting antibodies from erythrocytes such as heat, high concentrations of salt or urea, and alkalinization were used, they did not give as high yields as acid elution. Eluates have been stored frozen at −20° C. for periods up to 6 months with no greater than 50 per cent loss of activity. Lyophilized eluates, kept at 5° C., did not lose activity over a period of a year and when kept at room temperature retained full activity for at least several months.

Sometimes it was impossible to adsorb the final 5 to 10 per cent of antibody from particular sera even with repeated addition of the same number of cells that had adsorbed the initial 90 per cent of antibody. This apparently was due to the relatively low affinity of occasional antibodies. Antibody remaining in these sera could be removed more effectively in the presence of C′.

Sometimes antibodies that fixed C′ were masked by blocking or incomplete antibodies of the same specificity. The two forms of antibodies frequently had different adsorption and elution properties and could be separated by this procedure (see Serology).

Inhibition of Clot Retraction

This rapid screening test was similar to a clot retraction test described by Lucia et al.[196] Fresh whole blood and serum containing antibody were mixed in siliconized tubes by inverting the tube twice on parafilm; wooden applicator sticks were placed in each tube; tubes were incubated for at least 2 hours at 37° C., and then clots were withdrawn on the end of the applicator sticks. Normally the volume of free fluid expressed from the clot was about 50 per cent of the original volume of blood. Sera containing potent platelet isoantibodies completely inhibited clot retraction at dilutions as high as 1/28 in the plasma of the tested blood.[32] Sera that did not produce complete inhibition of clot retraction at 1/5 dilution in plasma (approximately 1/10 the volume of whole blood tested) were not suitable for phenotyping. Most platelet isoantibodies did not inhibit clot retraction or did so only partially (see Serology). Tests in which partial inhibition of clot retraction occurred could be used to detect antibody activity[32, 45, 54] but were not sufficiently clearcut for use in rapid phenotyping tests. Tests with antibodies that gave complete inhibition were run in duplicate, using 1 or 2 ml. of whole blood and antiserum not exceeding 1/10 the volume of blood. Duplicate control tubes contained AB serum instead of antiserum.

REFERENCES

1. Harrington, W. J., Sprague, C. C., Minnich, V., Moore, C. V., Aulvin, R. C., and Dubach, R.: Immunologic mechanisms in idiopathic and neonatal thrombocytopenic purpura. Ann. Int. Med. 38: 433, 1953.

2. Stefanini, M., Plitman, G. I., Dameshek, W., Chatterjea, J. B., and Mednicoff, I. B.: Studies on platelets. XI. Antigenicity of platelets and evidence of platelet groups and types in man. J. Lab. & Clin. Med. 42: 723, 1953.

3. Payne, R.: Leukocyte agglutinins in human sera. A.M.A. Arch. Int. Med. 99: 587, 1957.

4. —: The association of febrile transfusion reactions with leuko-agglutinins. Vox Sang. 2: 233, 1957.

5. Van Loghem, J. J. Jr., van der Hart, M., and Borstel, H.: The occurrence of complete and incomplete white cell antibodies. Vox Sang. 2: 257, 1957.

6. Brittingham, T. E., and Chaplin, H. Jr.: Febrile transfusion reactions caused by sensitivity to donor leukocytes and platelets. J. A. M. A. 165: 819, 1957.

7. Payne, R., and Rolfs, M. R.: Fetomaternal leukocyte incompatibility. J. Clin. Invest. 37: 1756, 1958.

8. Van Rood, J. J., van Leeuwen, A., and Eernisse, J. G.: Leucocyte antibodies in sera of pregnant women. Vox Sang. 4: 427, 1959.

9. Moulinier, J.: Iso-immunisation maternelle antiplaquettaire et purpura néo-natal. Le système de groupe plaquettaire "duzo". *In* Proceedings of the Sixth Congr. of the European Soc. of Haematol. Basel, S. Karger, 1957, p. 817.

10. Dausset, J.: Iso-leuco-anticorps. Acta haemat. 20: 156, 1958.

11. —: Présence des antigènes A et B dans les leucocytes, deceleé par des épreuves d'agglutination. C. R. Soc. Biol. 148: 1607, 1954.

12. Coombs, R. R. A., and Bedford, D.: The A and B antigens on human platelets demonstrated by means of mixed erythrocyte-platelet agglutination. Vox Sang. 5: 111, 1955.

13. Gurevitch, J., and Nelken, D.: A B O groups in blood platelets. J. Lab. & Clin. Med. 44: 562, 1954.

14. Ashhurst, D. E., Bedford, D., and Coombs, R. R. A.: Examination of human plate-

lets for the ABO, MN, Rh, Tjᵃ, Lutheran and Lewis system of antigens by means of mixed erythrocyte-platelet agglutination. Vox Sang. 1: 235, 1956.

15. Ducos, J., Broussy, J., and Ruffie, J.: Peut-on affirmer que les antigènes de groupes sanguins érythrocytaires existent dans les thrombocytes? Sang 30: 548, 1959.

16. Dausset, J., Colombani, J., and Evelin, J.: Présence de l'antigène Rh (D) dans les leucocytes et les plaquettes humaines. Vox Sang. 3: 266, 1958.

17. Moulinier, J., and Servantie, X.: Détection par le test de consommation d'antiglobu-line de l'antigène D sur les plaquettes des individus Rh-positif (D +). Vox Sang. 3: 277, 1958.

18. Gurevitch, J., and Nelken, D.: Studies on platelet antigens. III. Rh-Hr antigens in platelets. Vox Sang. 2: 342, 1957.

19. Swisher, S. N.: Nonspecific adherence of platelets and leukocytes to antibody-sensi-tized red cells; a mechanism producing thrombocytopenia and leukopenia during incompatible transfusion. Sixth Congr. Internat. Soc. Hematol. New York and Lon-don, Grune & Stratton, 1958, p. 635.

20. Barnes, A. E., Sarasti, H., Mavioglu, H., and Jensen, W. N.: The detection and quanti-fication of Rh(D) antigen sites on human leukocytes. Blood 22: 690, 1963.

21. Bakemeier, R. F., and Swisher, S. N.: Mixed agglutination of leukocytes and erythro-cytes in relation to studies of leukocyte antigens. Blood 12: 913, 1957.

22. Lewis, J. H., Draude, J., and Kuhns, W. J.: Coating of "O" platelets with A and B group substances. Vox Sang. 5: 434, 1960.

23. Walford, R. L.: Leukocyte Antigens and Antibodies. New York and London, Grune & Stratton, 1960.

24. Killmann, S.-A.: Leukocyte Agglutinins, Springfield, Ill., Charles C Thomas, 1960.

25. Van de Wiel, Th. W. M., van de Wiel-Dorfmeyer, H., and van Loghem, J. J.: Studies on platelet antibodies in man. Vox Sang. 6: 641, 1961.

26. Dausset, J., and Malinvaud, G.: Influence de l'agitation sur l'agglutination thrombo-cytaire. Son utilité pour la recherche des Thrombo-Agglutinines et dans la pratique du test de Coombs plaquettaire. Sang 25: 847, 1954.

27. Van Loghem, J. J. Jr., Dorfmeijer, H., van der Hart, M., and Schreuder, F.: Serologi-cal and genetical studies on a platelet antigen (Zw). Vox Sang. 4: 161, 1959.

28. Van der Weerdt, Ch. M., Veenhoven-von Riesz, L. E., Nijenhuis, L. E., and van Loghem, J. J.: The Zw blood group system in platelets. Vox Sang. 8: 513, 1963.

29. —, van de Wiel-Dorfmeyer, H., Engelfriet, C. P., and van Loghem, J. J.: A new plate-let antigen. Proc. Eighth Congr. European Soc. Haematol. Basel, S. Karger, 1961, p. 379.

30. Dausset, J., and Berg, P.: Un nouvel exemple d'anticorps anti-plaquettaire Ko. Vox Sang. 8: 341, 1963.

31. Van Rood, J. J., and van Leeuwen, A.: Leukocyte grouping. A method and its ap-plication. J. Clin. Invest. 42: 1382, 1963.

32. Shulman, N. R., Aster, R. H., Leitner, A., and Hiller, M. C.: Immuno-reactions in-volving platelets. V. Post-transfusion purpura due to a complement-fixing antibody against a genetically controlled platelet antigen. A proposed mechanism for throm-bocytopenia and its relevance in "autoimmunity." J. Clin. Invest. 40: 1597, 1961.

33. —, —, Pearson, H. A., and Hiller, M. C.: Immunoreactions involving platelets. VI. Reactions of maternal isoantibodies responsible for neonatal purpura. Differentia-tion of a second platelet antigen system. J. Clin. Invest. 41: 1059, 1962.

34. —, Marder, V. J., Aledort, L. M., and Hiller, M. C.: Complement-fixing isoantibodies against antigens common to platelets and leukocytes. Trans. Assoc. Am. Physicians 75: 89, 1962.

35. Pearson, H. A., Shulman, N. R., Marder, V. J., and Cone, T. E. Jr.: Isoimmune neo-natal thrombocytopenic purpura. Clinical and therapeutic considerations. Blood 23: 154, 1964.

36. Shulman, N. R.: Mechanism of blood cell damage by adsorption of antigen-antibody complexes. In Immunopathology, IIIrd Int. Symposium. Grabar, P., and Miescher, P. A. (Eds.). Basel, Schwabe & Co., 1963, p. 338.

37. —: Mechanism of blood cell destruction in individuals sensitized to foreign antigens. Trans. Assoc. Am. Physicians 76: 72, 1963.

38. —: A mechanism of cell destruction in individuals sensitized to foreign antigens and its implications in autoimmunity. Ann. Int. Med. 60: 506, 1964.

39. —, Marder, V. J., and Weinrach, R. S.: Similarities between known anti-platelet antibodies and the factor responsible for thrombocytopenia in idiopathic purpura. Physiologic, serologic and isotopic studies. Ann. New York Acad. Sc. Conf. on Autoimmunity—Experimental and Clinical Aspects. Feb., 1964.

40. —, —, and —: Comparison of immunologic and idiopathic thrombocytopenia. Trans. Assoc. Am. Physicians 1964. In press.

41. Ford, E. B.: A uniform notation for the human blood groups. Heredity, 9: 135, 1955.

42. Harris, H.: Human Biochemical Genetics. London, Cambridge University Press, 1959.

43. Race, R. R., and Sanger, R.: Blood Groups in Man, 4th ed. Oxford, Blackwell Scientific Publications, Ltd., 1962.

44. Masouredis, S. P.: Relationship between $Rh_0(D)$ genotype and quantity of I^{131} anti-$Rh_0(D)$ bound to red cells. J. Clin. Invest. 39: 1450, 1960.

45. Zucker, M. B., Ley, A. B., Borrelli, J., Mayer, K., and Firmat, J.: Thrombocytopenia with a circulating platelet agglutinin, platelet lysin and clot retraction inhibitor. Blood 14: 148, 1959.

46. Steffen, C.: Results obtained with the antiglobulin consumption test and investigations of autoantibody eluates in immunohematology. J. Lab. & Clin. Med. 55: 9, 1960.

47. Shulman, N. R., Marder, V. J., Aledort, L. M., and Hiller, M. C.: Isoantibodies against platelets and leukocytes. Proc. IX Cong. Internat. Soc. Blood Transf. Basel, S. Karger, 1964, p. 439.

48. KILLMANN, S.-A.: A study of antigens of human leukocytes. Vox Sang. 3: 409, 1958.

49. Dausset, J., Colin, M., and Colombani, J.: Immune platelet iso-antibodies. Vox Sang. 5: 4, 1960.

50. Jensen, K. G.: Leucocyte antibodies in serums of pregnant women. Vox Sang. 7: 454, 1962.

51. Payne, R., and Hackel, E.: Inheritance of human leukocyte antigens. Am. J. Human Genetics 13: 306, 1961.

52. Engelfriet, C. P., and van Loghem, J. J.: Studies on leucocyte iso- and auto-antibodies. Brit. J. Haemat. 7: 223, 1961.

53. Harrington, W. J., Minnich, V., and Arimura, G.: The autoimmune thrombocytopenias. In Progress in Hematology, Vol. I. Tocantins, L. M. (Ed.). New York and London Grune & Stratton, 1956, p. 166.

54. Shulman, N. R.: Immunoreactions involving platelets. III. Quantitative aspects of platelet agglutination, inhibition of clot retraction, and other reactions caused by the antibody of quinidine purpura. J. Exper. Med. 107: 697, 1958.

55. Silber, R., Benitez, R., Eveland, W. C., Akeroyd, J. H., and Dunne, C. J.: The application of fluorescent antibody methods to the study of platelets. Blood 16: 958, 1960.

56. Vazquez, J. J., and Lewis, J. H.: Immunocytochemical studies on platelets. The demonstration of a common antigen in human platelets and megakaryocytes. Blood 16: 968, 1960.

57. Chambers, D. G., Coombs, R. R. A., and Gurner, B. W.: The mixed antiglobulin reaction in the detection of human iso-antibodies against leucocytes, platelets and HeLa cells. Brit. J. Haemat. 5: 225, 1959.

58. Kissmeyer-Nielsen, F.: Demonstration of platelet antibodies by haemagglutination of antigen coated tanned erythrocytes. Vox Sang. 3: 123, 1953.

59. Anderson, R. E., and Walford, R. L.: Detection of leukocyte antibodies by means of I^{131}-labelled, purified anti-human-globulin antibody. Problems of nonspecific adsorption of globulin by leukocytes. Blood 16: 1523, 1960.

60. Terasaki, P. I., and Rich, N. E.: Quantitative determination of antibody and complement directed against lymphocytes. J. Immunol. 92: 128, 1964.

61. Gräsbeck, R., Nordman, C., and de la Chapelle, A.: Mitogenic action of antileucocyte immune serum on peripheral leucocytes in vitro. Lancet I: 385, 1963.

62. Morgan, W. T. J., and Watkins, W. M.: Some aspects of the biochemistry of the human blood-group substances. Brit. Med. Bull. 15: 109, 1959.

63. Watkins, W. M., and Morgan, W. T. J.: Further observations on the inhibition of blood-group specific serological reactions by simple sugars of known structure. Vox Sang. 7: 129, 1962.

64. Flodin, P.: Dextran Gels and Their Applications in Gel Filtration. Halmstad (Sweden), Meijels Bokindustri, 1962.

65. Kramp, P.: Primatologia, Handbook of Primatology. Hofer, H., Schultz, A. H., and Stark, D. (Eds.). Basel, S. Karger, 1960, Vol. 3, p. 88.

66. Joysey, V. C.: The relation between animal and human blood groups. Brit. Med. Bull. 15: 158, 1959.

67. Landsteiner, K.: The Specificity of Serological Reactions. New York, Dover Publications, Inc., 1962.

68. Wiener, A. S., and Moor-Jankowski, J.: Blood groups in anthropoid apes and baboons. Science 142: 67, 1963.

69. Moor-Jankowski, J., Wiener, A. S., and Gordon, E. B.: Blood groups of apes and monkeys: I. The A-B-O blood groups in baboons. Transfusion 4: 92, 1964.

70. Aster, R. H., and Jandl, J. H.: Platelet sequestration in man. II. Immunological and clinical studies. J. Clin. Invest. 43: 856, 1964.

71. Shulman, N. R.: Immunoreactions involving platelets. IV. Studies on the pathogenesis of thrombocytopenia in drug purpura using test doses of quinidine in sensitized individuals; their implications in idiopathic thrombocytopenic purpura. J. Exper. Med. 107: 711, 1958.

72. Brittingham, T. E.: Immunologic studies on leukocytes. Vox Sang. 2: 242, 1957.

73. Dausset, J., Fonseca, A., and Brecy, H.: Élimination de certains chocs transfusionnels par l'utilisation de sang appauvri en leucocytes. Vox Sang. 2: 248, 1957.

74. Berson, S. A., and Yalow, R. S.: Quantitative aspects of the reaction between insulin and insulin-binding antibody. J. Clin. Invest. 38: 1996, 1959.

75. Shulman, N. R.: Immunoreactions involving platelets. I. A steric and kinetic model for formation of a complex from a human antibody, quinidine as a hapten, and platelets; and for fixation of complement by the complex. J. Exp. Med. 107: 665, 1958.

76. Craddock, C. G. Jr., Adams, W. S., Perry, S., and Lawrence, J. S.: The dynamics of platelet production as studied by a depletion technique in normal and irradiated dogs. J. Lab. & Clin. Med. 45: 906, 1955.

77. Corn, M., and Upshaw, J. D. Jr.: Evaluation of platelet antibodies in idiopathic thrombocytopenic purpura. Arch. Int. Med. 109: 157, 1962.

78. Jackson, D. P., Schmid, H. J., Zieve, P. D., Levin, J., and Conley, C. L.: Nature of a platelet-agglutinating factor in serum of patients with idiopathic thrombocytopenic purpura. J. Clin. Invest. 42: 383, 1963.

79. Cohen, P., Gardner, F. H., and Barnett, G. O.: Reclassification of the thrombocytopenias by the Cr[51]-labeling method for measuring platelet life span. New England J. Med. 264: 1294, 1961.

80. Bedson, S. P.: The effect of splenectomy on the production of experimental purpura. Lancet 2: 1117, 1924.

81. Elliott, R. H. E. Jr., and Whipple, M. A.: Observations on the interrelationship of capillary, platelet, and splenic factors in thrombocytopenic purpura. J. Lab. & Clin. Med. 26: 489, 1940.

82. Jandl, J. H., Richardson Jones, A., and Castle, W. B.: The destruction of red cells by antibodies in man. I. Observations on the sequestration and lysis of red cells altered by immune mechanisms. J. Clin. Invest. 36: 1428, 1957.

83. Cutbush, M., and Mollison, P. L.: Relation between characteristics of blood-group antibodies in vitro and associated patterns of red-cell destruction in vivo. Brit. J. Haemat. 4: 115, 1958.

84. Creger, W. P., Tulley, E. H., and Hansen, D. G.: A note on the effect of hydrocortisone

on the microelectrophoretic characteristics of human red cell-antibody unions. J. Lab. & Clin. Med. 47: 686, 1956.

85. Thorn, G. W., Jenkins, D., Laidlaw, J. C., Goetz, F. C., Dingman, J. F., Arons, W. L., Streeten, D. H. P., and McCracken, B. H.: Pharmacologic aspects of adrenocortical steroids and ACTH in man. New England J. Med. 248: 323, 1953.

86. Kass, E. H., and Finland, M.: Adrenocortical hormones in infection and immunity. Ann. Rev. Microbiol. 7: 361, 1953.

87. Packer, J. T., Greendyke, R. M., and Swisher, S. N.: The inhibition of erythrophagocytosis in vitro by corticosteroids. Trans. Assoc. Am. Physicians 73: 93, 1960.

88. Kaplan, M. E., and Jandl, J. H.: Inhibition of red cell sequestration by cortisone. J. Exp. Med. 114: 921, 1961.

89. Spaet, T. H., and Mednicoff, I.: The effect of cortisone on artificially induced thrombocytopenic purpura in rats. Bull. New England Med. Center 13: 201, 1951.

90. Craddock, C. G., Perry, S., Lawrence, J. S.: The dynamics of leukopenia and leukocytosis. Ann. Int. Med. 52: 281, 1960.

91. Bierman, H. R., Marshall, G. J., Kelly, K. H., and Byron, R. L. Jr.: Leucapheresis in man. II. Changes in circulating granulocytes, lymphocytes and platelets in the blood. Brit. J. Haemat. 8: 77, 1962.

92. Payne, R.: Neonatal neutropenia and leukoagglutinins. Pediatrics, 33: 194, 1964.

93. Braun, E. H., Buckwold, A. E., Emson, H. E., and Russell, A. V.: Familial neonatal neutropenia with maternal leukocyte antibodies. Blood 16: 1745, 1960.

94. Marsh, J. C., and Perry, S.: The granulocyte response to endotoxin in patients with hematologic disorders. Blood 23: 581, 1964.

95. Perry, S., Weinstein, I. M., Craddock, C. G. Jr., and Lawrence, J. S.: The combined use of typhoid vaccine and P^{32} labeling to assess myelopoiesis. Blood 12: 549, 1957.

96. Yunis, J. J., and Yunis, E.: Cell antigens and cell specialization. I. A study of blood group antigens on normoblasts. Blood 22: 53, 1963.

97. Brittingham, T. E., and Chaplin, H. Jr., Production of a human "anti-leukemic leukocyte" serum and its therapeutic trial. Cancer 13: 412, 1960.

98. Snell, G. D.: Incompatibility reactions to tumor homotransplants with particular reference to the role of the tumor. Cancer Research 17: 2, 1957.

99. Kaliss, N.: Immunological enhancement of tumor homografts in mice. Cancer Research 18: 992, 1958.

100. Whang, J., Frei, E. III, Tjio, J. H., Carbone, P. P., and Brecher, G.: The distribution of the Philadelphia chromosome in patients with chronic myelogenous leukemia. Blood 22: 664, 1963.

101. Bronson, W. R., McGinniss, M. H., and Morse, E. E.: Hematopoietic graft detected by a change in ABO group. Blood 23: 239, 1964.

102. Schwarzenberg, L., Duplan, J. E., Maupain, B., Latarjet, R., Larrieu, M. J., Kalic, D., and Djukic, Z.: Transfusions et greffes de noelle osseuse homologue chez des humains irradiés à haute dose accidentellement. Rev. franc. Etudes clin. biol. 4: 226, 1959.

103. Hungerford, D. A., Donnelly, A. J., Nowell, P. C., and Beck, S.: The chromosome constitution of a human phenotype intersex. Am. J. Human Genetics 11: 215, 1959.

104. Borel, Y., Baldini, M., and Ebbe, S.: Isoimmunity to blood platelets in the rabbit. Blood 21: 674, 1963.

105. Medawar, P. B.: Iso-antigens. In Biological Problems of Grafting. A Symposium. Oxford, Blackwell Scientific Publications, 1959, p. 6.

106. Green, H., Barrow, P., and Goldberg, B.: Effect of antibody and complement on permeability control in ascites tumor cells and erythrocytes. J. Exper. Med. 110: 699, 1959.

107. Green, H., and Goldberg, B.: The action of antibody and complement on mammalian cells. Ann. New York Acad. Sc. 87: 352, 1960.

108. Sears, D. A., Weed, R. I., and Swisher, S. N.: Differences in the mechanism of in vitro immune hemolysis related to antibody specificity. J. Clin. Invest. 43: 975, 1964.

109. Baldini, M., Costea, N., and Ebbe, S.: Studies on the antigenic structure of blood

platelets. *In* Proc. of the Eighth Congr. of the European Society of Haematol. Basel, S. Karger, 1962, p. 378.

110. Salmon, Ch., and Schwartz, D.: Analyse statistique d'une série de 639 malades poly-transfusés: Essai d'interprétation des conditions de l'iso-immunisation. Revue d'Hématologie 15: 162, 1960.

111. Payne, R., and Rolfs, M. R.: Further observations on leukoagglutinin transfusion reactions. Am. J. Med. 29: 449, 1960.

112. Kevy, S. V., Schmidt, P. J., McGinniss, M. H., and Workman, W. G.: Febrile, non-hemolytic transfusion reactions and the limited role of leukoagglutinins in their etiology. Transfusion 2: 7, 1962.

113. André, R., Dreyfus, B., and Salmon, Ch: Iso-immunisation antileucocytes après transfusions anticorps antileucocytes et leucopénies. Revue Francaise d'Etudes Cliniques et Biologiques 3: 33, 1958.

114. Anthony, B., and Krivit, W.: Neonatal thrombocytopenic purpura. Pediatrics 30: 776, 1962.

115. Moulinier, J.: Les purpuras "immunologiques" du nouveau-né. Nouvelle Revue Francaise d'Hematologie 4: 164, 1964.

116. Lalezari, P., Nussbaum, M., Gelman, S., and Spaet, T. H.: Neonatal neutropenia due to maternal isoimmunization. Blood 15: 236, 1960.

117. Jaeger-Draafsel, E., Wiegman, D., and van Loghem, J. J. Jr.: Detection of incomplete platelet antibodies by means of the indirect anti-human globulin test. Vox Sang. 1: 78, 1956.

118. Swisher, S. N.: Studies of the mechanisms of erythrocyte destruction initiated by antibodies. Trans. Assoc. Am. Physicians 67: 124, 1954.

119. Fudenberg, H., and Allen, F. H. Jr.: Transfusion reactions in the absence of demon-strable incompatibility. New England J. Med. 256: 1180, 1957.

120. Marchal, G., Dausset, J., Colombani, J., Bilski-Pasquier, G., and Jaulmes, B.: Im-munisation anti-leucocytaire et anti-plaquettaire provoquée par l'injection répétée du même sang. Sang 29: 549, 1958.

121. Brittingham, T. E., and Chaplin, H. Jr.: The antigenicity of normal and leukemic human leukocytes. Blood 17: 139, 1961.

122. Freireich, E. J., Kliman, A., Gaydos, L. A., Mantel, N., and Frei, E. III: Response to repeated platelet transfusion from the same donor. Ann. Int. Med. 59: 277, 1963.

123. Silver, T. T., Utz, J. P., Fahey, J., and Frei, E. III: Antibody response in patients with acute leukemia. J. Lab. & Clin. Med. 56: 634, 1960.

124. Desai, R. G., and Creger, W. P.: Maternofetal passage of leukocytes and platelets in man. Blood 21: 665, 1963.

125. Allison, A. C., and Blumberg, B. S.: An isoprecipitation reaction distinguishing human serum-protein types. Lancet i: 634, 1961.

126. Mollison, P. L.: Blood Transfusion in Clinical Medicine, 3rd ed. Oxford, Blackwell Scientific Publications, 1961.

127. Dameshek, W., and Neber, J.: Transfusion reactions to plasma constituent of whole blood: their pathogenesis and treatment by washed red blood cell transfusions. Blood 5: 129, 1950.

128. Mendes de Leon, D. E., and van der Hart, M.: A severe plasma reaction after trans-fusion of blood and serum. Vox Sang. 5: 30, 1955.

129. Chaplin, H. Jr., Brittingham, T. E., and Cassell, M. Methods for preparation of suspensions of buffy coat-poor red blood cells for transfusion. Am. J. Clin. Path. 31: 373, 1959.

130. Kaplan, E.: Congenital and neonatal thrombocytopenic purpura. J. Pediat. 54: 644, 1959.

131. Hugh-Jones, K., Manfield, P. A., and Brewer, H. F.: Congenital thrombocytopenic purpura. Arch. Dis. Child. 35: 146, 1960.

132. Robson, H. N., and Walker, C. H. M.: Congenital and neonatal thrombocytopenic purpura. Arch. Dis. Child. 26: 175, 1951.

133. Wiener, A. S.: Rh factor in immunological reactions. Ann. Allergy, 6: 293, 1948.

134. Kochwa, S., Rosenfield, R. E., Tallal, L., and Wasserman, L. R.: Isoagglutinins associated with ABO erythroblastosis. J. Clin. Invest. 40: 874, 1961.

135. Barclay, A. E., Franklin, K. J., and Prichard, M. M. L.: The Foetal Circulation, Springfield, Charles C Thomas, 1944.

136. Reepmaker, J., and van Loghem, J. J.: Anti-A and anti-B immune antibodies in pregnancy. Vox Sang. 3: 143, 1953.

137. Hitzig, W. H., and Gitzelmann, R.: Transplacental transfer of leukocyte agglutinins. Vox Sang. (N.S.) 4: 445, 1959.

138. Jensen, K. G.: Transplacental passage of leucocyte agglutinins occurring on account of pregnancy. Dan. Med. Bull. 7: 55, 1960.

139. Rossi, J. P., and Brandt, I. K.: Transient granulocytopenia of the newborn associated with sepsis due to Shigella alkalescens and maternal leukocyte agglutinins. J. Pediat. 56: 639, 1960.

140. Ackroyd, J. F.: The pathogenesis of thrombocytopenic purpura due to hypersensitivity to sedormid. Clin. Sci. 7: 249, 1949.

141. —: The immunological basis of purpura due to drug hypersensitivity. Proc. Roy. Soc. Med. 55: 30, 1962.

142. Neter, E.: Bacterial hemagglutination and hemolysis. Bact. Rev. 20: 166, 1956.

143. Lamanna, C.: Adhesion of foreign particles to particulate antigens in the presence of antibody and complement (serological adhesion). Bact. Rev. 21: 30, 1957.

144. Nelson, D. S., and Nelson, R. A.: On the mechanism of immune-adherence. II. Analogy to mixed aggregation of sensitized antigens in the presence of complement. Yale J. Biol. Med. 31: 201, 1959.

145. Boyden, S. V., and Andersen, M. E.: Agglutination of normal erythrocytes in mixtures of antibody and antigen, and haemolysis in the presence of complement. Brit. J. Exper. Path. 36: 162, 1955.

146. Miescher, P., and Cooper, N.: The fixation of soluble antigen-antibody complexes upon thrombocytes. Vox Sang. 5: 138, 1960.

147. Alexander, M. M., Wright, G. G., and Baldwin, A. C.: Observations on the agglutination of polysaccharide-treated erythrocytes by tularemia antisera. J. Exper. Med. 91: 561, 1950.

148. Berthrong, M., and Cluff, L. E.: Studies of the effect of bacterial endotoxins on rabbit leucocytes. I. Effect of intravenous injection of the substances with and without induction of the local Shwartzman reaction. J. Exper. Med. 98: 331, 1953.

149. McKay, D. G., and Shapiro, S. S.: Alterations in the blood coagulation system induced by bacterial endotoxin. I. In vivo (generalized Shwartzman reaction). J. Exper. Med. 107: 353, 1958.

150. Bennett, I. L. Jr., and Beeson, P. B.: The properties and biologic effects of bacterial pyrogens. Medicine 29: 365, 1950.

151. Wolff, S. M., Rubenstein, M., Mulholland, J. H., and Alling, D. W.: Comparison of hematologic and febrile responses to endotoxin in man. Blood. In press.

152. Kopeloff, N., and Kopeloff, L. M.: Blood platelets in anaphylaxis. J. Immunol. 40: 471, 1940.

153. Lee, L.: Reticuloendothelial clearance of circulating fibrin in the pathogenesis of the generalized Shwartzman reaction. J. Exper. Med. 115: 1065, 1962.

154. Hardaway, R. III, McKay, D. G., Wahle, G. H., Tartock, D., and Edelstein, R.: Pathologic study of intravascular coagulation following incompatible blood transfusion in dogs. I. Intravenous injection of incompatible blood. Am. J. Surg. 91: 24, 1956.

155. Miescher, P., and Straessle, R.: Experimentelle studien über den mechanismus der thrombocyten-schädigung durch antigen-antikörperreaktionen. Vox Sang. 1: 83, 1956.

156. Dixon, F. J.: The pathogenic significance of antigen-antibody complexes. In Immunopathology, Symposium 1958. Grabar, P., and Miescher, P. (Eds.). Basel, Benno Schwabe & Co. 1958, p. 299.

157. Waksman, B. H.: Auto-immunization and the lesions of auto-immunity. Medicine. 41: 93, 1962.

158. Third Tissue Homotransplantation Conference. Ann. New York Acad. Sc. 73: pp. 539–868, 1958.

159. Biological Problems of Grafting. Oxford, Blackwell Scientific Publications, 1959, pp. 1–453.

160. Fourth Tissue Homotransplantation Conference. Ann. New York Acad. Sc. 87: pp. 1–607, 1960.

161. Transplantation, Ciba Foundation Symposium. Wolstenholme, G. E. W., and Cameron, M. P. (Eds.). Boston, Little, Brown & Co., 1962, pp. 1–426.

162. Fifth Tissue Homotransplantation Conference. Ann. New York Acad. Sc. 99: pp. 335–942, 1962.

163. Gorer, P. A.: Some recent work on tumor immunity. Advances Cancer Res. 4: 149, 1956.

164. Brent, L.: Tissue transplantation immunity. Progr. in Allergy 5: 271, 1958.

165. Medawar, P. B.: The homograft reaction. The Croonian Lecture. Proc. Roy. Soc. London, Series B, 149: 145, 1958.

166. Amos, D. B.: The use of simplified systems as an aid to the interpretation of mechanisms of graft rejection. Progr. in Allergy 6: 468, 1962.

167. Billingham, R. E., and Silvers, W. K.: Sensitivity to homografts of normal tissues and cells. Ann. Rev. Microbiol. 17: 531, 1963.

168. Medawar, P. B.: Immunity to homologous grafted skin. II. The relationship between the antigen of blood and skin. Brit. J. Exper. Path. 27: 15, 1946.

169. Friedman, E. A., Retan, J. W., Marshall, D. C., Henry, L., and Merrill, J. P.: Accelerated skin graft rejection in humans preimmunized with homologous peripheral leukocytes. J. Clin. Invest. 40: 2162, 1961.

170. Ebbe, S., Baldini, M., and Dameshek, W.: The antigenic structure of blood platelets. I. Demonstration in the rabbit of antigens in common between skin and blood platelets. Blood 19: 537, 1962.

171. Brent, L., Brown, J., and Medawar, P. B.: Skin transplantation immunity in relation to hypersensitivity. Lancet 2: 561, 1958.

172. Merrill, J. P., Friedman, E. A., Wilson, R. E., and Marshall, D. C.: The production of "delayed type" cutaneous hypersensitivity to human donor leukocytes as a result of the rejection of skin homografts. J. Clin. Invest. 40: 631, 1961.

173. Waksman, B. H.: Delayed hypersensitive reactions: a growing class of immunologic phenomena. J. Allergy 31: 468, 1960.

174. Jandl, J. H., and Tomlinson, A. S.: The destruction of red cells by antibodies in man. II. Pyrogenic, leukocytic and dermal responses to immune hemolysis. J. Clin. Invest. 37: 1202, 1958.

175. Stone, H. B., Owings, J. C., and Gey, G. O.: Transplantation of living grafts of thyroid and parathyroid glands. Ann. Surg. 100: 613, 1934.

176. DeWitt, C. W., Huser, H.-J., Moor-Jankowski, J., Shulman, N. R., and Wiener, A. S.: Some immunological aspects of homo- and heterotransplantation in man and other primates. (Abstract) Xth Cong. Internat. Soc. Blood Transfusion, Stockholm, 1964.

177. Herzenberg, L. A., and Herzenberg, L. A.: Association of H-2 antigens with the cell membrane fraction of mouse liver. Proc. Natl. Acad. Sc. 47: 762, 1961.

178. Davies, D. A. L.: H-2 histocompatibility antigens of the mouse. In Transplantation, Ciba Foundation Symposium. Wolstenholme, G. E. W., and Cameron, M. P. (Eds.). Boston, Little, Brown & Co., 1962, p. 45.

179. Peer, L. A.: Behavior of skin grafts exchanged between parents and offspring. Ann. New York Acad. Sc. 73: 584, 1958.

180. Billingham, R. E., and Sparrow, E. M.: The effect of prior intravenous injections of dissociated epidermal cells and blood on the survival of skin homografts in rabbits. J. Embryol. Exper. Morphol. 3: 265, 1955.

181. —, Brent, L., and Mitchison, N. A.: The route of immunization in transplantation immunity. Brit. J. Exper. Path. 38: 467, 1957.

182. Steinmuller, D., and Weiner, L.: Evocation and persistence of transplantation immunity in rats. Transplantation 1: 97, 1963.

183. Hašek, M., Hašková, V., Lengerová, A., and Vojtíšková, M.: Mother-foetus immunological relationship as an exceptional homograft model. *In* Transplantation, Ciba Foundation Symposium. Wolstenholme, G. E. W., and Cameron, M. P. (Eds.). Boston, Little, Brown & Co., 1962, p. 118.

184. Simmons, R. L., and Russell, P. S.: The antigenicity of mouse trophoblast. Ann. New York Acad. Sc. 99: 717, 1962.

185. Schmidt, P. J., and Hertz, R.: Blood group factors in women with choriocarcinoma as compared with those of their husbands. Am. J. Obstet. & Gynecol. 82: 651, 1961.

186. Doniach, I., Crookston, J. H., and Cope, T. I.: Attempted treatment of a patient with choriocarcinoma by immunization with her husband's cells. J. Obstet. Gynaec. Brit. Emp. 65: 553, 1958.

187. Hackett, E., and Beech, M.: Immunological treatment of a case of choriocarcinoma. Brit. Med. J. 2: 1123, 1961.

188. Itoh, T., and Southam, C. M.: Isoantibodies to human cancer cells in healthy recipients of cancer homotransplants. J. Immunol. 91: 469, 1963.

189. Möller, E., and Möller, G.: Quantitative studies of the sensitivity of normal and neoplastic mouse cells to the cytotoxic action of isoantibodies. J. Exper. Med. 115: 527, 1962.

190. Brecher, G., and Cronkite, E. P.: Morphology and enumeration of human blood platelets. J. Appl. Physiol. 3: 365, 1950.

191. Chaplin, H., Jr., Crawford, H., Cutbush, M., and Mollison, P. L.: Preservation of red cells at −79° C. Clin. Sc. 15: 27, 1956.

192. —, Schmidt, P. J., and Steinfeld, J. L.: Storage of red cells at sub-zero temperatures, further studies. Clin. Sc. 16: 651, 1957.

193. Kabat, E. A., and Mayer, M. M.: Complement and complement fixation. *In* Experimental Immunochemistry. Springfield, Ill., Charles C Thomas, 1961, pp. 133–240.

194. Chudomel, V., Jezkova, Z., and Libansky, J.: Detection of leukocyte antibodies by the complement consumption test. Blood 14: 920, 1959.

195. de Nicola, P., Rosti, P., and Zangaglia, O.: Complement fixation test due to the interaction of specific antiplatelet serum and heterologous platelet antigen. J. Lab. & Clin. Med. 45: 725, 1955.

196. Lucia, S. P., Aggeler, P. M., and Hamlin, L. M.: Blood clot retraction; significance of extracorpuscular volume of clot and its clinical application. Am. J. Med. Sc. 204: 507, 1942.

Index

305